COMPREHENSIVE NEUROLOGIC REHABILITATION
Volume 1

The Management of High Quadriplegia

Comprehensive Neurologic Rehabilitation

COMPREHENSIVE NEUROLOGIC REHABILITATION
Volume 1

The Management of
High Quadriplegia

EDITORS

Gale Whiteneck, Ph.D.
Daniel P. Lammertse, M.D.
Scott Manley, Ed.D.
Robert Menter, M.D.

Craig Hospital
Englewood, Colorado

Carole Adler, O.T.R.
Conal Wilmot, M.D.

Santa Clara Valley
Medical Center
San Jose, California

R. Edward Carter, M.D.
Karen A. Wagner, Ph.D.

The Institute for Rehabilitation
and Research
Houston, Texas

$\mathcal{D}emos$

Demos Publications, 156 Fifth Avenue, New York, New York 10010

© 1989 by Demos Publications, Inc. All rights reserved. This book is protected by copyright. No part of it may be reproduced, stored in a retrieval system, or transmitted in any form or by any means, electronic, mechanical, photocopying, recording, or otherwise, without the prior written permission of the publisher.

Made in the United States of America

Great care has been taken to maintain the accuracy of the information contained in this volume. However, the Editors and Demos Publications cannot be held responsible for errors or for any consequences arising from the use of the information contained herein.

ISBN: 0-939957-19-1
LC: 88-71753

Preface

High-level spinal cord injury (SCI) with complete paralysis below the fourth cervical neurologic level is one of the most devastating catastrophes that can befall an individual. The person with high quadriplegia not only loses the use of all extremities, but every other body system is radically affected as well, and ventilatory function often is lost or severely compromised.

The resources required to address the array of issues presented by the person with high quadriplegia are enormous. The cost of care in the initial hospitalization is high but modest by comparison to the cost of lifetime maintenance. However, with adequate resources, a specialized multidisciplinary team and a comprehensive program of care can both sustain life for the high quadriplegic and help the individual achieve a satisfying quality of life as well. Unfortunately, few centers in the world have the experience or expertise to produce this result.

Three SCI centers with long-standing experience in high quadriplegia care (Craig Hospital in Englewood, Colorado; Santa Clara Valley Medical Center in San Jose, California; and The Institute for Rehabilitation and Research in Houston, Texas) recognized the need to develop and share information regarding the acute medical management, rehabilitation, discharge, and outcome of this uncommon catastrophe. The collaboration of these three centers has produced three workshops on high quadriplegia (San Francisco, California in 1980; Houston, Texas in 1985; and Vail, Colorado in 1988), two publications of conference proceedings, and a research study investigating the long-term outcomes of high quadriplegia. This book represents the culmination of these collaborative efforts in an attempt to thoroughly examine the complexities of high quadriplegia management.

The many perspectives that must be integrated in the management of high quadriplegia are presented in this book. It is organized in four major sections beginning with acute care, moving through rehabilitation, delineating the process of discharge, and finally addressing lifetime issues in the real world. The authors represent the many team members involved in this continuation of care including physicians directing care; consulting physicians; nurses; physical, occupational, respiratory, and recreational therapists; nutritionists; social workers; psychologists; counselors; educators; case managers; third-party payors; attorneys; ethicists; researchers; and consumers.

It is assumed that readers have a working knowledge and background in spinal injury at the lower quadriplegic and paraplegic levels. The focus of this book, therefore, is on the aspects of high-quadriplegia care that differ from basic SCI care. Elements of care that are quite similar to the care of lower-level SCI are not emphasized. Although each of the collaborating centers has a slightly different approach to various issues, every effort has been made to include the perspectives of all three centers.

The four physicians on the editorial board reviewed initial drafts of each chapter in their roles as section editors: R. Edward Carter, M.D., *Acute Care;* Conal Wilmot, M.D., *Rehabilitation;* Daniel P. Lammertse, M.D., *Discharge Planning;* and Robert Menter, M.D., *The Real World.* Collaboration on this book was organized by the three center coordinators: Carole Adler, O.T.R., Santa Clara Valley Medical Center; Karen Wagner, Ph.D., The Institute for Rehabilitation and Research; and Gale Whiteneck, Ph.D., Craig Hospital. Considerable peer review also occurred to insure that the perspectives of all three centers were included in each chapter.

It is our hope that this book will lay the groundwork for more SCI respiratory centers in the United States. In addition, we hope that this volume will foster an understanding of the unique medical needs and treatment techniques of this unusual catastrophic injury. Finally, may it help all health care professionals who work with high quadriplegic persons to reach beyond the medical crisis to the individual and his potential for an active, meaningful life.

Robert Menter, M.D.

Acknowledgments

Encouragement for this book came from the American Spinal Injury Association and financial support from the National Institute on Disability and Rehabilitation Research, Dr. J. Paul Thomas, Project Director.

In addition to peer review by fellow authors, chapters were reviewed by several individuals whose contributions were invaluable: Terry Carle, M.D.; Susan Charlifue, M.A.; Kathy Davis, R.R.T., R.C.P.; Jane Henderson Eversole, M.A., R.P.T.; Theresa Gregorio, O.T.R.; Sara Herber, M.S., P.T.; Frances Pendergraft, M.S.W., C.S.W.-A.C.P.; Lois Schaetzle, R.N., B.S.N., C.R.R.N.; and Evelyn Thomas, C.R.T.T.

Special thanks are extended to the Honorable Charles Buss, J.D., Kathy DeSilva, J.D., and Giles Scofield, J.D., for their contributions to Chapter 22 on ethics, and to Kathy DeSilva, J.D., Brian Hogan, and Leslie Peer for their contributions to Chapter 23 on consumer perspectives. Gratitude is also expressed to the many individuals in clinical education and the research departments at the three collaborating institutions who contributed to the production of this book. Finally, we acknowledge the hundreds of individuals with high quadriplegia who have informed us and have motivated us in this effort.

The Editors

Contents

III. DISCHARGE PLANNING

IV. THE REAL WORLD

Contributors

Carole Adler, O.T.R., Clinical Supervisor, Spinal Cord Injury Unit, Santa Clara Valley Medical Center, San Jose, California.

Joan Anderson, M.S.W., L.C.S.W., Supervisor, Social Service Department, Santa Clara Valley Medical Center, San Jose, California.

Sam Andrews, C.T.R.S., Director, Therapeutic Recreation, Craig Hospital, Englewood, Colorado.

Lester Butt, Ph.D., Clinical Psychologist, Craig Hospital, Englewood, Colorado.

R. Edward Carter, M.D., Professor of Clinical Rehabilitation, Baylor College of Medicine, Houston, Texas.

Maureen A. Cox, M.S.W., Medical Social Worker, Santa Clara Valley Medical Center, San Jose, California.

William H. Donovan, M.D., Director, Model Regional Spinal Cord Injury Center; Vice President, Medical Affairs, The Institute for Rehabilitation and Research, Houston, Texas.

Gail Gilinsky, O.T.R., Occupational Therapy Supervisor, Craig Hospital, Englewood, Colorado.

Karyl Hall, Ed.D., formerly Project Director, Northern California Regional Spinal Injury System, Santa Clara Valley Medical Center, San Jose, California; currently Director, Traumatic Brain Injury Project, Institute for Medical Research, San Jose, California.

Dolores Hynes, R.N., Senior Rehabilitation Claims Consultant, North American Reinsurance Corporation.

Cindy Kelly, T.R.S., Therapeutic Recreation Specialist, Craig Hospital, Englewood, Colorado.

Daniel P. Lammertse, M.D., Medical Director, Craig Hospital, Englewood, Colorado.

Sam Maddox, Author and Publisher, *Spinal Network,* Boulder, Colorado.

Scott Manley, Ed.D., Vice President, Craig Hospital, Englewood, Colorado.

Janet McIntyre, R.P.T., Physical Therapy Supervisor, Craig Hospital, Englewood, Colorado.

Virginia McKay, R.N., Flight Nurse, Craig Hospital, Englewood, Colorado.

Kevin McVeigh, M.A., Director of Education, Craig Hospital, Englewood, Colorado.

Robert R. Menter, M.D., Director of SCI Grant, Craig Hospital, Englewood, Colorado.

Rene L. Monforton, Director of Claims, Automobile Club of Michigan.

Suzanne Nyre, Director of Admissions and Coordinator of High Risk Admissions, Craig Hospital, Englewood, Colorado.

Peter Peterson, M.D., Medical Director, Department of Respiratory Therapy, Craig Hospital, Englewood, Colorado.

Phyllis M. Syers, R.N., M.S.N., formerly Nurse Educator and Clinical Nurse Specialist, Department of Nursing, The Institute for Rehabilitation and Research, Houston, Texas; currently Clinical Director for Rehabilitation, St. Joseph's Medical Center, South Bend, Indiana.

Patricia Tracy, M.S.W., L.S.W., Family Services, Craig Hospital, Englewood, Colorado.

Barbara R. Vaughn, R.N., Head Nurse, Spinal Cord Injury Unit, The Institute for Rehabilitation and Research, Houston, Texas.

Sue Frazior Vizuete, M.S., R.D./L.D., C.N.S.D., Nutritional Support Dietitian, St. Luke's Episcopal Hospital, Houston, Texas.

Karen A. Wagner, Ph.D., Vice President for Education, The Institute for Rehabilitation and Research; Assistant Professor, Department of Rehabilitation, Baylor College of Medicine, Houston, Texas.

Gale Whiteneck, Ph.D., Research Director, Craig Hospital, Englewood, Colorado.

Allan B. Wicks, M.D., Pulmonary Consultant, Craig Hospital, Englewood, Colorado.

Conal B. Wilmot, M.D., Medical Director, Chairman, Department of Rehabilitation Medicine, and Director, Spinal Cord Injury Services, Santa Clara Valley Medical Center, San Jose, California; Associate Clinical Professor, Stanford University, Palo Alto, California.

Marsha Wood, C.R.T.T., Respiratory Care Supervisor, Craig Hospital, Englewood, Colorado.

Teresa Yoshimura, R.N., C.R.R.N., formerly Head Nurse, Spinal Cord Injury Unit; currently Admissions/Discharge Coordinator, Department of Rehabilitation, Santa Clara Valley Medical Center, San Jose, California.

1

Introduction to High Quadriplegia Care

Robert Menter

Craig Hospital, Englewood, Colorado, U.S.A.

Spinal cord injury (SCI) has been occurring since the earliest evolution of humans. Only in the last 40 years has it come to mean something other than imminent death. Over the decades there has been a gradual change in patterns of survival from low level paraplegia in the 1950s, high level paraplegia in the 1960s, low quadriplegia in the 1970s, and finally high quadriplegia in the 1980s. Associated with each advancement has been the evolution of a medical milestone: limited antibiotics in the 1950s, full-spectrum antibiotics in the 1960s, improved respiratory care and cardio-pulmonary resuscitation (CPR) in the 1970s, and emergency medical services at the accident scene in the 1980s.

In this book, high quadriplegia refers to individuals with paralysis initiated at the fourth cervical neurologic level or above. It is usually associated with respiratory insufficiency at the scene of the accident or soon after. Often, there is a dramatic slowing and stoppage of the heart, which may also cause death if not reversed. Beyond respiratory and cardiac concerns lie many other life-threatening physiologic imbalances.

Only in the last decade have there been significant numbers of high quadriplegic survivors. Reasons for this recent increase in survival are multiple. First, more people have been trained in CPR. Second, most hospitals have the capability of inserting endotracheal tubes and using ventilators. Third, medical diagnosis and treatment in intensive care units has evolved to control nearly all medical complications.

Specific data relating to this group of people with SCI have been limited due to the low incidence, the limited numbers of SCI facilities admitting and treating ventilator-dependent patients, and the inability to separate this subgroup out of general quadriplegic data. The informa-

1

tion in the National Spinal Cord Injury Statistical Center in Birmingham, Alabama, estimates the incidence of C1 to C3 spinal injuries to be 0.75 per million per year. The C4 level SCI incidence is 2.4 million per year. Using the most recent United States census of 225 million (1980), the occurrence would be 166 cases of C1 to C3 and 540 cases of C4 quadriplegia per year.

The most extensive study to date of high quadriplegia was conducted by the centers the editors of this book are affiliated with (1). The 1985 study focused on 216 patients treated in these three centers from 1973 to 1984 and followed them from 1 to 11 years postinjury. Seventeen patients died during the initial hospitalization. The remaining 199 cases were divided into two categories at discharge: ventilator-dependent (63) and nonventilator-dependent (136). The survival status at 9 years postinjury was 63% for ventilator-dependent patients and 73% for nonventilator-dependent patients. It is important to acknowledge that these figures represent a selected population that first had to live long enough and qualify for transfer to one of the three study centers and, second, survive the initial hospitalization at the study center.

The 1985 study (1) not only demonstrated that individuals with high quadriplegia were surviving, but that they were leading fulfilling lives. They were living at home, interacting socially, getting out of their homes regularly, and participating in a wide variety of activities. They had high self-esteem, reported a good quality of life, and indicated they were glad to be alive. Furthermore, the assessments of ventilator-dependent individuals were just as positive as the assessments of nonventilator-dependent cases. These data are in marked contrast to the belief frequently held by health care professionals that the lives of these individuals are hopelessly full of suffering no one would want to endure.

Clearly, a specialized comprehensive program of care can produce genuinely positive outcomes for individuals with high quadriplegia. However, the resources required to produce positive results are substantial. Institutional commitment is necessary for this highly specialized program. Adequate numbers of patients with high quadriplegia are needed in the program for them to learn from each other and for staff to gain experience. Due to the infrequent occurrences, many otherwise experienced qualified SCI centers never develop the experience to establish a team approach to high quadriplegia. Special high quadriplegia-oriented SCI centers with experienced multidisciplinary teams are therefore needed to address the needs of this population.

The cost of such specialized care is high (1). Medical expenses for acute care and initial rehabilitation average approximately $300,000 for ventilator-dependent cases and approximately $100,000 for nonventilator-dependent cases. The comprehensive continuing care of individuals with high quadriplegia averages over $50,000 annually for ventilator-dependent cases and over $20,000 annually for nonventilator-dependent cases. Given the incidence and survival rates already discussed, a reasonable estimate of the total annual cost to society for the care of all persons in the United States with high quadriplegia might exceed $250,000,000.

What is it that makes the care of high quadriplegia different from other levels of SCI? Foremost is the lifelong need for greater amounts of attendant care and its associated costs. The C4 group, although not on ventilators, have similar physical dependency needs to the C1 to C3 persons who are ventilator dependent. Both groups are dependent in bowel, bladder, and skin care, activities of daily living, body handling, etc. Although attendant needs for the C4-level persons allow some time alone, they need potential physical assistance 24 h per day. The C1 to C3 group, being ventilator dependent, has even more critical needs and must have someone immediately available to respond to alarms 24 h per day.

Another unusual feature of this group is the problem of obtaining funding for equipment and attendant care after discharge. Due to the unusual extent and expense of equipment, financial sponsors often will delay authorization and defer to lengthy review processes that postpone discharge planning. Funding for attendant care is frequently nonexistent or inadequate to effect a discharge. Even discharge to a nursing home facility is difficult because of the increased costs of care for these individuals.

The combination of these factors creates typical hospital stays of 6–8 months after injury, far in excess of the typical 3–4 months for most quadriplegic and paraplegic persons. This inability to effect a discharge due to inadequate financial support is occurring with increasing frequency, leaving SCI facilities to provide domiciliary long-term care.

Although the difficulties of high quadriplegia care are many, they are not insurmountable. The key to success is a comprehensive, specialized program with experienced, creative, multidisciplinary team members committed to the challenge. Hopefully, the ensuing pages will give the reader some insight into the interactions of a team focusing on the needs of high level quadriplegia.

REFERENCES

1. Whiteneck GG, Carter RE, Charlifue SW, Hall KM, Menter RR, Wilkerson MA, Wilmot CB (1985): *A Collaborative Study of High Quadriplegia* (Rocky Mountain Regional Spinal Injury System, Northern California Regional Spinal Injury System, and Texas Regional Spinal Cord Injury System). Englewood, CO: Craig Hospital.

I

Acute Care

Introduction

Karen Wagner

The Institute for Rehabilitation and Research, Houston, Texas, U.S.A.

Perhaps the most significant medical advances in the management of persons with high quadriplegia have occurred in emergency and acute care. Extensive training has been conducted with emergency medical technicians and ambulance personnel throughout the country. There has been vast improvement in the skills of extraction, stabilization, and transport of persons with spine injuries resulting in fewer complete spinal cord injuries and more survivors of injuries at the C1 to C4 levels.

The chapters in this section address the initial issues faced by the acute care team as they manage the patient with high quadriplegia. These patients are best managed in spinal cord injury systems of care that have had sufficient numbers of patients to have developed the comprehensive resources to handle the complexities involved. However, accidents resulting in high quadriplegia do not always occur at a location or at a time convenient to a medical center involving such a system of care. Although transfer to a system hospital often occurs within a relatively short time, initial management is frequently done in a community hospital.

As the following chapters discuss, the initial medical issues involve insuring survival of the patient by maintaining respiration and stabilizing all body systems. The key elements to maximizing long-term potential then become the prevention of secondary injury. The spine is evaluated and appropriately stabilized, respiratory conditions are mechanically normalized, and nutritional status is assessed to ensure that the system is receiving the essentials to withstand the physiological stress of major trauma. The emphasis in nursing is on the maintenance of range of motion, skin integrity, and the management of bowel and bladder functions so that secondary complications in these areas do not prevent the patient from beginning rehabilitation as soon as possible. In addition, as presented in Chapter 8, the entire acute care team is cognizant of the long-term psychological issues surrounding the trauma. It is critically important that the patient and family are given factual information as test results become available. It may be necessary to repeat the prognosis and long-term considerations throughout the acute care hospitalization.

Not all patients have the option of participating in a comprehensive rehabilitation program. Some are never discharged from the acute care hospital but are maintained in intensive care units. Some are discharged to nursing homes. For those who are able to obtain financial resources to participate in rehabilitation, discharge can be to the family or to live independently with attendant care. The person with high quadriplegia who is able to participate in rehabilitation does have the potential for a productive, quality life, and it is for these individuals that we continue to justify extensive efforts in acute care.

2

Medical Issues in Acute Care

R. Edward Carter

The Institute for Rehabilitation and Research, Houston, Texas, U.S.A.

Acute care in ventilator-dependent quadriplegia should focus simultaneously on survival, secondary prevention, and maintaining as many of the patient's future options as possible. The crucial period in the management of the ventilator-dependent quadriplegic patient in an acute trauma center begins immediately postinjury. Initial preoccupation with patient survival can outweigh the long-term program, and early medical complications may leave their permanent mark. It is during this period that the spinal-cord-injury physician should be consulted and methods of secondary prevention initiated. Because the spinal-cord-injury physician has more experience with the long-term outcome of these patients and of their potential, irreversible complications frequently can be avoided.

GENERAL METABOLIC RESPONSE

The physiologic stress imposed by severe spinal cord injury together with associated injuries is complicated by the factors of bed rest, paralysis, and the additional stresses that may come from surgical procedures and/or exogenous steroids. These factors may be compounded further by fever associated with the secondary complications of infections and decreased nutrition. Management must be anticipatory in nature and started as early as possible. The spinal-cord-injury incident rates are highest in young individuals, and most are in a very good state of health immediately preinjury. At the moment of injury, these patients have normal stress responses such as corticoid release. Young patients generally tolerate this stress fairly well. For the initial 48-h period, there is a tendency to retain fluid. After this, there is a diuretic stage that begins 48–72 h posttrauma and may persist for some 7–10 days posttrauma.

9

Because of the body's continued normal response to stress, the patient can usually tolerate additional stress, i.e., surgery, without too much difficulty. After the initial 36–72 h, the patient goes into a state of hypercatabolism with rapid loss of albumin and total protein in addition to a decrease in the anabolism of proteins. There is also a rapid and marked decrease in the patient's general endurance. In addition, due to many of the factors already mentioned, the patient undergoes a variable period of relative anergy in which the immune responses are diminished or absent, leaving the patient vulnerable to the secondary complications of infections that may be quite severe at this stage.

Calcium loss from the bones begins in approximately 72 h and is accompanied by phosphorus and nitrogen loss through the urine. Quadriplegic persons tend to lose approximately one-third more of these values than do neurologically normal individuals placed on bed rest for similar lengths of time. Muscle strength tends to deteriorate at the rate of 15% per week. The first major medical goal is to halt and then plateau the downhill hypercatabolic process. Hemoglobin, due to both decreased anabolism and increased catabolism, tends to drop to approximately 11 g. Hemoglobin values below 10.5 g warrant an extensive workup to identify other reasons for this decrease. General treatment consists of range of motion techniques, a beginning exercise program, and appropriate attention to secondary prevention of the many complications of immobility, paralysis, and bed rest. An adequate diet that is high in calories and protein together with fluid replacement during the diuretic stage are implemented. If necessary, hyperalimentation should be initiated as early as possible. The respiratory tract, urinary system, and skin should be watched extremely closely.

NUTRITION

The initial diet needs to be high in protein and calories. The average caloric requirement of quadriplegic patients in the early stage postinjury is approximately 3,500–3,700 calories per day. Alimentation should not be delayed. If necessary, dietary supplements via a nasogastric tube or via a subclavian catheter should be initiated quite early. For chronic cases as well as those with dysphagia and/or aspiration, a gastrostomy or nasogastric tube is used for continual feedings, particularly throughout the night.

POSITIONING AND TURNING

The quadriplegic patient should be turned a minimum of every 1½–2 h to prevent pressure ulceration, excessive soreness in the shoulders, and most importantly, to promote better pulmonary drainage. The upper extremities should be externally rotated and placed away from the sides and, especially in quadriplegia, the crucifix position should be used for several hours intermittently during the day. In patients with skeletal traction, the head of the bed may be elevated slightly for countertraction if the lower extremities are elevated at least 15° higher than the level of the heart and the knees are slightly flexed to promote better venous drainage. As soon as the patient is orthopedically cleared, range of motion should begin immediately with isometric exercises to the muscles of the neck, which may continue for months to years. If possible, a gradual program of tilting should be employed while the patient is in tongs and traction to reestablish postural control of blood pressure as early as possible. To diagnose early atelectasis and/or cephalad extension of the spinal cord lesion that may involve one or both diaphragms, ventilator-dependent patients should be followed with serial vital capacities on each nursing shift for the first 7–10 days, followed by monitoring several times weekly. Intermittent positive pressure breathing and incentive respirometry should be employed prophylactically, particularly in smokers, and should be followed by chest physical therapy, postural drainage, and assisted coughing and/or suctioning. Further issues of respiratory management will be addressed in Chapter 12.

GASTROINTESTINAL SYSTEM

The initial period postinjury may be associated with gastric dilatation or ileus and the patient may have to be fed intravenously during this period. Hyperalimentation should be begun if the ileus persists for more than 2 days. Care should be taken not to overhydrate the patient to the point of pulmonary edema, which is the most common problem during the first several days postinjury. If continuation of intravenous feeding is necessary and oral feeding is delayed more than 3 or 4 days, hyperalimentation should be considered. Daily bowel programs should be initiated with stool softeners for stool softness management and a laxative medication for increased motility, followed by a suppository-triggered bowel movement at a time when convenient. Abdominal distension can frequently occur in the early stages posttrauma secondary to ileus or acute gastric dilatation. The abdominal distension may further compromise respiratory function by upward pressure on the diaphragms.

GENITOURINARY SYSTEM

Initial management should be with a closed-system Foley catheter using a catheter as small as possible to allow drainage of urethral mucus around the catheter. Intermittent catheterization should begin immediately after the diuretic phase when the patient is able to restrict fluid intake and achieve an average output of 400 ml every 4 h. The catheter should be taped to the appropriate area as required by male or female anatomy. Intermittent catheterization can be continued until the patient develops reflex voiding or has been found to have a low motor neuron problem with the bladder. This management also covers the period of relatively low patient energy and low host resistance, during which time urinary tract infections can be severe.

SKIN

In addition to turning every 1½–2 h, the skin should be inspected for reactive hyperemia where body pressure on bony prominences may exceed the capillary pressure for too long a time. The reactive hyperemia should disappear within 20 min or all pressure should be removed from this area until the discoloration has disappeared. In the event that reactive hyperemia takes longer than 3 or 4 days to heal, direct pressure should also be avoided until any subcutaneous induration has also disappeared.

FUNCTIONAL THERAPY (OCCUPATIONAL AND PHYSICAL)

In addition to all of the above, range of motion and appropriate positioning by occupational therapists and physical therapists should begin as soon as possible. From a muscular standpoint, the higher the level of the patient's lesion, the more important it is to concentrate activities on the remaining musculature. Strengthening and retraining of the remaining musculature of the neck with emphasis on any remaining respiratory musculature are critical. Maximizing the remaining accessory musculature may allow the patient some degree of time off from ventilator support, which benefits the patient with easier physical transfers and ultimately increases patient confidence for the goal of a home program. In addition, strengthening may help with head control, allowing the use of a powered wheelchair with a chin control at some point in the future.

PSYCHOSOCIAL ASPECTS

This is one of the major areas of potential problems during the early stages. The patient and family should be given accurate and repetitive information concerning medical tests and the reasons for each portion of the therapy program. Initially, it is important not to deny all hope with a severe prognosis. Later, when rapport has been established and there is further time for observation and caution, a more detailed prognosis may be discussed. It is especially important to explain the different parasthetic types of pain and hypersensitivity in the early stages posttrauma. It is important that psuedosensations not be confused with recovery. Concentration should be on the present and future short-term goals and not on the past. With the equilibration of patient care supplied by a spinal-cord-injury specialist consultant in the acute trauma center, it is hoped that transfer from a trauma center to a spinal-cord-injury center becomes virtually a matter of convenience. The patient and family should be appropriately oriented in the transfer process as the goal changes from one of survival to one of restoration of function.

3

Neurologic and Orthopedic Considerations

William H. Donovan

The Institute for Rehabilitation and Research, Houston, Texas, U.S.A.

This chapter deals with the pathophysiologic changes caused by trauma to the spinal cord and spinal column, the means currently employed to diagnose the neurologic level of the lesion, the means by which the extent of the bony and soft-tissue injuries are classified, and finally the treatment recommended during the initial and definitive stages of care.

PATHOPHYSIOLOGY: SPINAL CORD

The structural and ultrastructural changes that occur after damage to the spinal cord have been studied in both laboratory animals and postmortem human subjects. Laboratory experiments have been carried out primarily on the cat. In experimentally induced spinal cord injury (SCI), these animals are seen to develop scattered petechial hemorrhages in the central gray matter within the first 15 min, and these enlarge and coalesce by 1 h (1). The extrusion of blood into the gray matter generally reaches a maximum in 3–4 h, and by 24–36 h the gray matter has undergone hemorrhagic necrosis. The white matter begins to show petechial hemorrhages at 3–4 h. Myelinated fibers show enlargement of the periaxonal space and fraying of the myelin. By 24–36 h, long tracts show extensive structural degeneration (2).

Kakulas (3) has studied hundreds of severely traumatized spinal cord specimens obtained from people who were dead on arrival at a medical facility. He found that despite its delicate semifluid nature, the spinal cord may appear normal to the naked eye after trauma despite significant damage to the adjacent bony structure, ligaments, and muscles.

15

This is particularly true in patients who died instantly on impact. In others, the spinal cord showed petechial hemorrhages, edema, and disruption of the parenchyma. In many specimens, some continuity of long tracts appeared to be preserved. Complete dehiscence of the spinal cord was a rare finding from closed trauma. In patients who survived for a period of 12–24 h, vascular changes became prominent, and hemorrhages in the white and gray matter were noted similar to those described in the cat.

Animal experimentation has yielded information concerning blood flow to the spinal cord after injury and vasospasm, and constriction of the arterial supply has been a constant observation. The cause of the vasoconstriction has not been fully defined but serotonin, catecholamines, and prostaglandins have each been implicated as causal agents (4). In addition to being potent vasoconstrictors, norepinephrine and serotonin potentiate platelet aggregation. The decreased cord perfusion after injury therefore may occur from platelet aggregation coupled with chemically mediated large vessel vasoconstriction and thrombosis (5).

In his study of patients with SCI who died weeks to months after their injury, Kakulas described macrophage activity removing debris and the establishment of the process of gliosis. Macrophages were seen actively engaging in ingesting necrotic spinal cord tissues, mainly in the central areas of the cord and the adjacent posterior columns. A glial meshwork was seen beginning to demarcate the lesion from the tracts (3). One could infer that concomitant changes must be occurring in the various neuropeptides and other neurotransmitters, but no information of this nature is available.

The study of the human material affords the ability to learn of chronic changes after SCI, by studying changes seen in patients who died months to years after their injuries. This stage is characterized by the presence of multilocular cysts with thick glial walls, sensory nerve root regeneration, and a residuum of descending and ascending central nervous system fibers at the level of the lesion. Often, the subarachnoid space is obliterated by fibrous tissues, which may also enter and mix with the glial network. These glial scars may also be the source of abnormal neuropeptide release. Regenerating nerve roots, which are a feature of the chronic stage, rarely enlarge sufficiently to form a neuroma with compression of the cord remnant (3).

It is known that a small percentage of patients may develop posttraumatic syringomyelia, which may cause clinical deterioration with involvement of higher spinal cord segments. This becomes extremely critical in the cervical region where the loss of one segment adds significant impairment, particularly when the C3 and C4 areas become involved. In patients whose injuries occur in the cauda equina, some patients demonstrate a continuing active fibrosis of the nerve roots, which may persist after many years.

At the present state of the art, medical science can do virtually nothing to reverse the vascular and cellular reactions that occur after trauma to the spinal cord. It can, however, play an important role in minimizing further injury, which may be caused by improper handling of an unstable spinal column. In addition, by appropriate care it can reduce aggravating factors such as hypotension and hypoxia. In essence, the extent of the destruction and the potential for any recovery depends on the magnitude of force that has been impacted on the neural tissue within the spinal cord at the moment of injury. It is generally true that whether the trauma be minor or major, the spinal cord loses its ability to conduct action potentials. The only factor that will reveal how much neurotrauma actually occurred is time itself, for if the injury was indeed very minor, recovery will occur quickly and totally. If it was major, it will never recover at all. However, between these two extremes there are significant gradations that may result in incomplete SCI. In general, the sooner recovery occurs the more will occur, and the later it is noted, the less it will occur.

Incomplete lesions to the spinal cord may take the form of several syndromes based on the anatomical relationships of the neural tracts and gray matter. These syndromes of incompleteness (Figs. 3-1–3-5) include the following (6):

1. Anterior cord syndrome: This syndrome displays a neurologic picture that reflects the destruction of the anterior two-thirds of the cord. This includes the central gray and white matter in the anterior and lateral columns of the cord. Thus, dorsal column function is preserved and the individual has position and vibratory sense below the level of the lesion but lacks pain, temperature, and motor function.

2. The central cord syndrome: In this lesion, the central gray matter is damaged far more than the peripheral white matter. It occurs primarily in the cervical region and one sees a pattern of paralysis in the upper extremities due to the destruction of the anterior horn cells that serve this region of the body. There is often sparing of some or all of the more peripheral white matter, allowing these tracts to conduct past the area of injury. They are thus able to energize the motor neurons in the lumbar and sacral areas. Therefore, depending on the magnitude of the injury and the involvement of the white matter, the individual will be left with impairment of the upper extremities and less impairment of the lower extremities and, very possibly, preservation of bowel, bladder, and sexual function.

3. Brown-Séquard syndrome: This reflects the presence of function in

Incomplete Spinal Cord Syndromes

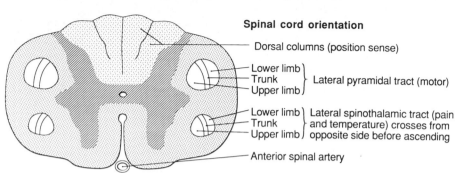

Spinal cord orientation

Dorsal columns (position sense)

Lower limb ⎫
Trunk ⎬ Lateral pyramidal tract (motor)
Upper limb ⎭

Lower limb ⎫ Lateral spinothalamic tract (pain
Trunk ⎬ and temperature) crosses from
Upper limb ⎭ opposite side before ascending

Anterior spinal artery

FIG. 3-1. Cross section of the spinal cord shows the dorsal columns, lateral corticospinal (pyramidal) and lateral spinothalamic tract, the central gray matter with its ventral and dorsal horns, and anterior spinal artery.

only one-half of the spinal cord. This syndrome is manifested by ipsilateral loss of motor function and ipsilateral loss of vibration and position sense. The unique feature here is the loss of pain and temperature on the contralateral side of the body. Therefore, the injured person retains the feelings of pain and temperature on the paralyzed side.

4. The posterior column syndrome: This consists of the loss of position

Anterior spinal artery syndrome

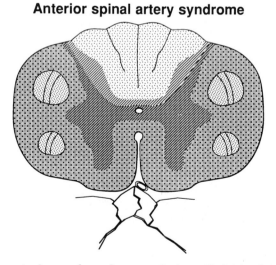

FIG. 3-2. The anterior cord syndrome reflects pathologic changes such as ischemia, infarction, or direct trauma to the anterior and lateral two-thirds of the cord (this coincides with the area supplied by the anterior spinal artery—hence, anterior spinal artery syndrome).

Central cord syndrome

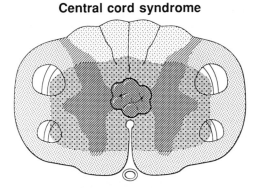

FIG. 3-3. The central cord syndrome reflects pathologic changes such as hemorrhage within the central gray matter and extending in some cases peripherally into the white matter and its major tracts (as shown here).

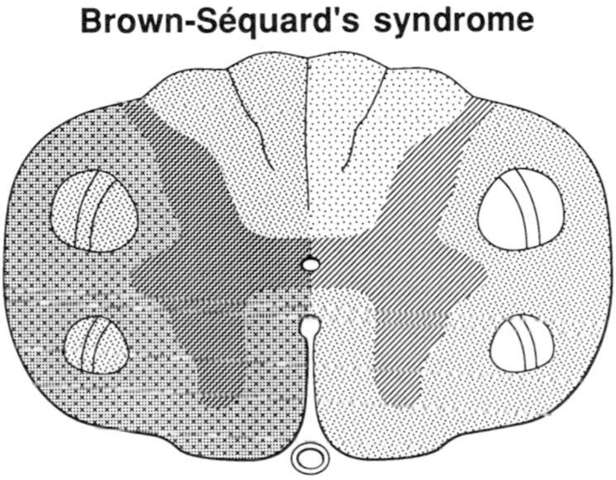

Brown-Séquard's syndrome

FIG. 3-4. The hemicord or Brown-Séquard syndrome reflects pathologic changes to primarily one side of the cord—shown as the darkened left side of the figure.

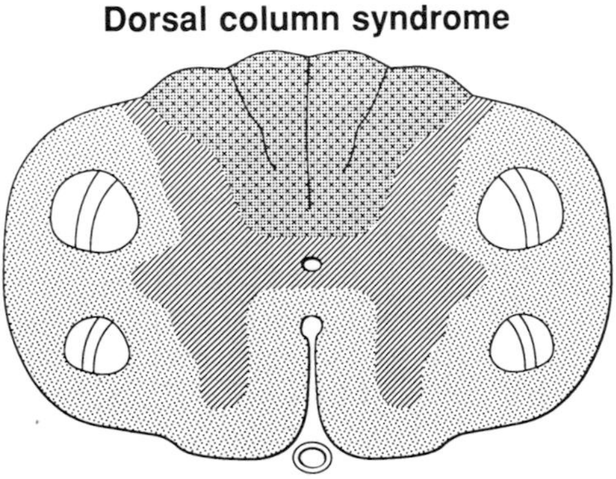

Dorsal column syndrome

FIG. 3-5. The dorsal column syndrome reflects pathologic change involving the dorsal columns.

and vibratory sense only, with preservation of the other motor and sensory modalities. This is rarely seen as a result of trauma.

It is important to remember that these syndromes are rarely "pure." That is, closed trauma rarely causes an exact manifestation of any one of the above syndromes. For example, someone will usually not manifest a Brown-Séquard syndrome in the pure form but rather will manifest an impairment of both sides of the spinal cord with one being more involved than the other.

Incomplete syndromes may also be described and classified on the basis of the function remaining below the level of the lesion. In 1969, Frankel (7) described a functional grading system for incomplete lesions of the spinal cord. He designated the letter "A" to describe a complete lesion, "B" described a lesion with only the preservation of sensation regardless whether it was perceived normally or in a diminished manner, and "C" described a lesion with preservation of some sensation and some motor function but the motor function was insufficient for functional activities such as ambulation. "D" described an injury in which the degree of motor function was useful. A patient with a cervical lesion in which ambulation is possible even though it requires braces and crutches would be classified as D. "E" described a lesion that was marked by complete recovery although the persistence of hyperreflexia did not preclude an E grade.

In high cervical lesions, the degree of completeness is indeed a very important issue, because preservation of motor function below the level of injury may well include some preservation of respiratory muscle function. The latter will be totally absent in a person who has a complete lesion above C3. Therefore, preservation of some diaphragmatic or intercostal muscle function may mean the difference between breathing and ventilator dependency.

PATHOPHYSIOLOGY: SPINAL COLUMN

The next important consideration in SCI relates to the injury to the bony column. Injuries to the spinal column are best analyzed from the point of view of the mechanism of injury. Although more elegant classification systems have been developed (8–10), a simple classification of flexion, compression, extension, and shearing has continued to survive (11). Although it is sometimes possible to ascribe a single mechanism to a vertebral injury, there are many instances in which combinations of these mechanisms occur. Disruption of the spinal column may therefore result from one or more directional force vectors. However, the mechanism(s) can usually be deduced from the appearance of the x-ray film.

Flexion injuries. This type occurs when a force from behind the upper part of the person's body pushes one vertebra forward on the vertebrae below, usually resulting in angulation or displacement. This can be due to an anteriorly directed blow to the back of the head or back, or could be caused by an individual falling backward and striking the head or back against a fixed object such as a wall. The resultant radiograph shows an anterior displacement or an anterior angulation of the superior vertebra relative to the inferior one in the affected part of the body.

A flexion injury is the kind most likely to cause disruption of the spinous ligaments, particularly when it is combined with some rotational and distraction forces. Because spine stability is directly related to the integrity of the ligaments, this mechanism is more likely to create a potentially unstable spine. Instability is defined for these purposes as the abnormal movement of one vertebra on another. It is important to remember that normally some movement does occur between adjacent vertebrae but for most adjacent vertebrae (also called motion segments) it is a very small amount.

Compression. In these injuries, the force is essentially directed vertically downward or upward, that is, along the longitudinal axis of the spinal column. It is manifested by a crushing of the vertebral body and possibly the posterior elements. Generally no ligamentous disruption occurs, and therefore these injuries are generally quite stable.

Extension. In this type of injury, a posteriorly directed force is applied to the anterior surface of the person's body. It is seen primarily in cervical injuries. The radiograph may show a posterior displacement of the superior vertebral body on the inferior one, but more often one sees a separation of the disk space at one motion segment or an avulsion fracture of the anterior superior part of the inferior vertebrae. This is commonly called a teardrop fracture. Fractures of the posterior elements may also occur from this mechanism. Because little in the way of ligamentous disruption occurs, these fractures are also usually stable.

Shear. In this injury one sees a total displacement or translation of one vertebra on another in either the sagittal or coronal plane. The former is best seen on the lateral radiograph whereas the latter is noted on the anteroposterior (AP) film.

The important clinical considerations from this analysis of injuries to the spinal column are those of stability and deformity.

The potential for instability must be deduced from the radiographic examination because it is important to prevent any abnormal movement at the injury site for fear of causing further damage to the spinal cord. Some types of fractures are generally accepted as being unstable and require surgical stabilization whereas others are generally regarded as inherently stable and do not require it. There is, however, a large area in between that is contested by different schools of thought. Dennis (12) has tried to clarify this issue by proposing a three-column concept for

the spine. The anterior column includes the anterior longitudinal ligament, and the anterior two-thirds of the vertebral body and annulus;
the middle column consists of the posterior longitudinal ligament and
the posterior one-third of the vertebral body and annulus; and the posterior column contains the posterior elements and ligaments. Dennis believes that if two of the three columns are damaged, then the injury is
unstable. Further, it is also known that the presence of significant displacement or separation of bony elements implies ligamentous damage
and these kind of injuries are more likely to be unstable. In such instances, operative fixation and bony fusion are often indicated.

The second important aspect of these injuries is the presence of deformity. Deformity is measured in terms of angulation and/or displacement at the injury site. Although some minor degrees of deformity are
acceptable, it is undesirable to leave the patient with a significant deformity and therefore reduction of the deformity is warranted. If closed
reduction is impossible or fails, then open reduction is indicated.

Although the foregoing principles apply to all vertebrae, some specific
examples relative to C1 and C2 should be mentioned, because their ar-
chitecture is different from the rest.

Dislocations of the occiput on C1 and C1 on C2 are rare but may be
caused by severe rotatory forces resulting in either anterior or posterior
displacement of the occipital condyles on the atlas. Many of these injuries are incompatible with life owing to severe accompanying damage to
the spinal cord brainstem and/or the vertebrobasilar arterial system.
However, survival has been reported and high quadriplegia or the "locked-
in" syndrome may result (13).

Jefferson's fracture is a bursting or compression fracture of the ring
of C1 at more than one location. These are often seen best on computed
tomography (CT).

Fractures of the odontoid are classified according to the location of the
fracture on the dens. Type I is rare, involves the upper dens above the
transverse ligament, and probably represents an avulsion fracture where
the alar ligament attaches. Type II occurs at the junction of the dens
and body, whereas Type III extends down into the cancellous bone of the
body of C2. Both Types II and III can result from flexion or extension
mechanisms probably combined with rotation. Although the latter two
types can occur without displacement of the dens, when displacement
does occur it reveals the mechanism of injury: Anterior displacement
indicates a flexion mechanism (the more common of the two) whereas
posterior displacement reflects extension forces (14).

Hangman's fractures or traumatic spondylolisthesis of the axis is an
extension fracture through the pedicles of C2 causing the separation of
the neural arch from the body of the axis. As the names implies, the
lesion is usually seen in prisoners executed by hanging but is also com-

monly caused by rapid deceleration in automobile accidents where the head meets the windshield and is thrust back while the body is moving forward. The posterior arch of C2 remains with the rest of the spine while the anterior arch remains with the dens, atlas, and skull (15).

DIAGNOSIS

When a newly injured person with a SCI arrives at the emergency room, the neurological examination should be performed after one has established that the circulatory and respiratory systems have been truly stabilized. After that, attention can be turned to the neurological examination, which will disclose the neurological level (6, 16), and the degree of incompleteness as measured by the Frankel grade (7) and the motor index score (17).

The establishment of a sensory level depends on one's knowledge of the typical sensory dermatome maps (6, 16). The sensory level is designated as the lowest level in which all sensory modalities, i.e., sharp/dull, pain/temperature, proprioception, vibration, light touch, and deep pressure, are all perceived as normal. In patients with complete injuries, some of these modalities will be felt one to three dermatomes below the last normal one. This partial sparing of some neurologic function is referred to as the zone of injury. In incomplete lesions, some or all of the sensory modalities may be felt in a diminished or normal fashion for some distance below the level of injury. However, for a sensory examination to be designated as incomplete, this preservation of sensation must exist more than three segments below the last normal dermatome (16).

To determine the motor level, a knowledge of the "key muscles" as well as their innervation is crucial. It is important to remember that most muscles have a dual and sometime triple innervation. That is, usually two segments (via their corresponding nerve roots) innervate each muscle. Because of this, a muscle cannot perform at normal strength unless it has both segments contributing to its innervation. The biceps, for example, is a C5/C6 muscle. If all of its C5 but none of its C6 innervation were functioning, the muscle would not test as normal. It would more likely have enough strength to give a grade 3 or possibly a grade 4 level of performance but not a grade 5. (Conventional muscle grading is described as follows: 0, no movement; 1, trace movement; 2, poor movement through full range, gravity eliminated; 3, fair movement through full range, against gravity; 4, good ability to provide some resistance to movement; and 5, normal strength) (16). Therefore, the motor level is determined by knowing the lowest muscle that gives a normal grade, the next lower muscle that gives a fair grade, and finally the next lower muscle that gives a 0 grade. It is the muscle in this sequence that gives a fair grade, that indicates the lowest normal myotome (6, 16). The zone of injury may be reflected in the motor examination, as well as the sensory, by the finding of Grades 1–4 strength in muscles below the lowest normal myotome, but as with the sensory examination, this must be found in more than three myotomes below the last normal one before the lesion can be classified as motor incomplete.

The Frankel grade, as described above, is then determined and finally the motor index score is determined by testing the strength of specific muscles according to the muscle scale given above. Five muscles in each extremity are examined. A perfect score is 100 because each muscle is given a grade of 5 (Table 3-1).

The sensory and motor levels localize the lesion within the longitudinal axis of the spinal cord. The Frankel grade and the motor index score describe the degree of incompleteness. From this information, reasonable functional expectations can be predicted and reasonable comparisons can be made between patient groups.

In the high quadriplegic patient who happens to be complete, i.e., Frankel "A," the neurologic examination will likely be brief. However, it is still important to determine the precise extent of diaphragmatic function. The latter should be evaluated directly by fluoroscopic examination and indirectly using parameters such as the vital capacity and negative inspiratory force. As in all patients, a Frankel grade must never be assigned without examination of the sacral segments (anus and genitalia) for sensory and motor sparing. In addition, because patients with cervical spine injury may also sustain a head injury, careful documentation of mental status should be carried out as well as the Glasgow Coma Scale, if applicable.

It is often difficult to determine the existence and/or extent of a SCI in a patient with concomitant head injury (HI). There are several useful clues when examining the patient with impairment of consciousness which should be looked for, however.

1. Disparity of upper body/lower body tone. Acutely, SCI is marked by flaccidity (spinal shock) whereas HI is often marked by hypertonicity manifested by decerebrate or decorticate posturing.

2. Disparity of response to noxious stimuli. A painful stimulus administered to the head or upper part of the body may evoke arousal or response whereas stimulating the lower part of the body does not.

3. Disparity of reflex responses. Deep tendon reflexes, for example, may be elicited at the jaw and elbows but not the knees and ankles and Babinski's reflex may be unobtainable.

4. Disparity of autonomic findings. The combination of hypotension, bradycardia, and often hypothermia is in keeping with a picture of sympathetic blockade seen in quadriplegia but not HI. Also if sweating is

Table 3-1. *Spinal Cord Injury Motor Index Score*[a]

Suggested spinal cord injury motor index score[b]			Key muscles for motor level classification[c]	
Grade on Right	Muscle	Grade on left	C4	Diaphragm
5	C5	5	C5	Deltoid and/or biceps
5	C6	5	C6	Wrist extensors
5	C7	5	C7	Triceps
5	C8	5	C8	Flexor profundus
5	T1	5	T1	Hand intrinsics
5	L2	5		
5	L3	5	T2-L1	Use sensory level, abdominal re-
5	L4	5		flexes and Beevor's sign to help lo-
5	L5	5		calize lowest normal neurological
5	S1	5		segment
50		50		
	Total Score 100		L2	Iliopsoas
			L3	Quadriceps
			L4	Tibialis anterior
			L5	Extensor hallucis longus
Motor grading system:			S1	Gastrocnemius
0—absent	(total paralysis)			
1—trace	(palpable or visible contrac- tion)		S2-S5	Use sensory level
2—poor	(active movement through ROM with gravity elimi- nated)			
3—fair	(active movement through ROM against gravity)			
4—good	(active movement through ROM against resistance)			
5—normal				

[a]The key muscles, shown on the right, are tested according to the muscle grading system located on the lower left. A perfect score is illustrated on the upper left.

[b]This motor index score, when used accurately, provides a numerical grading system to document improvement or deterioration of motor function. Motor index score adapted from scoring system by Lucas and Ducker (17).

[c]This motor neurological level is considered the lowest intact segment when the muscle grade is fair (grade 3) or greater. Most of these key muscles have dual innervention. Therefore, if the listed level is fair, the given neurological level should essentially be normal.

present, it may be noted in the upper part of the body but not the lower. Finally, in the male patient, the presence of priapism strongly indicates the coexistence of SCI as well as HI.

After the neurological examination is concluded, x-ray films can then be obtained. Initially, AP and lateral films alone will suffice to provide a picture of the extent of the bony damage. It is important when taking cervical x-ray films, to be sure to see all seven cervical vertebrae. This will often necessitate the physician's presence in the x-ray suite or at the patient's side, if a portable film is taken, to supervise the taking of the lateral film. It will often necessitate the physician holding the patient's head while an assistant pulls down on the arms. If special views of the facets are necessary, this can be accomplished without turning the patient, but by simply angling the x-ray tube properly. In addition, "swimmer's" views can be taken to better visualize C7 in those patients for whom C7 cannot be visualized despite the maneuvers mentioned above. It is usually wise to x-ray the spine below the level of injury to rule out "silent fractures" (18) in insensate areas, and to x-ray the skull in patients with impaired consciousness.

When there are no contraindications, plain tomography and CT will afford the examiner with a much better picture of the extent of the bony damage. Magnetic resonance imaging (MRI) will also provide some information as to the extent of the soft-tissue damage.

It must be emphasized, in obtaining these special views that are afforded by CT and MRI, that the patient has to be placed in a confined area for an extended period. Therefore, anyone who is experiencing medical instability, particularly of the cardiovascular or respiratory systems, must be watched extremely closely and one must be prepared to delay the diagnostic procedure or remove the individual if the patient's distress becomes extreme. Also, the importance of pressure relief must not be ignored during this time. Ferromagnetic metal devices must be removed before obtaining either study. In the case of CT, they will obscure the image, and, in the case of MRI, they will not only obscure the image but also create a hazard within the magnetic field. The availability of the Monaghan 225 all-aluminum ventilator and a halo device now made from titanium has permitted the use of these devices in the MRI room.

INITIAL TREATMENT

Regardless of the position in which one finds the injured person, every effort must be made to stabilize the spine. This can be done with a backboard or neck brace and strapping the patient to the board while he/she is extricated, e.g., from the car or construction site.

If the respiratory status is extremely impaired and emergency tracheostomy or cricothyroidotomy becomes necessary, it may not be possible to apply a cervical collar. The same may be true if extensive bleeding is present in the cervical area. In such an instance, the head must be stabilized with sandbags applied laterally. It must be remembered that when the spinal cord has been damaged the patient is vulnerable to the development of pressure ulcers because of impaired sensation. Therefore, the patient must be turned at regular intervals, preferably every 2 h, *regardless* of the fact that the spine may be unstable and must be immobilized. Turning is also necessary to facilitate drainage of the bronchial tree. When turning is performed, the patient must be log rolled, keeping the chin, the sternum, and the symphysis pubis in a straight line at all times. When the patient is supine, the cervical and lumbar lordoses should be supported by towels or pillows. The backboard or splint of hard material must be removed as soon as the patient arrives at a hospital, where definitive care can be given.

It is generally agreed among experts in the field that patients with SCI should be taken to a trauma center that has the services of a neurosurgeon, orthopedic surgeon, or preferably both. In addition, only lifesaving and emergency measures should be applied before the patient is taken to such a center. A trauma center that is attached or closely affiliated with an SCI center is the most preferable place for an SCI person's initial care.

The patient should be transported in an ambulance or helicopter if at all possible and should only be given narcotics and other analgesics if the patient is actually complaining of severe pain. It is interesting that many individuals do not complain of pain as long as they are stabilized and handled with care.

On arrival at a trauma center, an intravenous line should be established if not already present and the circulatory and respiratory systems must be stabilized. An indwelling urethral catheter and, usually, a nasogastric tube should be placed; then the neurologic and radiographic examinations described above should be carried out.

In the case of cervical injuries, efforts at stabilization will usually center around the application of external support such as a cervical brace of one form or another, or the application of cervical traction by calipers or tongs such as the Gardner-Wells tongs. It is extremely important when dealing with a high-level cervical injury, such as those that may impair respiratory function, that the amount of traction be applied very cautiously, because it is possible to easily overdistract an injury in the upper cervical spine. Thus, frequent spine x-ray films should be taken if the amount of traction is increased.

In the past, most patients with high cervical injuries either had no neurological deficits or died. In recent times, due to the rapid advances in life-support systems and the wider availability of such services, many patients who would have died are now saved and are placed on artificial ventilation. This then creates the situation of the possible survival of someone who is not only paralyzed in the arms and legs but is also unable to breathe at all or unable to breathe adequately. Therefore, every effort must be made to foster conditions that will favor survival of as many cells as possible in the zone of injury within the spinal cord. In addition to careful rescue and immobilization referred to earlier, it is important to avoid complications that are known to affect neural tissue adversely such as hypoxia and hypotension. Therefore, the respiratory and circulatory systems must be assiduously supported.

It is important to realize that the advances in medicine that have taken place over the last 10–15 years have primarily dealt with issues that concern the biomechanics of the spine. In other words, much can be done to remedy the effects of the injury on the bony spinal column but this is not true for the spinal cord. Creditable research nevertheless has been done and is currently being done in the investigation of pharmacologic and surgical interventions aimed at reducing or ameliorating the effects of trauma on the spinal cord (19–22). Despite this, nothing has yet been developed that has proved to be of value to spinal man in the area of reversing the effects of trauma to the spinal cord. Despite some claims that "decompression" improves chances of recovery (19–23), this finding is unsupported and refuted by others (24–29). Therefore, in the following discussion the reasons whether to operate or not to operate are focused primarily around the issues concerned with the restoration of stability and normal alignment to the spinal column, rather than "curing" the paralysis.

In deciding whether a patient needs an operation or can be managed with conservative or nonoperative treatment, it is important to consider five factors.

The first is the individual's general medical condition. It would seem obvious that if the patient has circulatory or respiratory embarrassment, operative intervention on the spine is contraindicated. It is only after these and other visceral problems have been stabilized that consideration to surgery may be given.

The second is the likelihood of instability. It should be noted that instability is a relative term. The spine may be unstable when subjected to the forces of gravity and muscle action in the sitting position. However, it may be quite stable when the individual is supine and wearing an external support or in cervical traction. One may deduce the likelihood of instability from the x-ray films of the spine. In general, injuries that have been subjected to flexion, particularly with distraction and/or rotational mechanisms, are more likely to be unstable because they are more likely to disrupt the ligaments connecting vertebra to vertebra. Injuries that occur from compression or extension are less likely to produce such ligamentous damage. Injuries that occur from shearing produce a significant deformity but may be stable in the abnormal configuration.

For purposes of this discussion, we will define instability as the presence of abnormal movement between vertebrae. Normally there is a small amount of movement from one vertebra to another. Each pair of adjacent vertebrae is then considered a motion segment (30).

It may be concluded from the above discussion that some injuries that would demonstrate abnormal movement if the patient were allowed to sit can be managed conservatively as long as there is no compelling reason to get the patient out of bed. If the patient, for example, is quite ill and surgery is contraindicated anyway, there is usually no need to act quickly to stabilize the spine by operative intervention. In most cases, except for some flexion/distraction injuries, the injured vertebra(e) will heal by autofusion to the adjacent vertebrae (28). If the injury appears stable and the medical condition permits, the patient who has not undergone a surgical internal stabilization may be allowed to sit after 6 weeks in external support as long as the device insures the prevention of abnormal movement. In cervical injuries, particularly those involving the upper C-spine, a halo orthosis will often provide sufficient support to allow sitting even before 6 weeks postinjury. Before mobilizing a patient in other cervical orthoses such as a sterno-occipital mandibular immobilizer (SOMI) brace, cervicothoracic (Yale) brace, or Philadelphia collar (6, 24), many authorities prefer to wait 6 weeks to allow sufficient healing and they advocate the wearing of the external support chosen until the patient is 3 months postinjury (or operation if one was done).

As a rule, a halo orthosis gives the best external support to injuries to the upper cervical spine, particularly C1 and C2 (31), and its use may be advocated even in apneic patients with complete injuries at this level. Caution, however, is needed when managing such patients in a halo-vest orthosis because the vest makes respiratory therapy more difficult because it is harder to percuss and cough the patient.

For patients with C1 and C2 injuries described earlier, particularly those who have only minor neurologic deficit, the halo brace is generally considered the best form of external support. Exceptions to this general rule include the Type I odontoid fractures, which are inherently stable and can be treated symptomatically; the Type II odontoid fractures, which are prone to nonunion (36%) and therefore early fusion should be considered; and some undisplaced, stable hangman's fractures, which can be treated in a cervicothorocic brace (13–15).

Internal instrumentation used to stabilize the spine in the cervical area generally consists of wire. Fusions are usually done along with the instrumentation, the posterior approach being the more common type, in all areas of the spine.

A third factor influencing the decision whether to operate or not is the presence of deformity. If significant deformity is present, the spine must be reduced so that close to anatomical alignment may be obtained. Various authors will give different opinions as to the degree of deformity that is acceptable. If, however, there is angulation beyond 35° at the fracture site or if there is displacement beyond one-half of a vertebral body, the deformity has become significant. If reduction of the deformity cannot be effected by closed methods, then open methods are certainly justified if there are no contraindications.

The level of incompleteness is a fourth factor that also must be placed in the equation. The reason for this is that individuals who are very incomplete may need very little rehabilitation. Therefore, their hospitalization can be significantly shortened if they may be gotten out of bed. However, it is important that the spine be supported either by external stabilization methods, such as a halo device or other external support, or internal stabilization methods, such as wire and fusion. In most cases this will allow both the maintenance of alignment and stability and the assumption of the upright posture, if early mobilization is desired. The nature of the fracture will determine whether the stabilization must be done operatively or can be achieved with external support alone. However, the consideration of early mobilization, whether using internal or external support or both, must never come before the consideration of the recovering spinal cord. If the patient is showing signs of neurologic recovery, caution is advised before doing anything that will permit mobilization until one is sure the recovery has stabilized.

If, on the other hand, the patient is quite complete, i.e., Frankel A or B, early mobilization may be more difficult to achieve. This is particularly so in the case of the quadriplegic patient and more so in the case of the high quadriplegic patient. The quadriplegic patient has significant circulatory and respiratory pathophysiologic changes to deal with. Orthostatic hypotension will make the assumption of the upright, sitting position a very gradual process. In addition, even if the patient is not apneic but does have a marginal vital capacity, the latter is known to be less in the sitting position than in the supine position in quadriplegic persons and therefore respiratory fatigue must be looked for when sitting begins. Furthermore, it is harder to give assisted cough to patients in the sitting position and the patient is exposed to a greater risk of atelectasis and other respiratory complications during the transition to the sitting posture. Given these circumstances, surgery adds a significant additional stress in these patients and a halo may impede respiratory therapy and interfere with mobility training. In short, for the complete or nearly complete patients, particularly in the cervical region, the reasons for early mobilization are less compelling and therefore there is less indication to operate or apply halo fixation for this reason alone. However, this in no way implies that the rehabilitation of such patients should be delayed. If referred to a spinal center that is prepared to meet their needs, their rehabilitation can begin whether they are managed nonoperatively (bed rest or halo fixation) or operatively. The experience of spinal centers in Europe, Australia, and in some cases, North America has shown that the notorious complications of bed rest can be prevented even if the early treatment chosen for the spine is immobilization in bed, e.g., tongs and traction. It is neglected patients who are most prone to complications, be they at bed rest or involved in a sitting program (32).

The final factor that must be considered is the level of the lesion. As indicated above, the higher lesion levels have more pathophysiologic alterations of the circulatory and respiratory systems than do the lower injuries. Patients with lower injuries such as the dorsolumbar and lumbar injuries have normal arm function, better trunk balance, and are able to do more if they are mobilized early. In addition, another biomechanical factor comes into play, namely the weightbearing load across the fracture site if the patient is mobilized. In the cervical region, less weightbearing load passes through the fracture site. However, in the lower injuries more of the body weight passes through it and the force of gravity will exert a greater influence on the injury site. In addition, because more muscle tissue remains innervated, stronger forces from muscle contraction will be exerted around the fracture. Gravity and muscle action in combination will act as forces that may foster instability, increase deformity, impede fracture healing, and increase the usual pain and discomfort associated with mobilization. Therefore, it is more likely that injuries in this area will need internal stabilization if early mobilization is desired.

If all of the above five factors are considered, a rational decision can usually be made that will insure the patient's best chances for maintaining health, maintaining stability and alignment, and progressing along the path to rehabilitation in a period that is safe and also as soon as possible.

REFERENCES

1. Campbell JB, DeCrescito V, Tomasula JJ, Demopoulos HB, Flamm ES, Ortega BD (1974): Effects of antifibrinolytic and steroid therapy on the contused spinal cord of cats. *J Neurosurg* 40:726–33.
2. Koenig C, Dohrman GJ (1977): Histopathologic variability in "standardized" spinal cord trauma. *J Neurol Neurosurg Psychiatry* 40:1203.
3. Kakulas BA (1984): Pathology of spinal injuries. *Cent Nerv Syst Trauma* 1:117–129.
4. Osterholm JL (1974): Noradrenergic mediation of traumatic spinal cord autodestruction. *Life Sci* 14:1363–1384.
5. Naftchi NE, Demeny M, DeCrescito V, Tomasula JJ, Flamm ES, Campbell JB (1974): Biogenic amine concentrations in traumatized spinal cords of cats. Effects of drug therapy. *J Neurosurg* 40:52–57.

6. Donovan WH, Bedbrook GM (1982): Comprehensive management of spinal cord injury. *CIBA Clin Symp* 34:1–36.
7. Frankel HL, Hancock DO, Hyslop G, Melzak J, Michaelis LS, Ungar GN, Vernon DS, Walsh JJ (1969): The value of postural reduction in the initial management of closed injuries of the spine with paraplegia and tetraplegia. *Paraplegia* 7:179–192.
8. Braakman R, Penning L (1976): Injuries of the cervical spine. In: *Handbook of Clinical Neurology* (Vinken PJ, Bruyn GW, ed), Amsterdam: North Holland, pp. 227–380.
9. Allen BL, Ferguson RL, Lehmann TR, et al. (1982): A mechanistic classification of closed, indirect fractures and dislocations of the lower cervical spine. *Spine* 7:1–27.
10. Harris JH, Edeiken-Monroe B, Kopaniky DR (1986): A practical classification of acute cervical spine injuries. *Orthop Clin North Am* 17:15–30.
11. Holdsworth R (1970): Review article: Fractures, dislocations and fracture-dislocations of the spine. *J Bone Joint Surg [Am]* 52:1534–1551.
12. Dennis F (1983): The three column spine and its significance in the classification of acute thoracolumbar spinal injuries. *Spine* 8:817–831.
13. Pierce DS, Barr JS (1983): Fractures and dislocations at the base of the skull and upper cervical spine. In: *The Cervical Spine* (Bailey RW, ed), Philadelphia: JB Lippincott, pp. 196–206.
14. Anderson L (1983): Fractures of the odontoid process of the axis. In: *The Cervical Spine* (Bailey RW, ed), Philadelphia: JB Lippincott, pp. 206–223.
15. Garfin SR, Rothman RH (1983): Traumatic spondylolisthesis of the axis (hangman's fracture). In: *The Cervical Spine* (Bailey RW, ed), Philadelphia: JB Lippincott, pp. 223–232.
16. American Spinal Injury Association (1983): *Standards for Neurological Classification of Spinal Injury Patients*. Chicago: American Spinal Injury Association.
17. Lucas JT, Ducker TB (1979): Motor classification of spinal cord injuries with mobility, morbidity and recovery indices. *Am Surg* 45:151–158.
18. Shehata S, Adams J (1974): Spinal injuries—review of 168 patients with 224 fractures of the spine. *Orthop Rev* 3:29–33.
19. Jelsma RD, Rice JF, Jelsma LF, Kirsch PT (1982): The demonstration and significance of neural compression after spinal injury. *Surg Neurol* 18:79–92.
20. Wagner FC, Chehrazi B (1980): Spinal cord injury: indications for operative intervention. *Surg Clin North Am* 60:1049–1054.
21. Ducker TB, Bellegarrigue R, Salcman M, Walleck C (1984): Timing of operative care in cervical spinal cord injury. *Spine* 9:525–531.
22. Bohlman HH (1979): Acute fractures and dislocations of the cervical spine. *J Bone Joint Surg [Am]* 61:1119–1142.
23. Verbiest H (1969): Anterolateral operations for fractures and dislocations in the middle and lower parts of the cervical spine. *J Bone Joint Surg [Am]* 51:1489–1530.
24. Bedbrook GM (1979): Spinal injuries with paraplegia and tetraplegia. *J Bone Joint Surg [Br]* 61:267–284.
25. Munro D (1961): Treatment of fractures and dislocations of the cervical spine,

complicated by cervical cord and root injuries. *New Engl J Med* 264:573–582.

26. Maynard FM, Reynolds GG, Fountain S, Wilmot C, Hamilton R (1979): Neurological prognosis after traumatic quadriplegia. *J Neurosurg* 50:611–616.

27. Wagner FC, Chehrazi B (1982): Early decompression and neurologic outcome in acute cervical spinal cord injuries. *J Neurosurg* 669–705.

28. Donovan WH, Kopaniky DR, Stolzmann E, Carter RE (1987): The neurological and skeletal outcome in patients with closed cervical spinal cord injury. *J Neurosurg* 66:690–694.

29. Young JS, Dexter W (1978): Neurological recovery distal to the zone of injury in 172 cases of closed traumatic spinal cord injury. *Paraplegia* 16:39–49.

30. McNab I (1977): *Backache*. Baltimore, Williams & Wilkins, pp. 1–15.

31. Wolf JW, Johnson RM (1983): Cervical orthoses in the cervical spine. In: *The Cervical Spine Research Society* (Bailey RW, ed), Philadelphia: JB Lippincott, pp. 54–61.

32. Donovan WH, Carter RE, Bedbrook GM, Young JS, Griffiths ER (1984): Incidence of medical complications in spinal cord injury: patients specialized, compared with non-specialized centers. *Paraplegia* 22:282–290.

4

Pulmonary Physiology and Medical Management

Peter Peterson

Consulting Staff, Craig Hospital, Englewood, Colorado, U.S.A.

THE PROBLEM

Respiratory complications occur frequently in patients with quadriplegia. This is true both in ventilator-independent patients and in those requiring a ventilator.

Pulmonary complications in patients with quadriplegia have been reported to occur in 40–70% of the patients (1,2). Paralyzed patients have less mobility, and, therefore, drainage of lung segments is not accomplished as well as in nonparalyzed patients. The combination of impaired drainage and bronchial obstruction by mucus plugs may predispose to infection in these poorly drained, obstructed areas of lung. Mucus plugging and muscle weakness predispose to atelectasis (loss of aeration of lung, with accompanying loss of lung volume).

Much of this chapter is concerned with prevention and treatment of atelectasis. This is because atelectasis is related to many of the respiratory complications seen in quadriplegic patients. Infection in involved segments may result in pneumonia or bronchitis. Undrained pneumonia predisposes to abscess formation within the lung. Extension of the pneumonia to the pleural surface predisposes to empyema. Prolonged infection in obstructed bronchi may cause bronchiectasis, with the potential of a lifetime of recurrent infection. This pattern can lead to death in patients unable to keep a chronically collapsed segment clear of infection. In addition to the long-term medical problems and possible death, these medical complications prolong the treatment phase for the spinal-injured patients and delay the start of rehabilitation, thus increasing the cost of hospitalization.

The above-cited medical complications and cost factors dictate that it is vitally important to take preventive and therapeutic measures to prevent atelectasis and other respiratory complications, and if they occur, to treat in a timely fashion.

MEDICAL THERAPY

Whether the goal is to prevent respiratory complications, or to treat them if they have occurred, the best of medical management is imperative. The major medical therapies include theophylline derivatives, appropriate antibiotics, respiratory therapy, and oxygen.

Theophylline derivatives help to thin secretions, serve as bronchodilators, and have a positive effect on the heart and kidneys. Aminophylline may stimulate secretion of surfactant (3,4). Theophyllines have been shown to help prevent fatigue of the diaphragm (5–7). The latter has not been studied in quadriplegic patients but, by inference, should have a positive effect in quadriplegic patients with borderline vital capacities.

Antibiotics are a frequent requirement in quadriplegic patients. With mucus plugging and the threat of infection behind the plugs, there is the threat that infection will be spread if the mucus plugs are removed. This was dramatically exhibited in a patient who had a trapped lung after a hemothorax and a chest tube. He entered surgery with a clear left lung on chest x-ray film, and, after lying on his left side while the surgeon did a right thoracotomy and released the entrapped lung (and presumably released bacteria), his post-operative x-ray film revealed a left-sided pneumonia. This illustrates that the quadriplegic patient, with reduced muscle strength, may not be able to protect his uninfected lung by coughing out any intrabronchial spread of infection. Therefore, consideration should be given to administration of antibiotics before any bronchoscopic or surgical attempt to open atelectatic areas of lung.

Bronchodilators, such as albuterol, help moisten secretions, and also help relieve bronchospasm. In some patients, cromolyn sodium has been thought to be helpful in raising secretions and relieving bronchospasm. In addition, postural drainage is helpful in these paralyzed patients. Incentive spirometry would theoretically be helpful in strengthening the respiratory muscles and in opening atelectatic areas of lung. The usefulness of incentive spirometry may be limited by the mechanical factors inherent in the weakness associated with paralysis. Oxygen is an obvious therapy in patients who are hypoxic.

Other measures that fit in the category of desperation attempts at therapy but that are helpful in selected patients include glyceral guaiacolate to liquefy secretions, and various attempts at dietary manipulation. For example, some patients form mucus in response to milk products, and limiting such products in the acute phase may avoid exhaustion from coughing and help limit the formation of mucus plugs.

BRONCHOSCOPY

Bronchoscopy can be very helpful. This is true not only in ventilator patients, but also in nonventilator patients who have atelectasis. If the patient has a good vital capacity of >12.5 ml/kg, and still has atelectasis, daily bronchoscopy to clear out mucus plugs may help to avoid a ventilator. However, such patients need close observation, because they are apt to develop overwhelming mucus plugs, atelectasis, and cardiorespiratory collapse. Bronchoscopy should be done early in patients with atelectasis, and daily until the atelectasis clears. This is true whether or not the patient is being ventilated. Patients should be monitored during bronchoscopy with oximetry and telemetry. With these precautions, the risk is small, but the bronchoscopist must be watchful for hypoxia, arrhythmias, syncope, and trauma to the airway, and, if the patient is being ventilated, the bronchoscope may cause significant obstruction of the endotracheal or tracheostomy tube. In this regard, it is easier to do the bronchoscopy through a tracheostomy tube than through an endotracheal tube and is one reason for early tracheostomy in these patients.

MONITORING DURING ACUTE-PHASE ILLNESS

The problems previously listed in the introduction (respiratory insufficiency, mucus plugging, atelectasis, lung abscess, empyema, and bronchiectasis) all develop in quadriplegic patients as a direct effect of the respiratory muscle weakness, or are a secondary complication and indirectly the result of the respiratory muscle weakness. Pneumonia and bronchitis may be related to the muscle weakness but may occur for other reasons. In newly injured quadriplegic patients not requiring a ventilator, but being clinically monitored for respiratory insufficiency, mucus plugging, atelectasis, and the possible necessity for a ventilator, certain measurements should be made. In evaluating patients, it should be kept in mind that the functional level of injury may ascend in the first few days after injury. Hypothetically, this may occur because there is edema, hemorrhage, or hematoma formation in the spinal cord. Thus, a patient may arrive at the hospital a C5 quadriplegic and ascend to C3 over the next 48 h. This difference may be critical in the development of atelectasis and also respiratory insufficiency with respiratory acidosis, hypoxia, and death. Patients will not usually have atelectasis immediately, because the mucus plugging, fatigue, and ascending neurologic level take some time to cause the atelectasis. However, if patients develop atelectasis, they will also have worsening of hypoxia and may develop respiratory insufficiency and die. For these reasons, in high quadriplegic patients (C6 and above), an initial blood gas should be checked and the vital capacity should be checked every 4 h for the first few days. Patients who have a vital capacity < 12.5 ml/kg should be considered for placement on a ventilator. If the vital capacity is steadily deteriorating, and the deterioration cannot be reversed with medical measures and respiratory therapy, the patient should be intubated when the vital capacity reaches a low of 12.5 ml/kg, even if the blood gases and chest x-ray film remain normal. It is better if the patient never has atelectasis than to have to be intubated after developing it. There is more risk of death after atelectasis develops, primarily because of the risk of reperfusion pulmonary edema (or perhaps it should be called reexpansion pulmonary edema) with the attendant risk of adult respiratory distress syndrome (ARDS) and the high risk of death in this syndrome. Therefore, it is better to be aggressive and intubate early (if by so doing atelectasis can be prevented) than to wait for the development of atelectasis and respiratory arrest. In addition to the frequent vital capacity measurements, it is suggested that blood gases be determined and chest x-ray films be done at least daily early in the course of a high quadriplegic patient, and more often if the other parameters such as vital capacity, heart rate, or respiratory rate are unstable and deteriorating.

VENTILATOR-DEPENDENT PATIENTS

Intubation

In patients who need intubation but who have cervical spine fractures, the intubation should be done without extending the patient's neck. This can be accomplished by blind nasal intubation. If necessary, the posterior pharynx can be visualized after the nasal tube has been passed, and the tube's location relative to the epiglottis can be determined by pulling the tongue forward with the larnygoscope, without extending the patient's neck. In some cases, the fiberoptic bronchoscope will be needed. It is passed through the nasal tube to visualize the epiglottis and vocal cords. A nasal tube is preferred to the oral tube because it is easier to pass without extending the patient's neck, and can be secured more firmly than an oral tube. Once it is in place, the nasal tube is also more comfortable. Indications for intubation include low vital capacity (< 12.5 ml/kg), hypoxia, hypercarbia, intractable atelectasis, fatigue, tachycardia and arrhythmias, and trauma to the airway.

Tracheostomy

If the patient is going to need to be intubated for a prolonged period, perhaps longer than 5 days, it is best to perform a tracheostomy early. In expert hands, the risk of tracheostomy is small. The risk of serious bleeding is 1–2%, and an occasional patient may be hypoxic enough that he will develop syncope because of a lack of ventilation for the time it takes to insert the tracheostomy tube after the endotracheal tube has been removed. The author has had no patient deaths during the procedure in a series of 124 tracheostomies. This is similar to results reported in other series (8,9). With large-size tracheostomy tubes and soft cuffs, the pressure exerted on the trachea by the cuff is small, and the risk of tracheal stenosis is small. If the cuff becomes defective, or the tube occluded by mucus in the middle of the night, it is easier to change a tracheostomy tube than it is to change an endotracheal tube. It is easier to suction and do bronchoscopies through a tracheostomy tube than it is through an endotracheal tube. All of these factors favor early tracheostomy.

Aggressive Treatment of Atelectasis: Use of Large Ventilator Tidal Volumes and Frequent Bronchoscopies

Historical Perspective

Traditionally, pulmonologists have been taught to ventilate patients on ventilators with a tidal volume of 10 ml/kg of body weight. However, the vast majority of patients managed in this fashion are patients who are not quadriplegic. Spinal-cord-injury patients require different approaches because of their paralyzed diaphragms and intercostal muscles. For example, in the setting of the quadriplegic patient, atelectasis is more of a concern than in a nonparalyzed patient.

In conventional therapy, bronchoscopies are sometimes done to evacuate the mucus. However, there remains an impression that daily bronchoscopies are not done, perhaps because daily bronchoscopy seems to be overly dramatic, as well as hard on the patient. Also, the atelectasis may clear with appropriate medical management and vigorous respiratory care, in which case daily bronchoscopy is not necessary. Conversely, if the atelectasis does not clear, the repeated bronchoscopies seem to be accomplishing nothing. One treatment for atelectasis has evolved over the past several years and is based on a retrospective study (unpublished data) and on a prospective study now in progress. This treatment involves frequent bronchoscopies combined with increasing ventilator tidal volumes.

Current Therapy

In a current study protocol, all ventilated quadriplegic patients with atelectasis are started on ventilator tidal volumes of 15 ml/kg. In calculating the weight, ideal body weight is used. This is done because many of the patients have lost a considerable amount of weight since injury. The weight loss is due to muscle atrophy and the catabolic factors associated with acute injury and illness. Assuming that the ventilator pressures are not excessive, the tidal volume is progressively increased. It would not be unusual to ventilate an average-size man with tidal volumes of 1,700–1,800 ml, and in very tall men, tidal volumes of 2,200 ml have been used. If the patient has radiographic evidence of atelectasis, daily bronchoscopies are done until any atelectasis has cleared.

A Retrospective Study

A retrospective study of 24 patients with quadriplegia and atelectasis treated by mechanical ventilation over 39 months was done. These patients were treated before a protocol had been established for studying this problem. They were treated with various combinations of low and high ventilator tidal volumes, and with frequent and infrequent bronchoscopy. By chance, half of the patients were treated with tidal volumes <20 ml/kg, and half were treated with tidal volumes >20 ml/kg. Those treated with the smaller tidal volumes took an average of 23 days to clear, and those treated with the larger tidal volumes took an average of 10 days to clear (Table 4-1). The patients were also analyzed for frequency of bronchoscopy, and if the average time between bronchoscopy was over 3 days, the atelectasis cleared in an average of 36 days, whereas if the average time between bronchoscopy was under 3 days, the atelectasis cleared in an average of 9 days (Table 4-2). In those patients who had both frequent bronchoscopy and large tidal volumes the average time for clearing of atelectasis was 8 days, as opposed to 39 days in those with infrequent bronchoscopy and small tidal volumes (Table 4-3).

Table 4-1. *Clearing of Atelectasis and Tidal Volume*

Treatment	No. of patients	Average days to clearing
On ventilator at tidal volumes <20 ml/kg	12	23
On ventilator at tidal volumes <20 ml/kg	12	10

p = 0.05.

Table 4-2. *Clearing of Atelectasis and Bronchoscopy*

Treatment	No. of patients	Average days to clearing
Infrequent bronchoscopy	7	36
Frequent bronchoscopy	11	9

p = 0.001.

Thus, a month of medical therapy can be saved if the patients are treated aggressively. This amounts to tens of thousands of dollars per patient.

In the retrospective study, there were no cases of pneumothorax in 1,064 days of continuous ventilation (patient not being weaned from the ventilator).

Scientific Basis for Large Volumes and Frequent Bronchoscopies

Given the observation that frequent bronchoscopies and large tidal volumes improve results in atelectasis in quadriplegic patients, what are the scientific reasons for this observation?

In 1976, Bynum et al. (10) reported that ventilation and perfusion of the basilar lung regions were compromised by the supine position, and that ventilation and perfusion of the basilar lung regions were further compromised by prolonged positive pressure breathing. They concluded that larger tidal volumes on the ventilator improved both ventilation and perfusion at the lung bases in supine patients, but that spontaneous large breaths were more effective in preventing atelectasis. The mean resting tidal volume and large tidal volume they referred to were 556 and 1,718 ml, respectively. In quadriplegic patients, however, spontaneous large breaths are not mechanically possible, secondary to their paralysis. Based on the findings of Bynum et al., the use of large tidal volumes while avoiding excessively high pressures seems a logical ap-

Table 4-3. *Combined Therapy and Days to Clearing*

Type of therapy	No. of patients	Average days to clearing
Nonaggressive	7	39
Aggressive	8	8

p = 0.001.

proach, especially in supine, paralyzed patients with the inability to spontaneously generate a large breath. Cane and Shapiro (11) have also stated that use of large tidal volumes on the ventilator helps to minimize the development of atelectasis. However, they were talking in general terms, as far as ventilator patients are concerned, and they were suggesting tidal volumes of 15 ml/kg. Although it seems appropriate to start the quadriplegic patient at a setting of 15 ml/kg, it may be necessary to work the ventilator tidal volume up to one that may exceed 20 ml/kg.

Surfactant

Surfactant is a lipid that lines the surface of the alveoli. It helps keep the alveoli from collapsing. Several authors (12–19) have reported that large lung inflations are potent stimuli to surfactant secretion. This may be because the stretching of type 2 alveolar cells is the stimulus for release of surfactant, or it may be that in opening up additional alveoli by the larger volumes, more type 2 cells are recruited to secrete surfactant. Type 2 cells in atelectatic alveoli do not secrete surfactant. Hopefully, further answers to the mystery of surfactant will be forthcoming in the future.

Closing Volumes and Physical Forces Involved in Opening Alveoli

The closing volume is that point in exhalation in which the forces favoring collapse of airways—specifically, airways smaller than 1 mm in diameter (20)—are greater than the forces favoring keeping these airways open. This closure of airways occurs in the lower lung zones (21). In spinal-injured patients, the forces favoring the collapse of alveoli are loss of surfactant, water in the alveoli, pressure of subdiaphragmatic organs on the lung, and muscle weakness. The major force favoring the opening of alveoli is the negative pressure created by the respiratory muscles (including the diaphragm) during inhalation. In the spinal-injured patient, the closing volume may be adversely affected by the loss of respiratory muscle by the paralysis initially, and in the next few days, by the loss of the strength of the remaining respiratory muscles by fatigue. In addition, if the diaphragm is partially paralyzed, the abdominal contents will press on the basal portions of the lung. Many patients will develop abdominal distension, further aggravating this factor. In some patients the lungs may be "wet" because of fluid administration and the contribution of pulmonary edema from cerebral-pulmonary edema. These factors favor the collapse of terminal airways and progressive atelectasis. Added to this is the fact that the patient has collections of

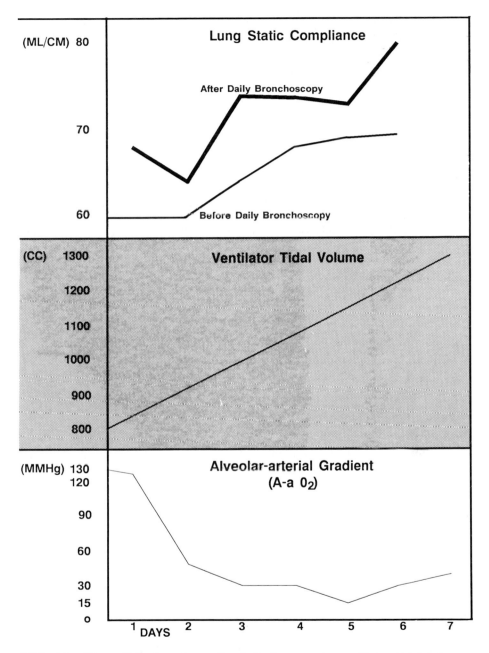

FIG. 4-1. The middle box shows the daily increase in ventilator tidal volume, starting at 15 ml/kg and increasing 1.25 ml/kg/day. The lower box shows the A-a (Alveolar-arterial) O_2 gradient. The upper box shows the lung static compliance before and after the daily bronchoscopy.

mucus in the airways. This is particularly true in the paralyzed patient, because their strength is insufficient to cough up the secretions. This serves to aggravate the closing volume, and adds to the progression of the atelectasis. The intrapulmonary pressure exerted by the ventilator in ventilator-dependent quadriplegic patients should be a factor serving to open the closed alveoli.

Observations in Patients

When bronchoscopies are done in quadriplegic patients with atelectasis, the usual finding is of mucus, sometimes in the form of occluding plugs. Anyone who has seen these occluding plugs realizes that the atelectatic lung will never reexpand until the plugs are removed. It is also observed that the compliance of the lung improves if the mucus plugs are first removed and then the tidal volume on the ventilator is increased. Figure 4-1 shows the improvement in one patient's compliance before and after the daily bronchoscopy, and the improvement in the A-a gradient over 1 week while on this protocol.

POSITIVE END EXPIRATORY PRESSURE

Positive end expiratory pressure (PEEP) means that there is continuous positive pressure being exerted on the lung by preventing the pressure inside the lung from going to zero at end of exhalation.

In the retrospective study, PEEP was used in 13 patients for a total of 157 days. There were two pneumothoraces in that time. The difference in pneumothoraces between the PEEP days and the non-PEEP days is statistically significant ($p = 0.002$). There was no evidence that PEEP speeded the resolution of the atelectasis. Use of PEEP in atelectasis has been studied several times and has not been found to be helpful in resolving atelectasis. The use of less than 5 cm of PEEP in trying to prevent atelectasis in quadriplegic patients has not been studied. Smaller levels of PEEP may avoid the barotrauma. However, the animal studies suggest that it is the alternative stretching and relaxation of the type 2 alveolar cells that is the stimulus for release of surfactant, rather than the constant stretching of the cells. Because of the evidence of barotrauma and the lack of evidence of a positive effect on atelectasis, PEEP should not be used in quadriplegic patients with atelectasis.

GAPS IN SCIENTIFIC BASIS FOR TREATMENT OF QUADRIPLEGIC PATIENTS WITH ATELECTASIS OR WITH THE POTENTIAL FOR ATELECTASIS

Although the available experimental evidence in animals supports the theory that more surfactant is generated in response to larger tidal volumes, and it is known that atelectatic areas of lung do not produce significant amounts of surfactant, and studies suggest that compliance is improved after bronchoscopy and higher inflation volumes, there are no scientific studies in humans to confirm the animal data. The reason we lack human data is that it is impossible to accurately collect human lung surfactant samples before and after bronchoscopy and before and after various tidal volumes on the ventilator. In animal studies the animals are killed to obtain the surfactant measurements. Physicians who care for quadriplegic patients need to do more measurements of compliance in their patients to collect the needed information, and perhaps it would help to measure the airway pressure at various points in the tracheobronchial tree.

Ventilator Triggering Not Recommended

Inductively, if the patient is allowed to trigger the ventilator cycle, this may have an adverse effect on the closing volume, actually exerting negative pressure inside the alveoli and terminal bronchioles, just as the ventilator valve opens in response to negative pressure generated by the patient. Usually, in normal breathing, negative forces are exerted outside the alveolus, causing improvement in the closing volume. In paralyzed patients who are allowed to trigger the ventilator, their muscle weakness may not allow for enough negative pressure to be exerted outside the alveolus, and with the ventilator attached, the negative pressure is exerted from the inside of the airway, acting to "suck" the air out of the alveolus and enhancing the process of producing atelectasis. For this reason, it is preferable not to allow the patient to trigger the ventilator. Triggering the ventilator can be prevented by eliminating the stimuli to breathe. This can be done by being certain the pO_2 is high enough, the pCO_2 is low enough, and the pH is high enough that the brain is not stimulated by any of these chemical stimuli to cause initiation of a breath by the patient. The stretch receptors in the lung also need to be satisfied. All of these things can be accomplished by giving large tidal volumes on the ventilator. Because of the above reasoning and because paralyzed patients may not be strong enough to keep their alveoli open, intermittent mandatory ventilation (IMV) should not be used in quadriplegic patients. The normal person requires 6–12 L of minute ventilation to maintain a normal pCO_2, and the paralyzed patient may not be able to generate enough spontaneous tidal volume and respiratory rate to maintain a minute ventilation of 6–12 L and a normal pCO_2. IMV requires voluntary ventilation on the part of the patient, and because the paralyzed patient may not be able to generate voluntary ventilation of the amount required, there may be very high levels of pCO_2 and a very low pH, which is a threat to the patient's life. This is another reason to never use IMV in the paralyzed patient.

Ventilator Settings

Suggested ventilator settings are as follows for the initial day: tidal volume 15 ml/kg, respiratory rate of 12, ventilator flow rate adjusted to obtain a peak inspiratory pressure between 35 and 40 cm water pressure, sigh 300–500 ml over the tidal volume, an oxygen to keep the arterial saturation over 92%. On subsequent days bronchoscopy should be done if the x-ray film shows atelectasis, and after the bronchoscopy, the ventilator tidal volume increased by 1.25 ml/kg, so long as the peak pressure does not exceed 40 cm H_2O. The pH can be maintained at 7.45–7.50 by adding or subtracting dead space. The pCO_2 level is irrelevant as long as the pH is in a good range. Patients are switched to uncuffed Jackson tracheostomy tubes as soon as the patient can tolerate it. The tidal volume on the ventilator is turned up to compensate for the air leak through the mouth. The metal Jackson tracheostomy tubes seem to cause less irritation and seem to stimulate less mucus secretion than do the plastic tracheostomy tubes. With the uncuffed tracheostomy tubes, however, it is impossible to keep the pCO_2 up to normal levels. One patient has been on a ventilator for 15 years, with an uncuffed Jackson tracheostomy tube in place. This long-time patient has run a pCO_2 of 15–18 for 15 years without ill effects. His (one) kidney has compensated and his pH is consistently between 7.40 and 7.45. In general, the patients can tolerate the above procedures without discomfort, and unless there is a complication such as atelectasis or pneumonia, supplemental oxygen will not be needed and the ventilator will not be triggered by the patient (see previous section on scientific basis for large volumes). Theoretically, the large volumes and relatively high inflation pressures should serve to overcome the forces causing deterioration of the closing volume. Very few patients on these settings develop atelectasis. Even with the uncuffed Jackson tracheostomy tubes in place, the goal is to achieve peak ventilator pressures of 35–40 cm. There is no evidence in the literature that "opening pressures" necessary to overcome the forces causing closure of alveoli have been studied. Pending such information, a peak pressure of 30–40 cm H_2O seems likely to avoid (or treat) atelectasis without causing barotrauma.

Associated Chest Injury

Quadriplegic patients often have other associated chest injuries. The most common of these are hemothorax, pneumothorax, flail chest, and sometimes they develop pleural effusions in association with atelectasis. They also develop reperfusion pulmonary edema (? reexpansion pulmonary edema), widespread respiratory infections, and ARDS. These other injuries are well treated with the principles outlined previously. The flail chest patients will heal very well with the large ventilator tidal volumes, and will not flail, because they are not triggering the ventilator. Those patients with hemo- or pneumothorax will do better with the large volumes because if they form pleural adhesions due to the chest tubes, the adhesions will be formed at full lung inflation and will not cause limitation of lung expansion after the patient has healed. The worst complication is reinflation pulmonary edema and ARDS. This occurs in trauma patients, but the common cause in the patient with quadriplegia is after reexpansion of atelectatic lung. Because of the high death rate in ARDS and because this occurs as a late complication in those patients who have had atelectasis, it is imperative that we not let patients develop atelectasis.

CONCLUSIONS

This chapter discusses techniques and theoretical reasoning involved in ventilating quadriplegic patients. Aggressive medical therapy is recommended both for those patients who are ventilator dependent and those who have potential for respiratory problems because of the level of spinal cord injury or other associated injuries. Large ventilator tidal volumes are recommended and, if the patient has atelectasis, frequent bronchoscopy is recommended. IMV should not be used in quadriplegic patients. PEEP should be used only for patients with ARDS. Using the techniques described will result in less morbidity and mortality and will save hundreds of thousands of dollars per year in the care of quadriplegic patients.

Acknowledgment: The author thanks the following: John Roberts, M.D., for reading the x-ray films in the retrospective study; S.-F. Hsu, M.D., and Janis Berend, M.S.N., C.N.P., for reviewing the charts; Gale Whiteneck, Ph.D., for his statistical analysis; and Ken McKay, R.R.T., for collecting and calculating the data on A-a gradients and compliance.

APPENDIX A: SAMPLE ORDER SET

1. Admit patient to quadriplegia protocol.
2. Do vital capacity (VC) every 4 h and call if VC is <1,000 ml (first 48 h).
3. Do VC every 6 h and call if VC is <1,000 ml (next 24 h).
4. Do VC every 12 h and call if VC <1,000 ml (next 48 h).
5. Thereafter do VC daily, and call if VC <1,000 ml.
6. Do VC each Monday (after first 3 weeks).

7. Do arterial blood gas, VC, chest x-ray film, complete blood count, and biochemical study on admission.

8. If NPO start aminophylline drip at 20 mg/h.

9. If taking oral medications, start theophylline (Theo-Dur) 200 mg p.o., b.i.d.

10. Culture sputum.

11. If O_2 saturation is <92%, start nasal O_2 and titrate to 92%.

12. Give albuterol 0.5 ml in 2 ml saline by nebulizer q.i.d., and p.r.n., followed by incentive spirometry, and chest clapping if indicated for secretions. May add cromolyn 20 mg to nebulizer if patient has excessive secretions. If patient is not able to do deep breath to use nebulizer, do intermittent positive pressure breathing (IPPB) "stretch" (start IPPB treatment at 15 cm H_2O pressure, and increase to as high as patient will tolerate during course of treatment, but do not exceed 40 cm H_2O pressure).

APPENDIX B: ALGORITHM (INJURY AT C6 OR ABOVE)

```
-------------------T----------------------+-----------------------T---------------

Admit and start medical Rx                   Monitor parameters

Theophyllines, bronchodilators,              Chest X-ray, blood gases,
O2, chest physical therapy,                  vital capacity, respiratory
and, if indicated, antibiotics,              rate, pulse, temperature,
and steroids.                                and fatigue.


-----------T------------------------------------------------------T---------------

       Atelectasis                  Vital capacity < 1000cc, low O2,
          |                         high CO2, respiratory acidosis,
daily bronchoscopy------->          or fatigue.

no respiratory failure,          ^------->  intubate
(low O2, high CO2,                          |
respiratory failure),                       set ventilator on 15cc/kg
vital capacity > 1000cc,                    ideal body weight, and
no fatigue.                                 adjust flow to achieve
          |                                 35-40cm H2O pressure,
No intubation.                              and do daily bronchoscopy
          |                                 for atelectasis.
Persistent atelectasis------->|
                                            increase ventilator tidal
                                 volume by 1.25cc/kg ideal
                              body weight, daily, until reach
                              point where 40cm H2O pressure
                              is exceeded, then reduce flow
                              or volume to maintain pressure
                              at 35-40cm H2O.
```

REFERENCES

1. Bellamy R, Pitts FW, Stauffer ES (1973): Respiratory complications in traumatic quadriplegia. *J Neurosurg* 39:596–600.
2. Carter RE (1987): Respiratory aspects of spinal cord injury. *Paraplegia* 25:262–266.
3. Barrett CT, Sevanian A, Phelps DL, Golden C, Kaplan SA (1978): Effects of cortisol and aminophylline upon survival, pulmonary mechanics, and secreted phosphatidyl choline of prematurely delivered rabbits. *Pediatr Res* 12:38–42.
4. Corbet AJ, Flax P, Alston C, Rudolph A (1978): Effect of aminophylline and dexamethasone on secretion of pulmonary surfactant in fetal rabbits. *Pediatr Res* 12:797–799.
5. Aubier M, De Troyer A, Sampson M, Macklem PT, Roussos C (1981): Aminophylline improves diaphragmatic contractility. *N Engl J Med* 305:249–252.
6. Viires N, Aubier M, Murciano D, Fleury B, Talamo C, Pariente R (1984): Effects of aminophylline on diaphragmatic fatigue during acute respiratory failure. *Am Rev Respir Dis* 129:396–402.
7. Aubier M, Roussos C (1985): Effect of theophylline on respiratory muscle function. *Chest* (supplement) 91–97.
8. Schusterman M, Faires RA, Brown D, Flynn MB (1983): Local complications and mortality of adult tracheostomy. *J Ky Med Assoc* 885–888.
9. Stauffer JL, Olson DE, Petty TL (1981): Complications and consequences of endotracheal intubation and tracheostomy. *Am J Med* 70:65–76.
10. Bynum LJ, Wilson JE, Pierce AK (1976): Comparison of spontaneous and positive-pressure breathing in supine normal subjects [abstract]. *Proceedings of American Thoracic Society/American Lung Association, Annual Meeting, May 16–19*, p. 150.
11. Cane RD, Shapiro BA (1985): Mechanical ventilatory support. *JAMA* 254:87–92.
12. Massaro GD, Fischman CM, Chiang M-J, Amado C, Massaro D (1981): Regulation of secretion in Clara cells. *J Clin Invest* 67:345–351.
13. Massaro GD, Massaro D (1983): Morphologic evidence that large inflations of the lung stimulate secretion of surfactant. *Am Rev Resp Dis* 127:235–236.
14. Klass DJ (1979): Dibutyryl cyclic GMP and hyperventilation promote rat lung phospholipid release. *J Appl Physiol* 47:285–289.
15. Faridy EE (1976): Effect of distension on release of surfactant in exercised dogs' lungs. *Respir Physiol* 27:99–114.
16. Faridy EE (1976): Effect of ventilation on movement of surfactant in airways. *Respir Physiol* 27:323–334.
17. Nicholas TE, Barr HA. Control of release of surfactant phospholipids in the isolated perfused rat lung. *J Appl Physiol* 51:90–98.
18. Nicholas TE, Barr HA (1983): The release of surfactant in rat lung by brief periods of hyperinflation. *Respir Physiol* 52:69–83.
19. Hildebran JN, Goerke J, Clements JA (1981): Surfactant release in excised rat lung is stimulated by air inflation. *J Appl Physiol* 51:905–910.

20. Murray JF (1986): *The Normal Lung*. Philadelphia: Saunders, pp. 112–114.
21. Tisi GM (1983): *Pulmonary Physiology in Clinical Medicine*. Baltimore: Williams & Wilkins, pp. 106–107.

5

Respiratory Therapy

Marsha Wood

Craig Hospital, Englewood, Colorado, U.S.A.

The respiratory therapist is a key member of the multidisciplinary rehabilitation team for the high quadriplegic patient. The respiratory therapist is intimately involved in early medical management of the injured person, and continues throughout the patient's hospitalization to help carry out the treatment team's management plan through discharge and reintegration into the community.

The respiratory therapist is important to the medical requisites of the unit, but as a staff person in close and constant contact with the patient and his or her family, the therapist assumes an important additional role as educator, coach, and, sometimes, cheerleader. Patient cooperation is maximized when anxiety is minimized. In the rehabilitation hospital setting, which is unknown and frightening to the newly injured high quadriplegic person and his or her family, the respiratory therapist is often a key resource for reassurance and psychological support.

The primary role of the respiratory therapist is to ensure that the patient's air passages are clear and that he or she is able to breathe at maximum capacity and comfort, whether with ventilator assistance or not. Moreover, the long-term health of the patient's respiratory system is often related to the self-care lessons learned from the respiratory therapy staff.

The respiratory therapist's role in the rehabilitation setting differs greatly from that of the respiratory therapist in the general hospital. The rehabilitation setting is typically more personal and less routine than general medicine. Although many of the therapist's duties and functions in either setting are interchangeable, the respiratory therapist in the rehabilitation unit assumes another important role, much more like that of teacher and coach.

TREATMENT OF HIGH QUADRIPLEGIC PATIENTS WHO ARE NOT VENTILATOR ASSISTED

For those newly admitted high quadriplegic patients not requiring ventilator assistance, the respiratory therapist assesses the person's vital capacity, comparing it with baseline readings reported at the acute care hospital, or to what is normal for age and body size. Typically, these patients have already been given tracheostomies. Some have reduced pulmonary function due to sedation or anxiety. If the vital capacity is 40% or less than the predicted normal, a "stretch" program is initiated. The stretch program uses intermittent positive pressure breathing (IPPB) to increase vital capacity by hyperexpanding the patient's lungs with high-pressure ventilation. The treatment begins with ventilation at the lowest pressure setting ($\sim$ 12 cm H_2O pressure). Every few breaths the pressure is increased; depending on patient tolerance, the maximum pressure is usually 30–40 cm H_2O. A stretch program is usually administered for about 10 or 15 min, four times a day. The effects of the stretching can typically be seen in a matter of days.

Treatments to boost vital capacity may also include incentive spirometry, a goal-oriented breathing exercise that measures and encourages patient success with deep breathing by exhaling against no resistance. Lung strength may also be enhanced by use of inspiratory muscle training, which is effected by way of a p-flex device. The device features an air hole that is adjustable in size from large to small; the smaller the air hole, the more the patient must use muscles to attain a full breath. The goal is to increase vital capacity, thereby increasing the ability of the lungs to pull in oxygen and move secretions from the alveoli and the air passages.

IPPB is usually accompanied by bronchodilation medication to keep the airways open. This is done by placing a nebulizer in line with the ventilator air circuits. The common medication used for dilation is albuterol; the dose is 0.5 ml with 2 ml saline, administered every 4–6 h for 5 or 10 min at a time. A nebulizer may also be indicated when the chest is tight, when secretions increase, or when either pneumonia or atelectasis (collapse of some of the small airways in the lungs) is present.

If the nonventilator patient is stable and lungs are clear, the respiratory therapist monitors progress without intervention. It may be necessary on occasion for the therapist to induce coughing to facilitate clearing of secretions. If the vital capacity drops, however, and x-ray films show that the chest is not clear, intubation may be indicated by the attending physician. The respiratory therapist keeps an eye on lung secretions, suctioning as needed to prevent infection or distress. Pneumonia or atelectasis can occur if secretions are not properly treated. If the patient's secretion amounts are especially high, the respiratory therapist may recommend more frequent turning.

TREATMENTS FOR PATIENTS USING A VENTILATOR

The initial assessment of a ventilator quadriplegic by the respiratory therapist begins immediately on admission, often before a full pulmonary consult by the physician staff. It is important for the therapist to be aware of a patient's vital capacity; those patients with zero or very low vital capacity demand much greater vigilance than a patient with a vital capacity of 1,000. For the most effective margin of safety, the therapist must be aware of the range of breathing capacities in high quadriplegic patients.

In the early assessment, an ear oximetry measure is obtained to gauge oxygen saturation in the capillaries of the ear. Oxygen is adjusted to the appropriate level for the individual and for the altitude. Ear oximetry has the advantage of being noninvasive and allows continuous or multiple sampling. It does not measure carbon dioxide. If this is needed, an arterial blood gas (ABG) sampling is made. Generally, the disadvantage of ABG is that it is an invasive, more time-consuming procedure, and is useful mainly for single samples.

A sputum culture is taken by the respiratory therapist as part of hospital protocol for patients with a tracheostomy. The therapist also auscultates the patient, listening to the lungs to assess air movement and secretion accumulation. A chest x-ray film is typically ordered. If the patient was admitted using a respirator, the respiratory therapist monitors the equipment and suctions excess secretions as needed.

THE THERAPIST AS TEACHER

The respiratory therapy staff are among the first members of the rehabilitation team to work with the newly admitted patient and his or her family. It is important to develop a personal and friendly relationship with the patient. Quite often, the injured person has many expectations—sometimes inappropriately high—and often has many anxieties about the new hospital situation. Patients using a respirator are frequently stressed and depressed. There are pressing medical issues to worry about, but the patient also has many unresolved emotions—feelings of dependency, financial uncertainty, and preoccupation, perhaps, with the futility of living. The respiratory therapist should be supportive. It is important to attempt to answer all questions regarding treatment, including what exactly is taking place and why things are done as they are. Peer support is a valuable tool for the rehabilitation team;

the patient often gets his or her most important support and information from those who have been in the same position.

The respiratory therapist's role as educator often extends to other members of the rehabilitation team. For example, the nursing staff, the physical therapists, occupational therapists, speech therapists, and recreation therapists should know how to "bag" or suction the patient when necessary. The respiratory therapist can assist the team in learning these functions. It is also important that the patient be taught all aspects of self-care; he or she, in turn, will need to teach these skills to caregivers, family members, etc.

Among the skills taught by the respiratory therapist are the following:

Assisted coughing: Coughing is very necessary to bring up mucus that normally accumulates in the lungs. Persons with high quadriplegia generally lack the necessary muscles—the intercostals, the diaphragms, the abdominals—to effect a good natural cough. Excess secretions can be dangerous, in that they increase susceptibility to infection. Other than working on exercises to strengthen the diaphragm (as noted above for nonventilator patients), it may be necessary for the respiratory therapist to initiative preventive decongestion treatments. One important method is the assisted cough, or "quad cough." Similar in appearance to the Heimlich maneuver, assisted coughing is the application of pressure under the patient's sternum/rib cage during expiration to expel secretions from the deep air sacs of the lungs (Fig. 5-1). The technique can be used while the patient is sitting or lying down. If the patient is in the wheelchair, be sure to lock the wheels. Apply pressure only on exhalation. Do not apply force on top of the rib cage; this could cause damage. Sometimes quad coughing is followed by suctioning.

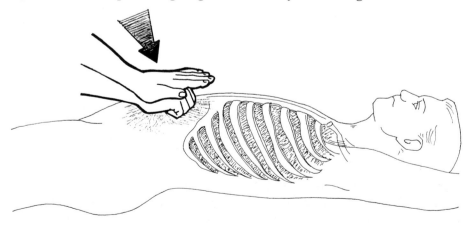

FIG. 5-1. Hand positioning for the quad-cough technique is shown. The arrow shows the direction of movement.

Postural drainage is a simple way to help clear lungs of excess mucus. Because the patient is upright for much of the day, secretions pool in the lungs. Postural drainage, using different positions and the force of gravity, allows secretions to drain to the central and higher areas in the chest for easier removal by cough or suctioning. Do not use postural drainage directly after meals (it may cause vomiting) or during autonomic hyperreflexia (postural drainage causes an increase in blood pressure).

Each position for drainage should be used for 5 or 10 min. To help drain posterior basal segments of the lungs, the patient lies face down with 18–20 inches of pillows beneath the hips. If a hospital bed is available, set it in Trendelenburg's position (head lower than feet). For the anterior basal segments, the patient lies face up with pillows under the hips. For drainage of the upper lung fields, the patient is in bed in an upright or semireclining position (45° angle) with the pillows below the knees. It may also be necessary to turn the patient from side to side.

To further loosen secretions in the lungs the respiratory therapist may need to call on other forms of chest physiotherapy. One very common method, known as chest percussion or "clapping," involves the firm application of the cupped hand to areas of the chest area above the congested lung. The motion is similar to playing a bongo drum. Percuss for 1 or 2 min, being sure to remove jewelry. Clapping is often used in conjunction with postural drainage.

Suctioning: It is common for secretions to build in the airways of ventilator-using quadriplegics. A primary task of the respiratory therapist is to remove excess secretions from the airways by way of a rubber catheter tube and a suction machine. In the hospital setting, most spinal injury centers prefer using a sterile suctioning apparatus. This reduces the chances of cross-infection. At Craig Hospital, a "clean" method is preferred; this is the method of choice outside the hospital, too. The clean method keeps the procedure as simple as possible, and is a major cost control consideration because the catheters are reused, and because paper cups and nonsterile gloves can be substituted for sterile equipment. After suctioning, rinse the catheter thoroughly with saline solution. Wipe it dry with gauze, and store it in a clean, dry container. In the hospital setting, the catheter, the saline, and the storage container are changed each shift.

The respiratory therapist often instructs family members and attendants in the proper techniques of suctioning. It is important to stress that suctioning is not limited to the clinical or even bedside environment. Family members and attendants must be instructed in how to suction the patient in the gymnasium, at the theater, at a picnic, or on an airplane. Battery-powered portable suctioning devices are a key piece of equipment for the high quadriplegic patient.

Generally, suctioning of the high quadriplegic patient is similar to standard respiratory therapy techniques used in the general hospital setting. It is important, however, to use much caution when suctioning a ventilator-using patient whose vital capacity is zero, or very low (<500 ml tidal volume). The apneic quadriplegic individual, who cannot draw any breath without assistance, must be suctioned with great speed. Such patients can become significantly hypoxic just 20 or 30 s after removing the ventilator. Therefore, the suction must not last longer than 15 s.

Therapists at Craig Hospital do not typically administer oxygen while suctioning the patient, although this is more common in other centers. Most patients are young and have healthy lung tissue; they are able to endure long suctionings. Some patients, however, may become hypoxic during suctioning. If this occurs, the time of each suction must be reduced, and preoxygenation may be necessary. The patient with preexisting pulmonary disease or infection may require extra care; older patients, or some who are heavy smokers, may be susceptible to increased secretions. The respiratory therapist must be aware of possible complications. If, for example, a patient is prone to having vagal reactions, or is susceptible to bradycardia, preoxygenation is often indicated.

Tracheostomy tubes. The pulmonologist writes the prescription for a patient's tracheostomy equipment, including choice of "trach" tubes. Most high quadriplegic patients begin with a cuffed trach (Fig. 5-2). This device allows for precise monitoring of air flow and vital capacity, and prevents aspiration in those patients who are unable to swallow. The main drawback to a cuffed device, which is inflated by syringe, is that a

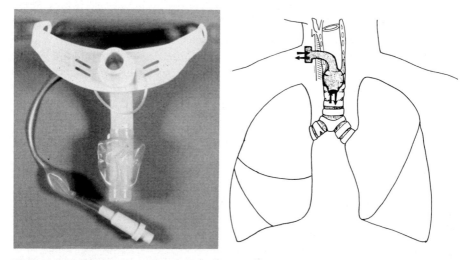

FIG. 5-2. A: Portex cuffed trach. **B:** The arrows show the direction of air flow through a cuffed trach. Note that the air passes both in and out through the trach tube. No air goes above the cuff, so the patient is not able to talk.

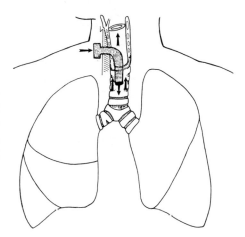

FIG. 5-3. This diagram shows direction of air flow with a cuffless trach, or a cuffed trach with the cuff down. Note that, on exhalation, the air is allowed to flow up past the trach tube, over the vocal cords, allowing the patient to talk.

person cannot vocalize when the cuff is activated. No air is passed by the vocal cords. The cuff pressure may also irritate, or cause stenosis or necrosis, to the sensitive tissue of the trachea. The cuff pressure should be adjusted so there is a minimal amount of air leakage; this is best done by slowly inflating the cuff until there is no air leakage, then backing the pressure off slightly until some air passes the cuff.

After a patient is able to swallow effectively, and the lungs are clear, the cuff is deflated for short periods (Fig. 5-3). For the first few minutes this is a rather unpleasant experience, because secretions that have accumulated above the cuff (sometimes making it necessary to suction above the cuff) will drain down the trachea into the lungs. The patient may cough a great deal, but soon learns to enjoy having the cuff down. The ability to vocalize is a major achievement. It is again important for the respiratory therapist to encourage the patient; also, it is beneficial to have other patients who have been through the process lend their peer support.

After the initial cuff deflation, the patient learns to eat and breathe with the cuff down for longer periods. When a patient can tolerate the cuff down for a substantial time, the respiratory therapist shifts to a stainless-steel trach; at Craig Hospital, a Jackson trach is used (Fig. 5-4). Some centers prefer using a plastic trach, but stainless steel is easier to clean, lasts longer, and is more cost effective. Patients are always glad to switch to the cuffless trach, because it allows them to vocalize at will.

For those patients who are not quite ready (because of high injury or lung congestion) for a cuffless trach, a "talking trach" may be used (Fig. 5-5). This trach uses an external air source that is controlled to pass air above the cuff so it may go up to the larynx. No ventilator volume is lost. Because the talking trach often produces a different-sounding voice,

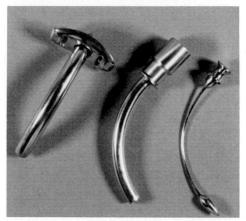

FIG. 5-4. Jackson trach outer cannula, inner cannula, and guide (for
inserting trach).

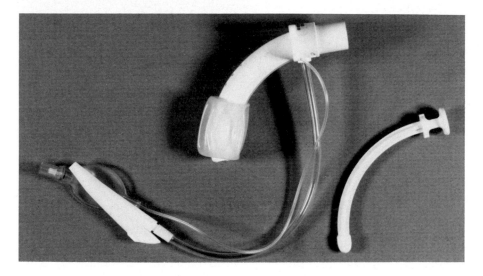

FIG. 5-5. Communitrach talking trach. White part is for hooking up to air
source (compressed air or O_2). Note holes above the cuff; this allows air from
the small tube to pass over the vocal cords, allowing the patient to talk.

and because it tends to dry out mucus membranes and cause a sore
throat, it is not tolerated by all patients.

Weaning: If the patient is attempting to breathe while not using the
ventilator, the therapist is at the bedside continually during the initial
weans. Typically there is great fear when the ventilator is first removed;
some patients have been told they would never be free of mechanical
ventilation. The therapist plays an important role in reassuring and
calming the patient. Until the patient is able to breathe without the
ventilator for more than half an hour at a time, the respiratory thera-

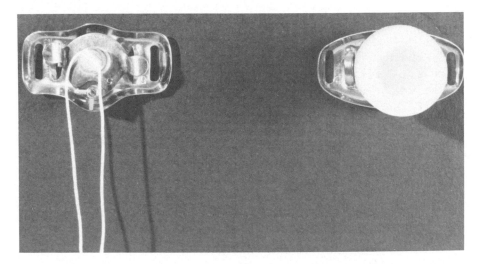

FIG. 5-6. Plugged trachs. The plug on the left is a pilling plug that is inserted into a flat Jackson trach. The plug on the right is a rubber plug that fits over a universal connector on a Jackson trach.

pist is always at the bedside; until the patient can breathe independently of the machine for 24 h, the therapy staff is never more than a moment's notice away. During the weaning process, some patients are fitted with a "trach-talk" tube, which features a one-way valve. Air enters the lungs through the trach tube, but must pass from the lungs via the vocal cords.

Once a patient begins to be weaned off the ventilator, the therapist begins to decrease the size of the Jackson trach. Also, once the patient is able to be weaned for at least 8 h, the therapist plugs the trach when the patient is off the ventilator (Fig. 5-6). Generally, a Jackson size 6 trach is the largest size that is plugged; trachs smaller than a Jackson size 4 won't accommodate the standard 14- or 16-gauge catheter tubing for suctioning. The adjustments in trach size are made with patient comfort and talking ability in mind; the ultimate goal is to gradually allow the stoma to close as the patient becomes clinically stable.

Glossopharyngeal Breathing (GPB): Although some centers do not stress GPB, or "frog breathing," the method has been effective to allow some high quadriplegic patients time off the ventilator. The technique has met with much greater success in patients with polio. The spinal-injured high quadriplegic patient, in many cases, cannot master GPB because of spasticity and impaired sensation. GPB, however, can act as a backup in case of mechanical breakdown or power failure. The GPB technique forces air into the lungs with 10–14 separate stoking or gulping maneuvers per breath. The method is not difficult to learn, although it is tiring in the initial training sessions. GPB exercises may strengthen cough, stretch the chest wall, and increase speaking volume. GPB is most useful for short periods, cannot be used while eating or sleeping, and is not possible unless the individual has good function of the lips, soft palate, mouth, tongue, pharynx, and larynx.

The respiratory therapist must be aware of many other management techniques in care and treatment of high quadriplegic patients. See Chapter 12 for details on ventilators, pneumobelts, phrenic nerve pacers, and other equipment.

The respiratory therapist plays an essential role in the successful rehabilitation of the high quadriplegic patient. While assuring that pulmonary functions are maximized, the therapist also brings to the process much of the human touch needed to restore patient confidence and motivation. The respiratory therapist embodies both the art and the science of modern rehabilitation technology.

6

Nursing Management

Teresa Yoshimura

Santa Clara Valley Medical Center, San Jose, California, U.S.A.

This chapter focuses on the nursing management of the high quadriplegic patient during the acute phase. Various methods will be described that will help the nurse, and other health professionals, to provide optimal critical and rehabilitative care and to provide psychological support for the patient, the family, and/or other nursing staff. Interventions used to promote optimal communication for the ventilator-dependent quadriplegic patient will also be discussed because lack of communication can be the biggest frustration for the patient as well as the family and staff. Finally, equipment and supply needs during the acute phase will be identified. Contrasted throughout the chapter will be the special needs of a respirator-dependent, spinal-cord-injured patient versus the needs of other acute trauma patients.

The role of the nurse will likely vary somewhat from one institution to another. Responsibilities may not pertain solely to the professional nurse. Often, other members of the treatment team are primarily involved with an aspect of the patient's care. The nurse is in a position to coordinate the patient's care and to integrate and support those activities that other disciplines may have introduced during treatment time.

There are four key responsibilities of the nurse during the acute phase. First, the nurse must fully assess the respirator-dependent quadriplegic patient to develop a plan of care. A careful and thorough assessment of all the systems must be completed, and an individualized plan of care must be developed using the nursing process and identifying nursing diagnoses.

Second, because cardiopulmonary complications rank among the highest causes of death in quadriplegic persons (1), especially during the acute phase, it is vitally important for the nurse to concentrate on promoting optimal respiratory care and to prevent further respiratory compromise. Acute problems will necessitate immediate intervention, but nurses must also bear in mind the long-term practices they may initiate. Thus, prophylactic care must be addressed during early phases of care.

Third, the nurse must support both the patient and the family in understanding and accepting the disability and help the patient increase independence. It is during this acute phase that the nurse must develop a caring and trusting relationship with the patient, one which will allow the patient to express feelings. It can be very frustrating for the patient to communicate while on a ventilator. It can be very frustrating for the family to try to understand what the patient is trying to say. The nurse may intercede to facilitate communication. Various communication aids are available and will be discussed later in the chapter.

Finally, the nurse must act as an educator and offer expertise as a practitioner to other team members. During the acute phase, the nurse becomes a key care provider and a key facilitator in patient adaptation. The nurse must be knowledgeable and willing to share information with the rest of the treatment team so the staff can successfully meet the challenges of caring for a ventilator-dependent quadriplegic.

EARLY NURSING CARE

The acute phase of nursing management begins when the patient is admitted to a hospital and continues until the patient is both medically and orthopedically stabilized. There are tremendous challenges facing a nurse, frequently a critical care nurse, caring for a ventilator-dependent quadriplegic patient. The nurse must incorporate all the fundamental nursing principles and skills of medical, surgical, and rehabilitation nursing supplemented by additional knowledge of spinal-cord-injury care. In addition to meeting the needs of a lower level quadriplegic patient, the nurse must reevaluate and reprioritize those interventions to promote optimal care to those patients requiring permanent ventilator support. This section will address the prominent issues dealing with the nursing care of the ventilator-dependent quadriplegic patient and should be used in conjunction with texts that address the nursing management of the spinal cord injury patient.

Aspiration

Paralytic ileus is a common cause of sudden respiratory arrest when the ability to cough is lacking and aspiration of stomach contents leads to respiratory distress. A quadriplegic patient may be admitted without any signs of respiratory distress; however, the patient's condition may deteriorate rapidly and require immediate intervention. Abdominal distension can also cause significant inhibition of diaphragm movement. Initially, nasogastric suction may be required to evacuate stomach contents. If aspiration of gastric contents occurs, the lungs will develop a severe inflammatory response.

As patients resume a full diet, they may tend to choke or gag on the food. Staff must be available and prepared to immediately suction or assist cough to clear the airway.

Respiratory Secretions

Retention of secretions is another major cause of respiratory distress. Pooling of secretions may lead to atelectasis and pneumonia in dependent areas of the lung. Small adjustments in the patient's position are enough to prevent accumulation of secretions. Percussion and vibration help to loosen and mobilize secretions in the bronchus. Postural drainage aids in gravity-assisted drainage of secretions; however, it should not be done if contraindicated for the patient, such as a patient with a head injury. Postural drainage can be done on specialty beds used with spinal-cord-injured patients, although some beds may require blocks to be placed under the wheels at the foot of the bed. All of these measures must be practiced diligently.

Suctioning

Although actual suctioning procedures may vary according to the institution, it is important to remember to initially preoxygenate the patient with a higher percentage of oxygen before attempting tracheal suctioning to prevent acute hypoxia. Once the patient has stabilized and is breathing room air, it may not be necessary to increase the oxygen percentage, but the patient should still be hyperventilated.

The irritation caused by excessive suctioning may actually increase tracheal secretions. It is important to choose the most effective times to clear the airway, such as after a respiratory therapy treatment or after repositioning. Excessive suctioning also increases the chances of introducing an infection into the respiratory system.

Bradycardia

Hypotension and bradycardia can occur after a spinal cord injury due to neurogenic shock. Although both neurogenic and hypovolemic shock are characterized by hypotension, they are treated differently. A slow bounding pulse accompanied by dry, warm skin is symptomatic of neurogenic shock, whereas hypovolemic shock is accompanied by a rapid, weak, and thready pulse. Treating a ventilator-dependent quadriplegic patient in neurogenic shock with increased fluids will lead to pulmonary edema and further complications for those in an already compromised respiratory state.

Bradycardia may also occur with activities that stimulate the vagus, such as deep tracheal suctioning and rapid changes in body positioning during turns. In addition to severe bradycardia, such activities may also cause asystole and a drop in oxygen saturation. Oxygen saturation and pulse may need to be monitored.

Bowel Dysfunction

Lack of bowel sounds indicates that paralytic ileus is still present. Laxatives, suppositories, or enemas should not be used until bowel sounds return. If stool needs to be removed, gentle manual evacuation may be done by the nurse. Once strong bowel sounds have returned, the patient may begin to increase oral intake, beginning with ice chips and progressing to a clear liquid diet and eventually to a full diet. A bowel program can also be initiated at this time. Using a bedpan while the patient is on bedrest will create a maladjustment of the spine, so the nurse should protect the bed linen with incontinence pads. Encouraging a high fluid intake will help to keep the stool soft and help liquefy respiratory secretions.

Immobility

In the acute phase, the nurse should recognize the hazards of immobility. It is important to maintain proper alignment and stabilization of the spine while maintaining skin integrity and preventing pulmonary complications. Once the life-threatening events after a spinal cord injury are over, the nurse must focus priorities towards preventing further deterioration and promoting psychological well-being. When caring for a patient with a high cervical spine fracture, it is very important to maintain skin integrity, proper alignment, and traction of the spine, and to prevent pulmonary complications.

Special Therapeutic Beds

There are many special therapeutic beds available that can assist in preventing complications (Table 6-1). The nurse must assess the patient's needs to determine the kind of bed needed and to understand the pros and cons of each bed. When choosing a bed, there are several issues the nurse must evaluate to determine the bed best suited for the ventilator-dependent patient. Some issues to consider are: (a) Can an unstable spinal-cord-injured patient be placed on the bed? (b) Can the skin be easily inspected? (c) Can the bed be manually turned in the event of a power failure? (d) Can the height of the bed be adjusted? (e) Will positioning further compromise the patient's respiratory status? (f) Can the patient be assessed and suctioned in all positions? (g) Can the bed be placed in Trendelenburg's position for postural drainage? (h) Is the field of vision limited, causing sensory deprivation?

Portable Suction Machines

Once a decision is made regarding the type of bed to be used, other equipment must be obtained. Because the ventilator-dependent patient is unable to remove secretions, a suction machine must be available at all times both for oral and tracheal suctioning. The nurse must be prepared with both a bedside suction machine and a portable suction machine. The portable suction machine can be used when the patient is taken off the unit for diagnostic tests. These portable suction machines must be able to run on internal and external batteries. Many can also be used in automobiles by attaching them to the cigarette lighter.

It is also vitally important that all members of the treating team have the ability to suction the patient. Respiratory distress can occur in a matter of seconds. The nurse may not be at the bedside during a therapy session, so all the staff must be able to suction the patient with both the bedside suction machine and the portable suction machine. It is also important for the staff to know how to use an Ambu bag (resuscitation bag) and where to find it quickly.

Transportation to Diagnostic Procedures

During the early stages of a spinal cord injury, many diagnostic procedures may be needed. Any procedures that can be performed without moving the patient should be done at the bedside. However, the patient may need to be safely transported between the ward and diagnostic procedures, such as computed tomography (CT) or magnetic resonance imaging (MRI). Transporting the patient may potentially cause further neurological damage; therefore, critical attention must be placed on maintaining spinal alignment. Transporting a patient who is ventilator dependent requires planning and preparation of equipment. Portable oxygen tanks, portable suction machines, ventilators, monitors, and stretchers need to be available and ready. Specially adapted spine boards with cervical traction attachments are available and can be used in CT scans and MRIs. If this specialized equipment is not available, the patient may be transferred using a five-person lift. One person stabilizes and provides cervical traction at the head and neck. Another person

Table 6-1. *Therapeutic Beds*

Therapeutic bed/description	Advantages	Disadvantages
Rotorest bed™—Equipped with removable, adjustable supportive packs that support the body in proper alignment while continuously rotating about the longitudinal axis in a cradle-like fashion.	Less back strain for staff since patient is mechanically rotated and alleviates the need for the patient to be turned. Reduced pulmonary, urinary, and venous stasis. Unstable spinal cord injuries may be placed on this bed.	Skin breakdown may occur due to shearing or pressure if the patient is not fitted properly in the packs or if the bed is stopped in the flat position. "Coffin effect" may occur due to sensory deprivation. Staff acceptance may be difficult due to the many moving pieces and highly technical-looking control panel.
Stryker frame™—An anterior and posterior frame with canvas covers and thin padding over each. Frame has a pivot apparatus that allows the patient to be turned from supine to prone while remaining packed between the frames.	Bed does not depend on electricity to be turned. Bed can be easily moved into the gym for therapies. Bed can be used for unstable spinal cord injuries.	Prone position further compromises respiratory status and makes it difficult to assess the patient's respiratory status and anxiety level. Cannot be easily placed in Trendelenburg's position. Must place shock blocks under the wheels. Bed is narrow and cannot accommodate patients >200 lb or >6′ tall comfortably.
Circle bed™—This bed rotates 210° in a circular motion. There is an anterior and posterior mattress between which the patient is packed.	Bed is wider than a Stryker frame and can accommodate a slightly larger-built patient. Can be used for unstable spinal cord injuries.	Traction is not constant and varies with turns. Postural hypotension frequently occurs during the turn and cardiac arrest may result. Difficult to assess pulmonary status in prone position, similar to Stryker frame.

Clinitron℗—An air-fluidized bed support system consisting of small silicone-coated glass beads, covered by a closely woven sheet to help contain the beads. The beads are fluidized by a flow of warm, pressurized air, which floats the polyester sheet. The patient is positioned on the sheet.

Useful for treating patients with skin problems due to the reduced skin contact pressure.

Moving and positioning the patient when the bed is "fluidized" allows one person to position the patient.

Bed will mold to the patient's body in the "defluidized" state.

Cannot be used with unstable spinal cord injuries.

Patient may become dehydrated due to the temperature and the warm air system.

Bed cannot be easily moved to other areas due to the weight of the bed.

Low air loss flotation beds—(Kin-Air℗, Flexi Care℗, Mediscus℗)

Air circulates within sacs. The pressure in each set of sacs can be independently adjusted.

Pliable air sacs follow patient's body contours to provide support in all positions.

Low friction surface of the sacs allows patient to be moved easily.

Can be easily moved into other areas without deflating cushions due to battery packs.

Requires a trained person to correctly adjust the air sacs to achieve maximal usage and correct pressures.

Patient needs to be closely monitored to avoid "bottoming out" if leak occurs or if pressures are not correctly adjusted. Patient will be lying on a hard bed frame and skin breakdown will occur.

Cannot be used with unstable spinal cord injuries.

Biodyne bed℗—A new specialty bed that provides the continuous oscillation of the Rotorest bed with the low-air-loss fluidized bed system. The cushions inflate and deflate according to the individual patient's programmed needs. This bed has not yet been used extensively to adequately assess its advantages and disadvantages.

—

—

continuously ventilates the patient with a resusitation bag. The other three lift the patient's body. In a smooth and coordinated lift, the patient is removed from the resusitation bag and transferred to a stretcher. Once on the stretcher, the patient is again ventilated and cervical immobility is maintained with sandbags or taping the head to the stretcher. Once the patient has reached the final destination, the ventilator may be reattached.

INITIAL CRISIS ISSUES

With the onset of a sudden neurologic trauma, such as a high cervical spinal cord injury, the prognosis for survival is uncertain and the condition is considered serious or critical. The family is immediately struck with a feeling of futility and hopelessness. Then, they are asked by the medical staff to decide whether or not to resuscitate their loved one should complications arise. They must deal with the fear that their loved one may not survive. It is a major trauma for both the patient and the family, and all are in a crisis situation. In an instant, a spinal cord injury has changed lifelong physiologic, emotional, social, and economic plans that affect not only the patient, but the entire family (2). These changes may not yet be recognized by the family because they are only able to focus on the fact that the patient may die. Crisis intervention and ongoing support for the patient, family, and nursing staff need to be available. It is frequently the nurse that provides the assistance.

Support for the patient is the first concern. He or she has lost control and feeling of their entire body. Along with this loss comes a tremendous psychological dilemma, often exhibited through denial, anger, or withdrawal. "How could this happen to me?" is a frequently asked question during the initial days after injury. Denial is an effective coping mechanism during the first days after injury because it helps to "buffer" the reality of the situation. There is the hope that like a disease, the hospital will "cure" them and that the paralysis is only a temporary condition. The patient will ask the staff awkward questions like, "When will I walk again?" This question is often answered by the staff with a long silence, deferring to the physician, or changing the subject. It is important for the staff to allow the patient to express feelings. Often, the patient is looking for some reassurance. Many times, these questions will be directed to the nurse because a nurse is at the bedside 24 h a day giving direct patient care and because the nurse is the only professional remaining after the physicians, therapists, and social workers have left for the day. During these moments the nurse should be warm, caring, and, most importantly, honest. Do not give false hope. Be realistic.

Due to the lack of sensation, the patient may frequently ask the nurse to verify the location of body parts. "Where is my hand?" and "Where is my leg?" are frequently asked questions. The nurse may need to lift patients' hands to their face so they can see them. Sometimes a Polaroid picture can calm patients' fears that they lost their legs. Sometimes a slight repositioning of the extremity can give the patient some relief.

Initially, patients become very anxious and obsessed with the fear that they will become disconnected from their ventilator, or that the ventilator may malfunction or something will go wrong and no one will be available to assist them. They can no longer shout for help or throw something against a wall to get attention. They are trapped within their body and feeling more and more helpless. They become more and more frustrated because they are on a ventilator and cannot verbalize thoughts or feelings without difficulty. They can no longer use hands for expression or emphasis. This is especially frustrating for those who had poor verbal skills before they were injured. Difficulty in expressing emotions may cause more difficulty in adjusting to their disability. It is very important for the nurse to provide an adequate call system so that the patient can have some peace of mind that in case an emergency arises, a nurse will be close at hand.

COMMUNICATION AND SUPPORT

There are several interventions that the nurse may initiate to assist the patient through this difficult period. The nurse should be readily available, especially in the initial stages, because the patient may feel very isolated and without any means of communication. The only way to get the attention of the staff is by clicking the tongue or smacking the lips. With the other noises around them (the "whooshing" of the ventilator and alarms), patients are often afraid that they will not be heard if they need someone immediately. They may react by making constant demands on the nurse or by asking an excess of questions to keep the nurse near the bedside. Establish a communication system early. Rather than relying on expensive communication aids that may be frustrating and discouraging, try patience, lip reading, and a simple spelling board for communication.

Family and friends should be encouraged to visit, but it is also important to limit the number of visitors to one or two at a time. Too many visitors at a time may cause too much stimulation. Allow flexible visiting hours to accommodate families and friends who must work. Allowing families to be at the bedside from the beginning reduces the anxiety of both the patient and the family. Explaining procedures and encouraging them to touch and participate in simple patient care activities, such as washing the patient's face or putting on foot positioners, makes them realize that although the patient has broken his/her neck, it is all right to touch them. This knowledge and expertise leads to greater comfort later during the rehabilitation phase when they will be asked to do more complex tasks for the patient.

Create a friendly environment for the patient. Encourage family and friends to bring in familiar objects, such as pictures, posters, or a favorite album or cassette. Placing pictures or posters on the ceiling makes them more easily viewed and will add more sensory stimulation than a blank ceiling. Cut flowers are nice, but not for patients who are immunocompromised. There is a danger of *Pseudomonas* growing in the stagnant water. A better idea would be a living plant or silk flowers.

Patients with high quadriplegia particularly feel as if they have lost all control. Procedures are done to them without their being able to see or feel what is happening. Explain procedures to the patient and give information as each step is occurring. Allow patients simple choices, such as when to brush their teeth or which limb to start with for range of motion, so there is some control.

FAMILY SUPPORT

Crisis intervention and emotional support are also needed by the family. It is important to listen to the family and allow them to express their feelings. It may be frustrating for the family to try to understand the patient because the patient can no longer vocalize and the family must try to lip read or rely on nursing staff to interpret for them. Encourage the family to talk to the patient. It is often easier for them to stay away and to avoid trying to have a meaningful conversation with the patient. The fact that the patient is no longer physically independent, but rather is dependent like a small child, will drastically change roles within the family structure. Parents who thought they were on their own again, having raised all their children, may now be placed back into a parental role. A wife who was responsible for raising the children may now need to be responsible for house modifications, paying the bills, etc. Like their loved one, they too may be feeling overwhelmed and helpless. When the family is ready, support groups can be made available to discuss issues with other family members of ventilator-dependent quadriplegic patients. They may also want to talk with stable ventilator-dependent quadriplegic patients. The patient or family may be in need of professional counseling. Inform them of the availability of professional assistance from a psychologist or social worker to assist them through this period of change. These professionals can assist the patient and the family in determining the impact of the disability on the relationships in the family.

STAFF SUPPORT

Caring for a ventilator-dependent quadriplegic patient is an enormous psychological challenge for all staff members. They need to deal honestly, directly, and effectively with a patient who has just suffered a devastating loss. It is important for the staff not to inflict their own values about grieving onto the patient. If the staff perceives that the patient is not grieving appropriately, they may believe that the patient is not coping well, when it may be the staff that is having difficulty dealing with the situation and projecting these feelings onto the patient. The staff may also closely identify with the patient's situation. Many nurses never wore a seat belt until they worked with spinal-cord-injured patients. Therefore, it is important for the staff to deal with their own feelings about a spinal cord injury and to understand their own reactions to this disability. Inservices may be needed when lack of information or skills leads to increased stress and inaccurate impressions.

Peer support through either formal or informal group discussions may be helpful to discuss feelings and reactions about caring for a ventilator-dependent quadriplegic patient. Social workers or psychologists may be needed to act as mediators for discussions. Many times, the nurses need to talk about the constant demands the patients seem to have and how to handle those demands and still get their work done. Another topic that frequently comes up is that the patient seems to manipulate the staff. Overprotective families and aggressive families have been the topic of discussion at many meetings. These discussions may become the forum to discuss ethical questions, such as "Why are we saving these people and are we doing them a disservice if their placement plans will not allow them to be as independent as we will train them to be?" Staff frustration may be vented because they feel a disproportionately small long-term benefit is being offered for the amount of energy spent to rehabilitate a ventilator-dependent quadriplegic patient.

There are no easy or simple answers and these sessions are used primarily for catharsis. Further discussion of many of these issues can be found in Chapter 8.

COMMUNICATION AIDS

As was discussed earlier, lack of communication is a major cause of frustration and emotional stress for the patient, family, and staff. Verbal communication is not possible because of the interruption of airflow to the larynx due to the tracheotomy or endotracheal tube. An endotracheal tube is good for a short period (7 days or less), but a tracheostomy is recommended for long-term pulmonary care. There are many methods

Table 6-2. *Oral Communication Approaches*

Voiceless approaches	Electrolarynges (*cont'd*)
Lip reading/mouthing and clicking	Oral tube type
Spelling boards	Cooper Rand™
Modified natural speech approaches	P.O. Vox™
Tracheo–stoma finger occlusion	Companion™
Tracheo–stoma buttoning/plugging	Robot™
Tracheostomy speaking valve	Venti-Voice™
Cuff deflation	Nasal tube type (invasive)
PITT™ tube; COMMUNItrach™	Venti-Voice™
Pneumobelt/exsufflation belt	Remote switches
Electrolarynges	Modified Cooper Rand™ (oral type)
Neck type	Venti-Voice™ (finger/eyebrow type)
Servox™	Electrical phrenic nerve stimulator
Western Electric™	

and aids available to establish communication. These different alternatives should be presented and explored with the patient and the staff.
Each method has its own advantages and disadvantages (Table 6-2). Lip
reading does not require extra equipment or cost, but it is difficult to
develop proficiency and it is almost impossible to lip-read in the dark,
when enunciation is poor, or when facial or head injuries exist. Spelling
boards are also inexpensive, but it is a tedious job to complete an entire
conversation using a spelling board. Modified natural speech approaches, such as tracheostomy occlusion or plugging, are also inexpensive and can promote normal vocalization, but tracheostomy occlusion
using a finger may lead to infections and many patients are unable to
plug or use a tracheostomy speaking valve. Electrolarynges are now
available. These electronically synthesized voices create an audible voice.
Some use an oral/nasal tube and others are placed on the neck. Several
can be activated by a finger or forehead switch, enabling the patient to
operate the device. However, these devices are expensive and may take
some practice for correct placement. Sometimes the patient is unable to
adapt to the artificial voice or to having a tube in their mouth/nose or
against their neck. Whatever the case, a careful evaluation should be
made to assist the patient in developing whatever form of communication they find most satisfying.

When a nurse is not at the bedside, an alarm or nurse call system
must be available to the patient. Standard nurse call systems cannot be
used by a newly injured high quadriplegic patient who cannot move any
part of their body, including their head, which is in cervical traction.

Current microchip and space age technology has made many new call systems available. They can be activated by microleafs, pressure-sensitive pads, sound stimulation, or puffs of air. The alarm system may be a stationary or flashing light or a buzzer, bell, click, or siren. The system selected for the patient must be safe, reliable, and comfortable for the patient to use.

INTENSIVE CARE UNIT SETTING VERSUS COMPREHENSIVE REHABILITATION SETTING

There has been much debate over whether or not a patient with an acute spinal cord injury should be initially placed in an intensive care unit (ICU) or in a comprehensive rehabilitation unit providing treatment from emergency care through follow-up care after discharge. Studies (3,4) have shown that early referral of patients to a spinal-cord-injury center will provide the patient with the most cost-effective management. Early referral is especially important for patients who require ventilation support because comprehensive management is provided within hours of the trauma. Emergency rooms in community hospitals usually do not have the resources available to provide the needed specialized level of care for spinal cord injuries. Even if the community hospital has a general ICU, the staff in these units is usually not ready to accommodate the prolonged stay required.

When a patient is admitted to a typical ICU, he/she is placed in a brightly lit room where the lights remain on 24 h a day to provide good illumination to make accurate assessments. ICU staff are rushing around at a frantic pace. Various machines and monitors are beeping and buzzing. This beehive of activity causes confusion and panic for both the patient and the family. The staff are concerned with crisis-oriented care for the critically ill and are usually unable to provide the physical and psychological support that spinal-cord-injured patients need to help them through the initial stages of their injury. The patient needs staff who have the time to listen to their fears about being left alone, the fears of dying, and the grieving over the loss of their independence. Communication with the patient and family is also very important. They need to be kept informed of the patient's progress.

An "ICU psychosis" may develop due to sensory deprivation. There are no changes in the level of lighting over 24 h, causing one day to merge with another. The patient sees only the same four walls, floor and ceiling, day in and day out. The rhythmic "whoosh" of the ventilator and beeping of alarms, in addition to the immobilization, sleep deprivation, and the medications the patient may be receiving add to the condition. Nursing should be especially sensitive to these issues. Lights should be dimmed throughout the nighttime. Allowing the patient to watch TV or listen to the radio will help orient the patient. Staff should explain all procedures to the patient. Teaching the family can begin during the early stages. Usually, in ICU settings, the nurse does not have the time or the space to accommodate family at the bedside for prolonged periods.

When patients are placed in a rehabilitation setting with other patients with similar diagnoses, they are able to see that all is not hopeless and that they are not the only patients like this. They are able to see other patients as role models in an active rehabilitation program.

The expertise of a few specialized rehabilitation centers offers programs designed for ventilator-dependent patients and achieves optimal results. These programs are able to provide total emotional, educational, and physical support for patients from the moment they reach the rehabilitation center, and coordinate the specialized medical–surgical support and the rehabilitation support. The role of the rehabilitation nurse in providing early patient and family support and education is of paramount importance during the acute stages.

However, when a patient cannot be referred to a spinal-cord-injury rehabilitation center, it is important for the community hospital to provide optimal and comprehensive care to prevent further complications until transportation to a specialized center can be arranged. It is exceedingly important for the nurse to obtain accurate information from the referring facility. The best option is to do an on-site assessment. However, many times an on-site visit is not feasible due to distance. The next best alternative is a telephone assessment from one nurse to the other. Discharge summaries, history and physical, consults, copies of all x-ray films and diagnostic procedures and treatment records should accompany the patient to assure a smooth transfer from one facility to the next. Often, if the patient is not transferred to a rehabilitation hospital, he or she spends the rest of the entire hospitalization in an ICU setting due to administrative policies regarding ventilator-dependent patients and the need for frequent assessments.

Comprehensive and specialized rehabilitation programs are very expensive to initiate and difficult to continue successfully. Early on, ventilator-dependent quadriplegic patients will need intensive one-to-one nursing care, with someone at their bedside almost constantly. Staffing will be similar to that used in ICUs. There must be strong nursing administrative support to continue this type of care. Working with a difficult patient day after day without any sign of discharge can lead to staff "burnout." Staffing in these high-stress areas of nursing can be a challenge. A key to retaining nursing staff is to keep them cognizant of the fact that they are assisting the patient in resuming control of his/her destiny and in developing future options.

CONCLUSIONS

The physical well-being and attitudes of the patient established during the acute phase will be the foundation for the individual's future well-being during the rehabilitation phase and through discharge.

Institutions may identify different specific responsibilities for the nurse and it is important to keep these requirements in mind when defining the role of the nurse. But no matter what role is defined for the nurse, it will be integral to the foundation of the multidisciplinary team in the acute phase.

REFERENCES

1. Hachen HJ (1977): Idealized care of the acutely injured spinal cord in Switzerland. *J Trauma* 17:931–936.
2. Bourdon E (1986): Psychological impact of neurotrauma in the acute care setting. *Nurs Clin North Am* 21:693–704.
3. Buchanan LE (1982): Patient preparation and transfer to a regional SCI center. *J Neurosurg Nurs* 14:137–139.
4. Gardner BP, Theocleous F, Watt JWH, Krishnan KR (1985): Ventilation or dignified death for patients with high tetraplegia. *Br Med J* 291:1620–1622.

7

Nutritional Management in Acute Spinal Injury

Sue Frazior Vizuete

St. Luke's Episcopal Hospital, Houston, Texas, U.S.A.

The fact that patients are entitled to food, as well as clothing and shelter, presents a special challenge to the health professional caring for the nutrition of spinal-cord-injured patients. The problems consist of: *how much* to feed this group who may have increased nutrient needs due to other extensive bone injuries, blunt trauma, or respirator dependency; *how* to feed the patients when adequate intake might be complicated by the inability to feed themselves, traction or C-collar, the nausea and anorexia of postural hypotension, or posttraumatic depression; and *what* to feed those patients when feeding route and formula selection may be complicated by ileus, decreased intestinal motility, facial fractures, or neurogenic dysphagia. When these nutritional risk factors are combined with the potential need for nutrients for continued growth and maturation in a young population or for management of chronic underlying disease, there is justification for an extensive nutritional plan of care. This chapter will discuss these issues and assist in the establishment of a plan for developing and monitoring nutritional care.

NUTRITIONAL IMPLICATIONS IN TRAUMA

Endogenous Stores

Individual response to trauma is influenced by the extent of traumatic injury as well as the state of nutritional health before injury. There are three primary endogenous fuel sources: carbohydrate, fat, and protein. There are only ~500 calories from carbohydrate that can be stored and used in an acute state in which exogenous support is not available: This is <12 h of calorie reserve. Approximately 150,000 calories are stored as fat but, unfortunately, there are some glucose-dependent cells that can only use carbohydrate as an energy source. Those include cells of the central nervous system, red blood cells, kidney tissue, and fibroblasts at the leading edge of wound healing. Protein is the third potential fuel source. However, it is important to remember that protein has a functional existence in the body such that using protein for energy sacrifices the function that it serves.

Hormonal Control

Hormonal responses to injury that dictate use of the endogenous fuels are different from normal hormonal regulation. In stress and injury, an increase in glucocorticoid, glucagon, and growth hormone secretion and a decrease in insulin activity result in an increase in catabolic activity. There is an increase in the breakdown of stored carbohydrate and in glucose made from protein (gluconeogenesis). Both processes provide for an increase in available glucose to meet increased energy demand. Body protein, however, is "wasted" for energy by releasing amino acids from skeletal muscle tissue protein for conversion to glucose. Gluconeogenesis plus a concomitant decrease in new protein synthesis can lead to protein depletion. In addition, lipolysis of fat stores results in the release of free fatty acids for energy.

A reference 70-kg man who is unstressed and completely at bed rest requires approximately 20 kcal and 0.8 g protein/kg body weight or 1,400 kcal and 56 g protein, per day. The standard 3 L of 5% dextrose intravenously (i.v.) per 24 h provides 510 kcal but no protein. Traumatic injury, sepsis, and wound healing increase nutrient needs well beyond the basic requirement. Due to the catabolism of lean mass and impairment of immune competency, failure to provide adequate nutritional support can result in a tremendous life-threatening insult to the injured person.

Nitrogen Wasting

The magnitude of protein losses seen in spinal cord injuries (SCI) in most cases can be quantified by laboratory measures of nitrogen. As stated earlier, the hormone responses resulting in gluconeogenesis release amino acids from skeletal muscle. The amino acids contain a carbon structure and nitrogen. In conversion to glucose, the carbon structure is used by the body and the nitrogen is given off as waste in the urine. In the author's experience, it is not unusual to see the nitrogen content of the urine of acute SCI patients as high as 20 g/24 h. In humans, each gram of nitrogen lost through the urine translates into 30 g of lean body mass (1). Thus, a loss of 20 g of nitrogen represents a loss of 600 g of lean body mass. In the SCI patient, nitrogen wasting continues beyond the acute postinjury phase and includes obligatory losses resulting from disuse atrophy. Because the 70-kg reference man is composed of 70% lean body mass, of which only 5% is skeletal muscle (1), this means that obligatory losses should not exceed 5% of the lean body mass or ~5.4 lb or nutritional status may be compromised. Providing exogenous energy and protein helps to blunt this catabolic response, so it is extremely important that these nutrients be provided in the acute phase.

MACRONUTRIENT REQUIREMENTS

Several methods have been devised for predicting energy and protein needs. Both are subject to change depending on the medical condition and stress level of the patient. Use of standard methods for calculating macronutrient requirements in trauma and stress can be applied in SCI and then evaluated through nutritional assessment.

Calculating Energy Requirements

The most specific method for determining caloric requirements is indirect calorimetry—the measure of gas exchange (O_2 and CO_2) and respiratory quotient. This method is not only specific for total energy expenditure, but also for showing the relative proportions of protein, carbohydrate, and fat that are being used for energy. Serial indirect calorimetry measurements are useful in calculating and monitoring current needs and changes in these needs as the patient progresses through rehabilitation. However, indirect calorimetry requires a mobile metabolic cart and staff trained in its operation and interpretation.

Without benefit of indirect calorimetry, the second approach, one more commonly used, is calculation of basal energy expenditure (BEE) by the Harris-Benedict equation (2) (Table 7-1). Percentage increases are added

Table 7-1. *Harris-Benedict Equations for Calculating Basal Energy Expenditure*

Male
    BEE = 66 + [13.7 × wt (kg)] + [5 × ht (cm)] − [6.8 × age (yr)]
Female
    BEE = 655 + [9.6 × wt (kg)] + [1.7 × ht (cm)] − [4.7 × age (yr)]

Reproduced from ref. 2, with permission.
BEE, basal energy expenditure.

to the BEE for the energy required in the digestion and absorption of food (10%, not used in parenteral), for stress, and for activity (5–15%) (3) to provide a predicted energy expenditure. One may question the activity factor in paralyzed patients but the literature suggests that transfers and remaining motor functions may be performed at a higher energy expenditure than normal (4).

There are several stress factors that affect the energy needs of spinal-cord-injured patients. These may include a 25% increase in metabolic activity due to infection or trauma and another 20% increase in cases involving multiple trauma in which the patient is on a ventilator (5). Control of body temperature below the level of the lesion may be difficult (poikilothermia) and the presence of prolonged fever increases energy expenditure (6). There is a 7% increase in energy expenditure for each degree of temperature above normal. Dopamine, which also increases metabolic rate, may be used to maintain adequate circulatory function in the first few postinjury days. Surgery, as may be required for stabilization of the fracture, can increase metabolic rate from 5 to 20%.

In a trauma center, the exact height and weight required for the Harris-Benedict equation is often not available; therefore, the extensive calculations may be futile. A simple method used for establishing initial repletion energy needs is to multiply current weight in kilograms by 40–45 (7). This method, however, may overestimate needs in the very aged population. For all methods of determining energy needs, analysis of actual nutrient intake compared with weight changes over time and other nutritional assessment parameters on repeated measure is essential in evaluating therapy and making changes as necessary.

Calculating Protein Needs

The recommended daily allowance (RDA) for protein in a nonstressed adult is 0.8 g protein/kg body weight (8). With SCI, that requirement may increase to 1.5–2.0 g protein/kg during acute phase care. In the reference 70-kg man, this translates into 105–140 g protein/day. Protein provided should be available for use in repletion. Usually a calorie-to-nitrogen ratio of 150:1 will spare protein so that it does not function as an energy source. The following formula may be used to calculate protein requirements after injury and allow protein sparing (3):

$$\text{Protein (g)} = 6.25 \times \frac{\text{Energy requirement}}{150}$$

Individual needs must be considered in establishing protein requirements. Protein losses from open draining wounds, hemolysis, and surgical intervention cannot be quantified but must be considered. However, protein losses from catabolism can be quantified by measuring nitrogen output in the urine and comparing that with exogenous nitrogen intake to come up with a nitrogen balance. Hence, in maintenance:

$$\text{Nitrogen intake } \frac{\text{(g Protein)}}{6.25} = \text{Nitrogen output} + 4 \text{ g}$$

where 4 g accounts for stool and nonurea nutrition losses. In catabolism, nitrogen output exceeds nitrogen input and adjustments should be made in amounts of protein provided. The goal of nutritional therapy in anabolism is a positive nitrogen balance of 4–6 g/day (9).

In addition to protein and energy, adequate water, usually 1 ml per calorie, electrolytes per individual need, vitamins, and minerals to meet RDAs are considered in designing a comprehensive nutritional care plan.

NUTRITIONAL ASSESSMENT PARAMETERS

A battery of parameters effective in establishing a descriptive statement about a patient's nutritional health have been collectively used and are extensively described elsewhere (10–12). Data for evaluation and development of that statement include a nutrition history, anthropometric and biochemical measurements, an estimation of energy and protein needs, and a plan for meeting those nutrient needs.

Nutrition History

The nutrition and weight history may be subjectively obtained from the patient or significant other. Answers to questions regarding food allergies, intolerances, preferences, difficulty chewing and/or swallowing, bowel patterns, and previous dietary intake are entertained and compared with medical status and level of injury to determine adverse effects on nutrient intake, digestion, and absorption. This type of information aids in selecting the physical mechanism best suited to get nutrients to the patient. For example, the patient may be intolerant but not allergic to eggs. Gastric stasis may also be a problem for this patient. Intravenous nutrition would be indicated and a fat source containing egg phospholipid would not be contraindicated.

Somatic Parameters

Anthropometric measurements include height, weight, frame size, arm circumference, triceps skinfold, and a calculated mid-arm-muscle circumference. These data are helpful in assessing baseline state of body composition and how that changes over time. Fatfold normally relates to adipose tissue and energy stores. Arm-muscle circumference relates to skeletal muscle mass. Data are compared with percentile of standard developed by Frisancho and can be interpreted as lean, below average, average, above average, or excessively fat depending on the value obtained (13). Due to expected tissue atrophy and redistribution of fat stores in SCI, interpretation is very quickly limited even in the acute-care setting. Until reference standards in the SCI population are established, interpretation of acceptable norms for body compartments will be somewhat subjective. Anthropometric measures taken serially may have greater application in a long-term care facility when patients are medically stable. Objective measures of strength and weight can be related to physical capabilities and may have application in goal setting and motivation. Anthropometrics and distribution of body compartments in SCI patients is an area in need of research and validation.

In SCI, weight change over time is the most valid somatic parameter. However, in acute stages of the injury before stabilization, the risk of weighing the patient may exceed the benefit. Initial hospital admission weight may be subjectively obtained from the patient or significant other but can still be used to aid in calculating nutrient requirements. Later, measured weights obtained may necessitate the reevaluation of nutrient needs. Bed scales must be used and a trained staff who have complete knowledge of the care of SCI patients should be available to provide consistency on repeated measures and to record all equipment that may influence the obtained value. The measure may not be actual, but can represent a valid comparative change.

Visceral Parameters

Metabolic parameters collected for use in evaluating visceral protein status may include serum albumin, prealbumin, transferrin, and hemoglobin (10–12). These function as transport proteins and are adversely affected by protein-calorie malnutrition but respond well to refeeding. Other derangements besides malnutrition can influence the values obtained for these parameters, such as fluid status, blood loss, and blood replacement. Therefore, it is important that a registered dietitian, skilled and trained in the area of nutritional support, is available for interpretation of these other factors as well as the battery of nutritional assessment tests.

Other parameters used to evaluate protein status can include antigen skin testing and total lymphocyte count for assessment of immune competence. There is an association between protein-calorie malnutrition and loss of immunocompetence or increased rate of infection.

All indices taken together as well as the nitrogen balance studies allow for the detection of depleted protein status and the evaluation of its severity. The objective evaluations are then used by the dietitian to help in goal setting and in determining the mode of therapy.

INDICATIONS FOR ROUTE(S) OF FEEDING

If the gastrointestinal tract is intact and functional, it should be used for delivery of nutrients. Taking food orally, then, would seem to be the route of choice. However, obstacles related to the injury can preclude adequate oral intake. If so, alternative feeding routes should be pursued without hesitation. The alternatives include central and peripheral i.v. nutrition, enteral tube feeding, or some combination of these feeding methods.

Central and Peripheral Parenteral Nutrition

Commonly, gastrointestinal stasis is exhibited in severe SCI. The ileus usually lasts only a few days, but if the ileus persists, parenteral nutrition should be implemented by the third postinjury day. This method bypasses digestion and absorption normally performed by the gastrointestinal tract. Because parenteral nutrition can consist of all elements of nutrition, it can be used as the sole source of support. Hydrolyzed nutrients are delivered directly into a vein for cellular uptake.

Central vein placement affords rapid dilution of a highly concentrated solution so that it can be used without precipitating phlebitis. Patients may already have an i.v. line inserted into the superior vena cava for use in monitoring cardiac pressure so parenteral nutrition can easily be initiated if the line has an unused port.

In addition to ileus, parenteral nutrition is indicated when decreased gastric motility interferes with delivering adequate amounts of enteral feeding. The gut may be functional but sluggish and tolerant to only small amounts of food or formula. Parenteral nutrition may also be desired if patients are on a rotorest bed where there could be increased potential for aspiration.

Peripheral i.v. nutrition can be used under similar circumstances but it is intended for short-term use (<2 weeks). One constraint is that fewer calories can be given peripherally than centrally. Lower dextrose concentrations are used to minimize risk of phlebitis. A sturdy peripheral vein is used when central vein access is not available. Deciding when to use central versus peripheral nutrition depends on the protocol and philosophy of the institution. There is need for research on application of parenteral nutrition in SCI. The degree of discrepancy in nutrients provided and predicted nutrients required should be considered. For example, a 25-year-old woman at 48 kg may meet 90% of required nutrients via the peripheral route in contrast to an 18-year-old 90-kg man, who may only meet 30% by the same route. Additionally, because foresight is limited, it is not known whether the ileus will resolve as predicted. Protein-calorie undernutrition in injury or sickness has never been the treatment of choice for the informed practitioner. Nevertheless, early resolution of gastric stasis is anticipated. In the interim and during progression of enteral feeding, peripheral parenteral nutrition may be the ideal way to provide nutrients. This early support can help to minimize the catabolic insult to body mass.

Enteral Nutrition

During the time the gastrointestinal (GI) tract is not functioning, a nasogastric tube for suctioning stomach contents is required. As the ileus resolves, progression is made toward using the alimentary tract. There should be a steady weaning from parenteral to enteral nutrition as soon as possible. Enteral nutrition uses the alimentary tract by way of oral and/or tube feedings. Decreased bowel motility may necessitate continuing the parenteral route or at least maintaining access until gastrointestinal tolerance is well established.

Feeding by tube is indicated any time the GI tract is functional but the patient cannot or will not eat enough. With SCI, mechanical and/or emotional barriers may exist, creating a situation in which intake is absent or insufficient.

Mechanical barriers are physical impediments to oral intake. The inconveniences of spinal traction and prone positioning have a negative impact both on the ability to chew and to swallow as well as on tolerating adequate volumes of food and liquid by mouth. Patients in traction may report early satiety. Another similar physical restraint to mastication exists when a cervical collar is worn. Nausea and anorexia due to postural hypotension, medications, and fever play a role in suboptimal intake. Intubation or tracheostomies can impose obstruction to eating by making swallowing uncomfortable and difficult. With concomitant fractures, surgical fixation and soreness can limit intake. Furthermore, oral bulbar or neurogenic dysphagia, resulting in weakness or paralysis of muscles of the jaw, tongue, pharynx, and larynx, may be evident. To compensate for absent or insufficient nutrient intake, tube feeding provides an alternative feeding route. In this manner, liquid nutrients are delivered to the alimentary tract and the mechanical obstructions are overcome. Therefore, complications (such as sepsis, wound dehiscence, respiratory failure, lethargy, and depression) related to protein-calorie undernutrition are minimized.

Psychosocial barriers may have an impact on sufficient nutrition intake at any time. In posttraumatic depression, patients may lack the will to eat at all. Grieving patients may pick at meals and appear to go through the motions while analysis of actual intake proves it to be scanty. The patient, frustrated with all elements of total dependency, may be emotionally unable to eat well. Others may find that the eating behavior is the one element that they can control and manipulate. Tube feedings bypass the oral cavity, precluding the element of patient input. The feedings can be the sole source of nutrition or used as a supplement to oral intake. These or enteral feedings are indicated during the acute phase when decreased intake can lead to the physical and emotional detriment of the patient.

Oral Diet

Oral intake is indicated as soon as possible to progress readily with rehabilitation. The GI tract must be functional and, if the patient is intubated or has a tracheostomy, the cuff must be inflated to provide a seal to prevent aspiration (14). If possible, a modified barium swallow may be recommended to determine risk of aspiration.

IMPLEMENTING TREATMENT

Malnutrition has been associated with poor wound healing, decreased resistance to infection, and loss of skin integrity. Because SCI patients are predisposed to multiple source infections and decubiti, adequacy of nutrient intake is integral to medical treatment. Therapy selections include parenteral, enteral, and oral diet.

Central and Peripheral Parenteral Nutrition

Central parenteral nutrition requires intravenous access into the superior or inferior vena cava or the jugular vein. Usually a hypertonic dextrose solution (30–70%) for energy is mixed with equal volumes of amino acids (5.5–10%) for protein. Initially 1–2 L of the dextrose/amino acid mixture is infused. The rate and/or concentration is adjusted to provide the necessary calories and fluid. A solution of 10 or 20% lipids is routinely provided as a source of essential fatty acids and calories three to seven times a week.

Calcium, phosphorus, magnesium, sodium, and potassium are added for maintenance of electrolytes. Multivitamins and trace elements are added once daily to the first liter of i.v. solution given. Vitamin K 10–15 mg is given twice weekly. A programmed instruction for calculating parenteral feedings has been published in the Journal of the American Dietetic Association, November 1984 (15).

The peripheral i.v. solution is similar to that used centrally; however, lower dextrose concentrations are given. A dextrose concentration of 20% (maximum 30%) is prescribed along with the amino acid source (usually 8.5%). Lipids are administered both centrally and peripherally separately from the base solution as a concentrated source of calories. They should be infused slowly and not exceed 1–2.5 g fat/kg body weight or

60% of total kcal (15). Heparin is sometimes added to the peripheral solution to decrease the risk of phlebitis.

Baseline body weight and laboratory data are noted. Serum glucose is closely monitored and hyperglycemia may necessitate the addition of insulin to the parenteral regimen. Electrolytes, triglycerides, liver function tests, prothrombin time, and serum levels of trace elements are monitored and adjustments are made as necessary.

Enteral Feeding

As peristalsis resumes, parenteral therapy is combined with enteral feedings. Usually this can be done by inserting a tube (soft No. 8 French) through the nose and into the duodenum. Duodenal placement is preferred to minimize aspiration risk from more proximal placement. Tubes should be radiopaque and weighted so that placement can be confirmed by x-ray film and maintained. If possible the patient's head should be elevated 30°. However, if oral bulbar or neurogenic dysphagia is seen, and long-term tube feeding predicted, patients can be fed by way of gastrostomy, or preferably jejunostomy, feeding sites.

A multitude of formulas are available to meet a battery of clinical conditions. Selection of the type of formula depends on the functional ability of the gut. Primarily, if initiated before any significant degree of malnutrition has occurred, a polymeric formula (a mixture of protein, carbohydrate, and fat) can be used. The formulas range from 1–2 kcal per milliliter and thus require that a specific volume is infused to supply adequate nutrition. The solutions vary in osmolality and protein content. Formula selection should be individualized according to patient needs. In addition, a select volume is required to meet the minimum RDA for vitamins, minerals, and trace elements. However, the micronutrients supplied are not sufficient to correct a deficiency if it is identified. Correcting a vitamin or mineral deficiency requires supplementation in therapeutic doses.

Other formulas that are elemental or "chemically defined" maximize absorption and are used with impaired pancreatic and small-bowel function, fistulas, and short-bowel syndromes. Defined formulas may be indicated for the malnourished patient in whom gut function and absorption capacity are markedly impaired.

Enteral feedings are best provided by continuous drip infusion regulated by a volumetric pump. Feedings should be colored blue so that they can be distinguished from body fluids (14). In this way monitoring secretions and contents of suctioning alerts personnel to overt and occult aspiration.

Oral Feeding

When oral feedings are considered, a clear liquid diet is provided and usually advances through standard hospital progression if tolerance is established. Due to volume intolerance, small frequent meals should be supplied. Foods should vary in taste, texture, and color to stay interesting. Additional moisture may be required to increase ease of swallowing. Individual food allergies, taste, and religious preference should be reflected in tray service. Nutrient analysis of intake should be maintained and supplements provided as necessary to meet nutrient requirements. A multitude of canned nutritional supplements intended for oral use are available. The supplements are convenient, can be provided at bedside, and ensure a specified delivery of nutrients per volume consumed.

Frequently patient and family education can begin as oral intake is initiated. Education should support the value of optimal intake in maintenance and repletion and may include information on dietary fiber and fluid. Fiber and fluid control can assist in rehabilitation when it involves bowel and bladder control. Fluid control needs to be a coordinated team effort so that the patient is educated on fluid intake and urine volume when intermittent catheterization is begun. However, fluid restriction should not be at the expense of adequate intake if patients are only capable of handling tube feeding or liquids by mouth. For the long term, patients should be counseled regarding adequate fluid intake because urological infections are common. Volume of intake should produce a dilute urine to decrease risk of forming calcium precipitates.

TRANSITIONAL FEEDINGS

Two goals of transitional feeding include maintaining the patient's nutritional status and returning to as near normal intake as possible (16). During this time, consideration must be given to social and psychological needs as well as nutrient requirements.

Transition from Parenteral to Oral Feeding

The process of changing from parenteral to oral feedings is simplified by the use of a graphic display of nutrient intake analysis (Fig. 7-1). As documented oral intake improves, i.v. feeding can be tapered (17). A stepwise method can be employed to assure consistency of intake. For example, as a patient consistently maintains an intake of 500 cal, for 4 days, parenteral nutrition then can be decreased by 500 cal. Therefore, if a standard solution (previously described) is used, providing ~1 calo-

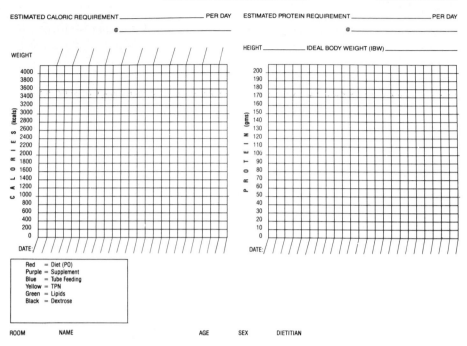

FIG. 7-1. Nutrient analysis graph displayed on patient door, St. Luke's Episcopal Hospital. (Reproduced with permission from ref. 10.)

rie per milliliter, its rate should be decreased by 500 ml in 24 h. The patient may be provided with frequent meals and given encouragement, striving for an intake well beyond the initial 500 cal. If it is sustained, the parenteral nutrition rate may again be lowered. The process continues until oral intake consistently meets 66% of the patient's total nutrient requirement. At that time it is appropriate to discontinue i.v. nutrition.

Transition from Parenteral to Enteral Feeding

The change from i.v. nutrition to tube feeding is made when the patient is not expected to eat in amounts sufficient to maintain or replete nutritional status. Usually, formulas are diluted to half concentration and the rate is advanced every 12–24 h to reach the goal rate. Then the concentration is advanced to full strength. This process may take 2–4 days or longer. Residuals are monitored to avert potential aspiration problems. Also, signs and symptoms of dehydration are noted, especially if the patient is unable to recognize or express thirst.

The rate of parenteral nutrition is reduced to decrease nutrients delivered from i.v. therapy in equal portions to that being provided from tube feeding. Again, actual intake from each source should be documented (17). Due to interruption of the infusion for various treatments and tolerance fluctuations, there can be a discrepancy between the amount of tube feeding prescribed and the amount received. Once adequate enteral intake is maintained, parenteral therapy can be discontinued.

Transition from Enteral to Oral Feeding

Again, a stepwise procedure is used in advancing intake from enteral to oral. Overlap of the two feeding routes should facilitate the reduction of enteral volume over 24 h in proportion to calories consumed orally. The rate of the tube feeding is diminished but continued over 24 h.

Other methods described include providing enteral tube feeding by night and oral intake during waking hours (17) or stopping tube feeding 60–90 min before consuming oral meals (18). As always, nutrient intake from all sources should be monitored, recorded, and reported to show adequacy of actual intake (17).

EVALUATION

Monitoring treatment mandates initial goal setting and determination of the mode and amount of nutrients required. The process is then repeated serially and therapeutic changes are made according to outcome. The application of the text of this chapter to a case presentation may help in delineation of nutritional assessment and calculations (Table 7-2).

It should be recognized that energy and protein requirements decline as stress level declines and as healing and repletion are accomplished. When the decline occurs depends on the clinical condition of the patient. Associated injuries, recurrent fevers, infection, or decubiti make nutrient provision dynamic in nature. As the patient stabilizes and enters into the rehabilitation phase, aggressive nutritional therapy also may be tapered. Suggestion has been made that ultimate ideal weight in the quadriplegic patient is 15–20 pounds below that of the Metropolitan Life Insurance Table (19). Nutritional support and/or education should reflect that goal and avoid excessive weight gain.

CONCLUSIONS

This chapter has been devoted to the physical management and delivery of adequate nutrition in the acute phase of spinal cord injury. The term physical management means employing all advances in technical

Table 7-2. *Case Presentation*[a]

Patient is an 18-year-old man, with C4 injury due to motor vehicle accident. Current status: respirator dependent, no bowel sounds. Fever: 100.4°F. Preinjury weight: 185 lb (84 kg).

Objective data
Somatic parameters *(81)*
 Height 5'11" (180 cm), weight 180 lb (81.8 kg); frame: medium
 Arm circumference: 25.2 cm
 Triceps skinfold: 4.5 mm
 Midarm muscle circumference (MAMC): 23.7 cm

Visceral parameters *(82)*
 Albumin: 2.4 g/dl
 Transferrin: 96 mg/dl
 Hemoglobin: 12.0 g/dl
 Total lymph count: 1,012 mm^3
 Antigen skin tests: *anergic*
 N_2 balance: -16 g *(81)*

Basal energy expenditure (BEE) $= 66 + (13.7 \times 81.8) + (5 \times 180) - (6.8 \times 18) = 1,964$ *(79)*

Predicted energy expenditure $= 1,964$ kcal (BEE) $\times 1.1$ (activity) $\times 1.14$ (fever) $\times 1.25$ (trauma) $\times 1.05$ (respirator) $= 3,232$ *(80)*

Crosscheck: 40–45 kcal/kg $= 3,272$–3,681 kcal *(80)*

Predicted protein needs (1.5–2 g/kg) $= 123$–164 g/24° *(80)*

Crosscheck: $6.25 \times \dfrac{\text{Energy requirement}}{135} = 135$ g *(80)*

Assessment
Somatic parameters: Lean man when compared with others his age. Baseline measures indicate minimal adipose tissue stores as fat, adequate lean mass.

Visceral parameters: Severely depleted visceral protein compartment. Decreased albumin; decreased transferrin; total lymph count is moderately depressed without the ability to recognize recall antigens—may relate to poor immunocompetence.

Goals
 3,270–3,681 kcal
 123–164 g protein
 ≤588 g carbohydrate (maximum oxidative capacity 4–5 mg·kg^{-1}·min^{-1})
 ≤81.8–204 g fat (1–2.5 g/kg) *(85)*

Problems: Unable to use alimentary tract. Attention to preservation of fat stores. Needs catabolism reversed and visceral protein repleted.

Resulting dietary Rx: parenteral nutrition
  500 ml 20% intralipid—over 12 h (100 g fat, 1,000 kcal)
  500 ml 40% dextrose (576 g cho, 1,958 kcal/24 h)
  500 ml 10% amino acid solution (144 g protein/24 h)
Rate: 120 ml/h ultimately
Rx: 3,534 kcal, 144 g protein, 1:154 kcal:N_2 ratio; 28% total fat kcal

---

Reevaluation
Current status: Fracture surgically stabilized, remains on ventilator, now with positive bowel sounds. Past 10-day average intake: 3,178 kcal/125 g protein.

Objective data
Somatic parameters *(81)*
  Height 5′11″ (180 cm), weight 185 lb (84 kg), frame: medium
  Arm circumference: 119 cm
  Triceps skinfold: 33 mm
  MAMC: 10.8 mm

Visceral parameters *(82)*
  Albumin: 2.3 g/dl
  Transferrin: 136 mg/dl
  Hemoglobin: 11.2 g/dl
  Total lymph count: 1,272 cells/mm^3
  Antigen skin tests: *anergic*
  N_2 balance: +1 g *(81)*

Assessment
Somatic parameters: Arm circumference and weight increased without corre sponding change in lean or fat mass indices relates to a fluid weight increase. Crosscheck of fluid intake and output data confirms positive fluid balance.

Visceral parameters remain hypoalbuminemic, some improvement in transferrin. May indicate beginning of anabolism. Nitrogen intake balances with output. Total lymph count depressed but *stable;* still anergic—may reflect continued poor immunocompetence.

Problems: May need slightly more protein and/or energy to promote anabolism.
Unable to tolerate oral intake. Needs advancement to enteral feedings.
Resulting dietary Rx: Continue parenteral, same rate. Begin enteral.
  Half strength 2 cal/ml formula 20% protein via nasoduodenal tube at 30 ml/h
  Day 2, advance to 55 ml/h, if tolerated, × 12 h; decrease parenteral rate to 75 ml/h

---

*a*The italic numbers in parentheses throughout the table refer to page numbers in the text where topic is discussed in detail.

skills and in the industry of nutritional care to maximize the survival and nutritional health of the patient in the immediate postinjury phase. The aim is that the patient can emerge with the physical means to begin to cope emotionally and adapt to necessary changes.

Protocols for nutritional care should be developed and used in institutions with acute SCI patients to communicate to all staff the plan of care and decision tree. In this way the nutritional health of the patient is not sacrificed while trying to decide how, how much, and what to feed.

REFERENCES

1. Goldfarb IW, Yates AP (1980): *Total Parenteral Nutrition Concepts and Methods*. Pittsburgh: Synapse Publications.
2. Harris JA, Benedict FG (1919): *A Biometric Study of Basal Metabolism in Man*. Washington, D.C., Carnegie Institute of Washington, Publication No. 279. Philadelphia: Lippincott.
3. Kinney JM, Long CL, Gump FE, Duke JH Jr (1968): Tissue composition of weight loss in surgical patients. I. Elective operation. *Ann Surg* 168:459–474.
4. Clarke KS (1966): Caloric costs of activity in paraplegic persons. *Arch Phys Med Rehabil* 47:427–435.
5. Wilmore D (1977): *The Metabolic Management of the Critically Ill*. New York: Plenum.
6. Stern J (1986): Nutritional care in physical medicine and rehabilitation. *News Dietetics Phys Med Rehabil* 5:4.
7. Spanier AH, Shizgal HM (1977): Caloric requirements of the critically ill patient receiving intravenous hyperalimentation. *Am J Surg* 133:99–104.
8. Food and Nutrition Board (1980): *Recommended Dietary Allowances, 9th ed.* Washington, D.C., National Academy of Sciences–National Research Council.
9. Kaminski M (1976): Enteral hyperalimentation. *Surg Gynecol Obstet* 143:12.
10. Dudrick SJ, et al. (1985): Nutritional assessment: indications for nutritional support. In: *Nutrition in Clinical Surgery* (Deitel M, ed), pp. 24–37.
11. Blackburn GL, et al. (1977): Nutritional and metabolic assessment of the hospitalized patient. *J Parenter Enter Nutr* 1:11–22.
12. Grant A (1979): *Nutritional Assessment Guidelines, 2nd ed.* California: Cutter Medical Laboratories.
13. Frisancho RA (1984): New standards of weight and body composition by frame size and height for assessment of nutritional status of adults and the elderly. *Am J Clinical Nutr* 40:808–819.
14. Treloar DM, Stechmiller J (1984): Pulmonary aspiration in tube-fed patients with artificial airways. *Heart Lung* 13:667.
15. Maillet JO (1984): Calculating parenteral feedings: a programmed instruction. *J Am Diet Assoc* 84:1312–1323.
16. Skipper A (1982): Transitional feeding and the dietician. *Nutritional Support Services* 2:45.
17. (1987): *Standards for Nutritional Support. Nutrition in Clinical Practice.* American Society for Parenteral and Enteral Nutrition.

18. Randall HT (1984): Sixth Annual Jonathan Rhoades Lecture on Enteral Nutrition: tube feeding in acute and chronic illness. *J Parenter Enter Nutr* 8:113–136.
19. Peiffer SC, Blust P, Leyson JFJ (1981): Nutritional assessment of the spinal cord injured patient. *J Am Diet Assoc* 78:501–505.

8

Psychological Issues Related to Ventilator-Dependent Quadriplegia

Joan Anderson

Social Service Department, Santa Clara Valley Medical Center, San Jose, California, U.S.A.

THE RACE[1]

When I got to the airport I rushed up to the desk
and they told me the flight was cancelled. The doctors had
said my father would not live through the night
and the flight was cancelled. A young man with a
dark blond mustache told me
another airline had a non-stop
leaving in seven minutes—see that
elevator over there well go
down to the first floor, make a right you'll
see a yellow bus, get off at the
second Pan Am terminal—I
ran, I who have no sense of direction
raced exactly where he'd told me, like a fish
slipping upstream deftly against the
flow of the river. I jumped off that bus with my
heavy bags and ran, the bags
wagged me from side to side as if to
prove I was under the claims of the material, I
ran up to a man with a white flower on his breast,
I who always go to the end of the line, I said
Help me. He looked at my ticket, he said make a
left and then a right go up the moving stairs and then

---

[1] Reprinted by permission. © 1985 Sharon Olds. Originally in *The New Yorker*.

run. I raced up the moving stairs
two at a time, at the top I saw the
long hollow corridor and
then I took a deep breath, I said
goodbye to my body, goodbye to comfort, I
used my legs and heart as if I would
gladly use them up for this, to
touch him again in this life. I ran and the
big heavy dark bags
banged me, wheeled and swam around me like
planets in wild orbits—I have seen
pictures of women running down roads with their
belongings tied in black scarves
grasped in their fists, running under serious
gray historical skies—I blessed my
long legs he gave me, my strong
heart I abandoned to its own purpose, I
ran to Gate 17 and they were
just lifting the thick white
lozenge of the door to fit it into the
socket of the plane. Like the man who is not
too rich, I turned to the side and
slipped through the needle's eye, and then I
walked down the aisle toward my father. The jet was
full and people's hair was shining, they were
smiling, the interior of the plane was filled with a
mist of gold endorphin light,
I wept as people weep when they enter heaven,
in massive relief. We lifted up
gently from one tip of the continent and
did not stop until we set down lightly on the
other edge, I walked into his room and
watched his chest rise slowly and
sink again, all night
I watched him breathe.

—Sharon Olds

The flight to the patient's bedside described by the poet Sharon Olds
in *The Race* (1) probably feels familiar to anyone who has been called
to a hospital in response to the medical crisis of a loved one. It is perhaps especially poignant for families of high quadriplegic patients. When
the injury occurs, the panic begins. The patient may know immediately
that his neck is broken. He may say later, "I heard my neck break, I
knew I couldn't move," or he may be unconscious or have sustained so
many injuries that he does not know the full extent of the damage.

This chapter seeks to review some common psychological experiences observed among newly injured ventilator-dependent spinal-cord-injury (SCI) patients and their families in an acute rehabilitation center, from the time of injury through medical stabilization to the beginning involvement in the full therapy program.

REVIEW OF THE LITERATURE

A large body of literature related to SCI exists. The psychological and social aspects have been discussed at some length. Comprehensive reviews of the issues can be found in Crewe and Krause (2), Trieschmann (3), and Woodbury and Redd (4). Because virtually no literature specific to the psychological aspects of ventilator-dependent quadriplegia exists, this chapter is based primarily on clinical experience.

Many theories of adaptation exist, some of which conflict with others. As with SCI in general, there is no proven, predictable pattern that occurs with every patient and family. Emotional reactions and accommodation to the injury vary with the individual and are influenced by the unique history of experience, coping styles, and resources that each family brings with them. Much remains to be studied in connection with this population.

ACUTE PHASE

Obviously, people who cannot breathe must receive rather immediate help from someone who knows cardiopulmonary resuscitation or they will not live to see the paramedics or the emergency room. One young woman fell over a cliff in a national park virtually into the lap of a physician who was hiking in the area, and thereby survived a C1 SCI. Once notified, families most immediately need information. They ask, "What has happened to my son? Will my husband live? What are you doing to my daughter?" Families, and the patient, if conscious, understandably display anxiety and distress. They are confronted with a medical emergency, an unfamiliar environment, and often questions of life or death. Few people are prepared to respond to such an overwhelming, catastrophic event.

Working through the maze of medical personnel to get answers to basic questions about the patient's condition presents a major challenge. Just getting near the patient can be difficult, with limited intensive care unit visiting hours and critical care procedures under way. The separation itself, the waiting, the unknown, and fear for the patient's life all engender a sense of helplessness.

Woodbury and Redd review several theories of adjustment that provide constructs for understanding human reactions to the trauma of SCI:

Seligman proposes that the helpless response occurs when the event is interpreted as uncontrollable. Shontz associates stress, anxiety, shock, detachment, helplessness, panic, disorganization, frustration, and depression with response to negative events (4).

In response to the crisis precipitated by the injury, families commonly stay near the patient 24 h a day, either sharing the watch or appointing one person to the task. If one person stays, it is typically the wife or mother. The vigil may last several weeks or months until the patient has stabilized. It may then decrease to a daytime shift or afternoon/evening visits. It is usually therapeutic for the patient and the family if the unit can accommodate this presence. Staff can let families know when they need more space or time to provide treatment.

One mother whose 19-year-old son had a C2 SCI stayed faithfully all day for months until one day, while walking down the hall in the unit, she thought to herself, "I have to get back to my own life in some ways." After that she attended more to the events of her life at home while maintaining appropriate contact with and support of her son. Her decision reflected her confidence that her son would survive.

Families may feel torn between their need to be at the hospital and their need to care for other children at home, or to attend to a job. They bear the burden of the emotional crisis plus all the mechanics of reorganizing their lives to accommodate the hospitalization. They put much "on hold" in their lives to attend to the injured.

One patient's mother could never be persuaded to take time out for herself, even after months of stabilization. Her 25-year-old son had never left home, and mother and son seemed to believe that their lives depended on one another's presence, even though their time together was filled with conflict. Before his injury, the son had decided that he would devote his life to the care of his mother, who had been abandoned by her husband years before. Rehabilitation never really changed that system and the patient was rarely willing to take initiative toward independence in his program.

At first, families may be unaware of their surroundings in the hospital because they are focused so intently on the patient. Some time may pass before they begin to absorb the activity beyond the bedside. Then they may notice other patients who are at different stages of rehabilitation, or begin to assimilate what people with injuries similar to their family member's are doing.

Some families begin to network with neighboring patients' families rather immediately, and vividly relate the progress of other patients to their injured relative. They seem to distinguish the different styles with which others cope, and deduce some possibilities that the future may hold for their family member, based on what they see on the ward. They also seem to be able to get support from the exchange with other patients and families.

If a patient and family can begin to reach out to other patients and families within a few days postinjury, it may be a good indication of their social skills and ability to empathize. For example, if a newly injured patient in a Rotorest bed can notice something his or her roommate needs and bring it to the attention of staff, it may show the patient's ability to look beyond his or her own needs. These qualities serve anyone well as they move through the rehabilitation process and into the community. Successful management of ventilator-dependent SCI depends on the patient's ability to relate well enough to other people to elicit their support to meet his or her needs.

The issue of breathing in high cervical lesions adds a profound aspect to the injury. Quite naturally, patients and families focus their apprehensions on the struggle for breath. The decision to place the patient on a ventilator may pose a dilemma for the patient, family, or medical team, but more often it is not an immediate question but a decision made in response to trauma.

At the time of injury the patient and family are rarely capable of comprehending the implications of the injury. It is hard to imagine what it will eventually take to live with it. Initially most patients and families accept the intervention of the ventilator as a life-sustaining treatment. It is not equivalent to the use of the machine to sustain someone who is terminally ill, where there may be more ambivalence about it. If there is significant brain injury, however, there may be more debate about whether to begin mechanical life-support.

Decisions are generally guided by the desire to do everything possible to care for the patient. The family's desire is personal; the medical team's is professional. Treatment is designed to offer state-of-the-art technology and to promote the patient's welfare. As the American Medical Association Judiciary Committee stated in December 1984: "Quality of life is a factor to be considered in determining what is best for the individual. Life should be cherished despite disabilities and handicaps, except when the prolongation would be inhumane and unconscionable . . ." (5).

Few families argue the use of the ventilator in the first few days or weeks after injury. At first, they are simply glad the patient is alive. Later, as the enormity of the situation sinks in, they must come to grips with how they will manage life under these conditions. At this point some patients express a wish to die. Others say much later, "I thought about whether I would be better off dead but I decided to live."

Families seem less likely to admit such thoughts immediately. They begin by saying, "We're so glad he's alive, it's OK." It is unusual for a family to say, "I can't handle this," even when they ultimately evade caretaking in various ways. Eventually, one person may confide the wish that the patient had died in the accident rather than have to go through the ordeal. This statement is generally not shared with the patient and is accompanied by feelings of guilt. Family members may also feel guilty about the circumstances of the accident (if they were driving, for example) or they may feel angry at the patient for getting hurt. These feelings can be difficult to express.

The use of the ventilator is a very tangible pro-life choice. Not everyone elects to make that choice. On one occasion, a few weeks postinjury, a teenage boy decided he did not want to live as a C1 quadriplegic. He was an avid baseball player and did not want a life so removed from his passion and experience. His parents agreed. After weeks of discussion among the patient, family, and staff, the family's wishes were respected and aggressive treatment was withheld. The patient died comfortably with his family at his side.

In another case, an older man who had been a sea captain all his life felt unequivocally that he did not want to be maintained on a respirator, so the machine was turned off and he died.

Recent court decisions (*Bartling* v. *Glendale Adventist Medical Center*, 1984) ruled that a patient's refusal of treatment is a "constitutionally guaranteed right which must not be abridged" (6). The 1983 President's Commission for the Study of Ethical Problems in Medicine and Biomedical and Behavioral Research (7) also reported that the principle of patient autonomy should guide treatment decisions.

The patient's decision to die can be an agony for staff. Rehabilitation, by its nature, promotes life and well-being. Deliberate death, when life is an option, disturbs the fundamental values on which staff rely. It also fails to reconcile the ethical dilemmas raised by the cultural mores prohibiting suicide and murder. Nonetheless, the reasons that move a patient to refuse treatment or request discontinuation of treatment must be carefully considered. Such considerations apply, of course, to the patient who is alert and competent to make informed consent.

The deliberation of these issues is well chronicled in the case of a 19-year-old man with a C1 SCI in Michigan who petitioned the County Circuit Court to be declared competent. He also asked "for the right to refuse further medical treatment, including mechanical ventilation, and for an order immunizing his parents from criminal liability or penalty for carrying out his desires" (8). The court granted his petition and 2 weeks later he asked his father to turn off his respirator and he died.

Most patients feel less certain that they want to die. One young woman with a C1 SCI and a mild head injury persevered for months on her wish to die yet she did not specify that the ventilator be discontinued. In fact, she agreed to a surgical procedure midrehabilitation and the night before surgery insisted on extra reassurance because she was worried that the anesthetic would kill her. In her case her desire to die was more a reflection of her anxiety and depression. It was her pattern to obsess on suicidal thoughts when under stress even before her injury. Intensive work with the psychologist in individual psychotherapy was effective in reducing her anxiety while in the rehabilitation program.

It is imperative that staff look for ambiguity and beyond the face value of a "wish to die" to give the patient the full opportunity to live.

For those who affirm their choice to live, the process of attuning to the breathing machine includes close attention to the detail involved. Patient and family may worry considerably about such things as tidal volumes, vital capacities, and blood gases. Questions about whether the patient is getting enough air or *feels* like he or she is getting enough air predominate. Sometimes the patient will be getting sufficient volume but will feel anxious and short of breath. "Holding their own breath" for the patient's breath continues for various lengths of time with various families. One mother realized in the acute phase that she "got to the point where I couldn't stand walking down the corridor waiting to hear a stat code called to my son's room. It had to be OK for him to live or *die* in order to relax enough to stop worrying about his breathing all the time."

A polio patient reports that years after he was stricken he understood that only when his mother finally let go of *his* breathing issue could he get on with his life. Other mothers confide that for a year or more after the patient came home they only half slept each night, keenly listening for the continual rhythm of the ventilator.

As learning about the technology involved proceeds, there begins the human exchange that builds trust between staff and family. Trust is a major issue for anyone in a hospital. The role of patient almost automatically places one at the mercy of strangers who are responsible for one's care. For high quadriplegic patients for whom that dependency is at a maximum, where every breath depends on the competence and reliability of other people, developing trust that the staff and machine will keep one alive is a critical matter.

Control is another privilege relinquished as one assumes the role of patient. As with trust, it is an issue magnified by quadriplegia. When at one moment a person enjoys the freedom to decide both the pivotal and trivial aspects of life, the next moment these freedoms are usurped by paralysis and medical regimen. Simple activities such as changing the TV channel or going out for a hamburger are stripped away by the injury.

In the midst of this monumental upheaval, families and patients naturally seek security, stability, and predictability. Separated from the familiar comforts of home and forced into the most stressful conditions, families may have difficulty distinguishing minute variations in treatment from actual causes for alarm. To the untrained eye, a 30-min delay in the turning schedule or medication delivery may cause as much fright as a ventilator alarm. When lost in the night in a foreign land, every noise may seem ominous.

Staff can do much to assuage anxiety with simple courtesies: appointing someone to convey information to families; explaining procedures before they are done; asking what the patient or family needs; establishing dependable routines; educating the patient and family about the relative value of treatments; forewarning them when there will be a delay or exception; reassuring them about which things have some latitude. Although these guidelines may be pertinent to any trauma, they are especially important with high quadriplegic patients, because every action, or nonaction, can be perceived as having life-or-death consequences.

In the administration of their duties, staff can all contribute to the emotional support of the patient and family, encourage trust, foster a sense of control, and nurture the opportunity for a positive outlook that will later assist the patient and family to see the options available for the reconstruction of a meaningful life.

In the first few days postinjury the family lives moment to moment, absorbing what they can about what has happened and what the treatment involves. Understanding comes at different rates for different people and almost all information will need to be repeated over several months. If the patient is incapacitated by surgery, medication, or hallucinations, the family can absorb information without the pressure of what to say to the patient at the moment (see Chapter 6).

As with any SCI, patients and families may continue to ask questions about the prognosis, even after it has been clearly explained several times. In high quadriplegic patients, the initial concentration on breathing may delay attention to the exigencies of the paralysis in general. Repetitions of questions or denial of the prognosis do not need to be considered problems unless they interfere with participation in therapy. If the patient refuses to do mouth exercises because he or she believes that they will recover fully and the exercises are unnecessary, treatment can stall. Otherwise, it serves the patient for the staff to repeat answers until they are heard. People assimilate tragedy as they can, and time alone will teach them reality. It is not useful to deprive people of the hope that will help them survive the ordeal.

MEDICAL STABILIZATION

Complications such as surgery or pneumonia may keep the family focused on the immediate. People attend to *basic* needs until they are met.

Once the patient has stabilized, it is possible for all involved to look toward the future, to imagine what life will be like in 6 months, or 5 years.

What information families use out of what staff members have given them may offer some clues about what they are able to imagine for the future. The parents of a 19-year-old college student with a C1 injury asked almost immediately, "Will he still be able to think?" They were well educated and considered a viable mind sufficient for a viable life. Because the patient shared that view, he was able to finish his graduate education and go to work.

As the family and patient begin to assimilate the injury and the hospital environment, begin to learn how to get their needs met, and see the patient stabilize, participation in the rehabilitation program can proceed. Setting up a basic communication system with the patient is important to engaging in the program. If possible, it should provide a way for him to express his needs, respond to people working with him, and to sound an alarm when in distress.

Acquiring comfort with the ventilator is an early task that will continue with adaptations such as the pneumobelt or phrenic nerve stimulators.

As the patient stabilizes, the staff can encourage the family to physically touch, especially where sensation is intact. Family can also begin to perform simple caretaking like washing the patient's face. Such tasks promote contact between patient and family, teach the family that the patient is not fragile, and initiate their education in the required care. This involvement can be expanded as the patient progresses, so that by the end of the hospitalization patient and family are familiar with all aspects of the patient's care.

When patient or family express anxiety or fear at new stages it can be helpful for staff to acknowledge feelings while remaining firm about cooperation. If anger predominates and cannot be ameliorated by ordinary means, staff should, while acknowledging the feeling, set limits against acting out and inappropriate social behavior. It is not a kindness to the patient to allow him or her to abuse others.

In one instance a young man with a C2/3 injury complained of pain incessantly, although his neurological tests indicated that he could not feel the parts of the body where he reported pain. His preoccupation interrupted most other social interaction with him, and prevented his participation in his scheduled therapy. The nurses requested a behavior modification program from the team psychologist. The psychologist advised the staff to turn away from the patient each time he complained about pain and to say, "I will not talk to you about pain." They were then to approach the patient with a question about a social activity he enjoyed, such as "Did you see the movie on TV last night?" The staff advised the patient before they began about what to expect. They also arranged for the good-natured resident physician to spend 15 min each morning with the patient while he catalogued his current pains. The patient agreed to the plan and within 24 h came to the psychologist to report his progress in limiting his complaints. His interactions centered more around social activities from then on, and his program continued.

INVOLVEMENT IN THE FULL PROGRAM

It is hoped that good working relationships with the staff have been established by the time the patient is able to participate in a full therapy program. Ideally, patient, family, and staff share mutually agreed-upon goals. If therapists encounter resistance to progress, it may be useful to review the goals in short-term, day-to-day steps; incorporate signs of progress into daily activities; communicate expectations to family; and hold regular team meetings to ensure consistency.

Patients may have a variety of responses to increased demands. Each new phase requires new behaviors and elicits deeper awareness of the injury. Many patients believe that once they are out of bed that they will recover, or that when their halo vest comes off they will be able to move. Each dashed hope has the potential to precipitate grief or depression.

The distinctions between grief and depression have been illuminated in rehabilitation literature by Stewart and Shields. They describe grief as "a normal reaction to the loss of a physical function. . . . Symptoms include a preoccupation with the lost object, somatic distress, inappropriate behavior, hostility and denial" (9). They differentiate grief from the affective disorder of depression which, "by definition, must manifest at least four of the following symptoms nearly every day for at least two weeks: poor appetite or significant weight loss, insomnia or hypersomnia, psychomotor agitation or retardation, loss of interest in usual activities, fatigue, sense of worthlessness, slowed cognition and suicidal thoughts" (9). Careful differential diagnosis allows for appropriate treatment and continuation in the rehabilitation process.

Passivity can pose a significant threat to the completion of a program. When efforts to engage the patient fail, when the patient refuses to talk, take initiative in directing his or her care, sit up, drive the power chair, leave their room, practice mouthstick activities, or socialize, staff feel frustrated and irritated and the patient feels hopeless. Self-imposed isolation intensifies depression, depression intensifies withdrawal, and withdrawal further impedes treatment in a vicious circle. At this point a psychologist may spend some time with the patient to explore the patient's possible wish for death. At times, the very act of exploring death as an option allows the patient to move through that aspect of grief.

Many people in the ventilator-dependent SCI population are teenagers or young adults who have just been preparing to leave home or have recently left. SCI often throws people back into the lap of the family, so that many developmental steps may need to be retraced (10). With any disability it is a demanding task to learn that independence is still possible and to figure out how to achieve it. With a respirator, it may seem impossible to imagine. If the leaving home process was not going well, or failing, the injury will underscore the enmeshment.

Those who are bright, verbal, social, and able to take initiative are more likely to fare well from the outset. Those who do not have those traits face the task of learning social skills to compensate for the loss of physical mobility and self care.

David, an 18-year-old with C2 SCI, was a gregarious sort. He eagerly anticipated each new step in the rehabilitation program. He adapted to sitting up and the use of the pneumobelt in record time. He went out of his room the moment he was able and instantly acquainted himself with everyone on the floor. He spent much of his time visiting other patients who were still in bed, encouraging them to tolerate the tedium of confinement and instilling hope about future progress. He not only served as a model for other people on ventilators, but patients with lesser injuries would look at him and say, "Gee, look at that guy. He can't even breathe by himself and he's up having fun!"

David was also very verbal about his feelings and talked freely with staff and patients about all aspects of his condition. He spoke of his wish, "If only I could breathe." He talked about life and death, and he looked forward to going home. David did go home. He had the good fortune to have an insurance policy that provided the best home care available. Even so, the first 2 years were difficult. He drank too much beer, smoked marijuana with his friends, and despite all his good traits, seemed to lack purpose. Not until his nurses issued ultimatums that he stop his substance abuse or get a new agency did he seek counsel.

After a few weeks of outpatient counseling he agreed to finish his general equivalency diploma and apply for a computer training program designed for the disabled. He passed the aptitude tests and became passionately involved in programming. His drug use decreased considerably and he completed his training.

Another patient, Jeremy, who also had a drug abuse history, managed to join a circle of patients who gathered behind the hospital at the end of the day to smoke marijuana. It was tempting to admire his social skills and to think, "Well, I guess he's been rehabilitated," except that drug use potentially jeopardized the programs of all the patients involved.

Many patients enter the hospital with preexisting drug and alcohol abuse problems. Many are under the influence at the time of injury, and some continue to use drugs while in the hospital and at home. High quadriplegic patients are not exempt from these problems, but it takes the help of other people to permit the abuse by physically providing the drink or drug.

Friends often mistakenly feel sorry for the patient and think drugs will offer escape or pleasure even when it is clear that the abuse compromises the patient's health in such ways as producing more mucus, which requires more suctioning and increases the risk of respiratory problems.

Drug use in the hospital or at home also poses a management problem for caretakers. They can be caught in a bind when they know that the patient has the right to choose, but that they are responsible for his care. It can be an untenable position for the caretaker to feel he or she must sit by while the patient becomes inebriated with friends or family. Attention to the issue in the hospital can be as important a component as any in the program and should be addressed with the patient and family. Teaching the family how not to enable the drug abuse is a standard drug treatment approach.

In the first few months of rehabilitation staff gear themselves toward mobilizing the patient, physically and mentally. The goal is to teach the patient every detail of his or her nursing care and how to assume responsibility for instructing others in such things as weight shifts, suctioning, transfers, bowel and bladder management, and trouble-shooting the ventilator.

What can be done when the patient refuses some aspect of the program? It is helpful to review the goals, break them into smaller components, and look for positive reinforcements for goal-oriented behavior. For example, staff may say, "The goal is to sit up without feeling dizzy by the end of the week" or "I'll put your makeup on while you are sitting up." The goal should be pursued consistently, even in the face of the patient's resistance. For example:

Sydney absolutely refused to leave her room to socialize. When the nurses did persuade her to vacate the room for a few hours each day, the patient did not socialize any more than before, but she used some of her time to sun herself on the patio, and the break relieved the tension between patient and staff.

Tiffany refused to have anything to do with a mouthstick, retorting, "I don't need that thing. It's ugly." She never would turn a page, which frustrated the staff, but offered them the opportunity to remember that one cannot always impose one's own values on someone else. The patient did not share the staff's value of mouthstick activities and it was her right to make that choice. She was entitled to her own style as much as anyone.

Such patients give the staff the opportunity to practice clear team communication. Teamwork can counteract attempts to sabotage therapy when patients try to confuse staff about the schedule, feign illness, pick fights with the occupational therapist, or pit day staff against night staff. Staff can respond effectively against these maneuvers with regular team meetings, anticipation of the behavior, and agreement on clear limits. The limits may have to include how hard to push toward a goal *and* when to give up. It is important for staff to know they have tried everything they can think of so they can stop exhausting themselves with vain efforts. The team may feel guilty about discontinuing such a patient's therapy program, but it is useful to know when to give up and to give up as a group.

It can also help staff to create a list of techniques for intervention in difficult situations, such as agreeing that each nurse will say, "I don't like it when you yell at me." Or, "If you continue to be rude I will walk away. I deserve to be treated politely."

Staff may need the chance to discuss their own feelings about their ventilator patients. Nursing this group is an intense experience because of the profound injury involved, the number of hours each nurse spends with the patient, and the critical nature of the care. It is quite different from nursing a paraplegic, who may only require an hour or so a day, and who is comparatively independent.

The social work and psychology staff can facilitate staff support groups where people can express their concern, sadness, frustration, anger, helplessness, and even homicidal fantasies. It is not unusual in such meetings for someone to admit, "I really want to throttle her," followed by, "I feel so guilty to think that."

People (families and staff) sometimes feel guilty if they get angry with the patient. They seem to believe that if a person has a disability he or she is too fragile to withstand normal human interactions. They think "I would really seem like a jerk to chew this guy out when he's got enough troubles already."

Such an attitude dehumanizes the disabled person and robs him or her of the normal exchange of feelings that keep our relationships mutual and balanced. To expect a patient to make a contribution toward keeping the relationship in good order is a step toward normalization and a critical survival skill. It is recognition that the patient is still a person. To permit the patient to behave abusively and then to consider such behavior manipulative can hardly be fair. If a staff member feels manipulated, it may indicate that they have failed to state their own needs or set their own boundaries clearly.

If not passively depressed, a patient may be actively demanding, calling for attention every few minutes, such as "Suction me . . . Move my hand . . . I'm thirsty . . .". If the situation reaches unmanageable proportions and the patient is unwilling to negotiate a more workable agreement, psychological consultation or a behavior modification plan may help. Some patients exhibit a euphoria initially, seeming unperturbed by reality. This state is not usually difficult to manage, and in time changes to a more congruent affect.

As in other kinds of SCI, empowerment can be an issue for patients. If personal identity has been rooted in physical prowess, the challenge is to reestablish a sense of mastery in the environment.

CONCLUSIONS

Many of the psychological issues pertinent to ventilator-dependent quadriplegia appear in other levels of SCI. These issues are well catalogued in the general SCI literature. The injury affects the patient and family in a catastrophic way, precipitating tremendous change and loss. As with any disability, the loss is ongoing, and awareness of specific aspects of it wax and wane in each life stage.

As with SCI in general, high quadriplegia affects a predominantly young, vital population, people whose lives lay uncharted in front of them.

Medicine now has the technology to manage the injury and sustain the body in relative health. Rehabilitation specialists have the knowledge to mobilize people and return them to the community.

The magnitude of the injury and the complexity of care can be a staggering burden to absorb, for the injured and the people who assume their care. The disruption of breathing—that primary, automatic function so fundamental to life—disturbs our assumptions about the minimum functions needed to survive and prosper, yet our experience with this population demonstrates that people can surmount the most grievous injury and, with adequate medical and community support, can continue to live vital, productive lives.

REFERENCES

1. Olds S (1985): The race. *The New Yorker* 61:44.
2. Crewe N, Krause J (1987): Spinal cord injury: psychological aspects. In: *Rehabilitation Psychology Desk Reference* (Caplan B, ed). Rockville, MD: Aspen, pp. 3–35.
3. Trieschmann R (1980): *Spinal Cord Injuries: The Psychological, Social and Vocational Adjustment*. New York: Pergamon Press.
4. Woodbury B, Redd C (1987): Psychosocial issues and approaches. In: *Spinal Cord Injury Concepts and Management Approaches* (Buchanan LE, Nawoczenski DA, eds). Baltimore: Williams & Wilkins, pp. 185–217.
5. American Medical Association (1984): *Current Opinions of Judicial Council of AMA*. Chicago: American Medical Association.
6. *Bartling* v. *Glendale Adventist Medical Center*, et al. (1984): Case No. C500735.

Superior Court, Los Angeles, CA (Dept. 86, Wadington J), June 22.

7. President's Commission for Study of Ethical Problems in Medicine and Biomedical and Behavioral Research (1983): *Making Health Care Decisions: Ethical and Legal Implications of Informed Consent in Patient–Practitioner Relationship*. Washington D.C.: U.S. Government Printing Office.

8. Maynard FM, Muth AS (1987): The choice to end life as a ventilator-dependent quadriplegic. *Arch Phys Med Rehabil* 68:862–864.

9. Stewart T, Shields C (1985): Grief in chronic illness: assessment and management. *Arch Phys Med Rehabil* 66:447–450.

10. Thompson D (1980): Psychosocial development of spinal cord injured persons. *SCI Digest* 2:6–43.

II

Rehabilitation

Overview

Conal Wilmot

Department of Physical Medicine and Rehabilitation, Santa Clara Valley Medical Center, San Jose, California, U.S.A.

The goals of rehabilitation are limited for high quadriplegic patients due to their total physical dependence. Cost-effective treatment necessitates a coordinated, comprehensive rehabilitation program with a staff who are well trained and experienced in the care of the individual with high quadriplegia. This is vital not so much for survival, which can now be accomplished at any progressive medical center, but for maximizing the potential of the patient and minimizing costs. This treatment is necessarily aggressive, with no margin for error. Because of the positive attitude of the rehabilitation team towards the high quadriplegic patient, the patient and family are optimistic that something can be done, that all is not lost. A high quadriplegic individual can ideally be discharged home when the experienced rehabilitation team is involved early in the care of the patient and when appropriate equipment, patient/family/attendant training, and home setup are arranged expeditiously.

It has been reported that 63% of respirator-dependent quadriplegic persons are expected to survive at least 9 years after injury (1). The major medical problem specific to the high quadriplegic patient, as contrasted to a quadriplegic patient in the C5/6 range, is the necessity for ventilated respiration (2). There is now an increased understanding of the respiratory physiology of the high quadriplegic patient, and an increased realization of the importance of a prophylactic program to render the lungs as clear as possible clinically. The accessory muscles of respiration must be strengthened if possible and there must be constant watchfulness for the development of complications, which will respond to early, vigorous, acute treatment (3). Specific achievable rehabilitation goals are addressed in Chapters 10 and 11 of this section. If the patient has progressed beyond acute care, i.e., the spinal fracture is united,

113

and the major medical problems have been stabilized, that is, the chest is clear, then the program of prescreening as outlined in Chapter 3 can be instituted.

The initial acute hospitalization length of stay will require 3–4 months, depending on the extent of associated injuries and complications. Another 3–4 months will be required for rehabilitation. Some centers combine the acute and rehabilitation phases into one hospital stay. If in addition to the above the patient is tested and proved suitable for the phrenic nerve stimulator, the fitting, i.e., surgery, postoperative conditioning, and teaching of patient and nurses the use of the phrenic nerve stimulator (PNS), will add at least an additional 3 months to the hospital stay.

The availability of new respiratory equipment, e.g., the PNS, has resulted in heightened interest in the high quadriplegic patient, as demonstrated by the increase in writings in the spinal injury and respiratory journals. The success of this program in properly selected cases has allowed the patient to be free of the respirator at least for some time each day and possibly all day, allowing more mobility. With use of the pneumobelt, a portable respiratory device, the patient can breathe by external compression, enabling him/her to communicate verbally (4). The advantages of these various respirators (PNS, pneumobelt, respirator, or a combination of these appliances) provides increased choices in respiratory care, and ultimately in quality of life (5). Chapter 12 includes the details and pros and cons of respiratory options.

Electric wheelchairs have evolved to better meet the needs of the high quadriplegic patient in the past few years. The patient can be fitted for a personalized seat cushion for balance and skin protection, have electronic control of recline and upright positions, and have numerous options for driving the chair, e.g., chin or pneumatic control. Computers and environmental control units provide a new generation of manipulative capabilities for the totally paralyzed individual. Voice control technology is improving rapidly and is expected to be a viable assistive aid in the near future (6). Chapters 14 and 15 discuss considerations for equipment and chairs.

The availability of sophisticated electronically controlled equipment allows the patient to look better, have more mobility and independence, have minimal complications, and be able to communicate. Although the care of the high quadriplegic patient remains very complex and requires special expertise, the new attitude on the part of the patient, family, and staff allows more aggressive treatment. This permits a seriously disabled patient to make many more decisions for himself/herself that result in feeling and actually being more independent. Because this sophisticated equipment is evolving and improving on a yearly basis, vocational applications are already in use and may have greater application in the future. Several patients now work part time or full time: computer programmer, financial analyst, and law student are specific examples of high quadriplegic individuals in the community that come to mind.

The rehabilitation team must have a realistic plan for discharge. Having imbued the patient and family with this positive, forward-looking approach, it is catastrophic for the patient not to be discharged home. That means having a suitable family or friends, having an adequate living situation, and most importantly, having sufficient money to pay for nursing/attendant care. The training of the patient, of the family, and eventually of the nurse/attendant has to start as soon as the triaging is over. This allows the patient to feel comfortable instructing people, it allows the family to feel comfortable handling the disabled person, and it enables both patient and family to train, under the supervision of the team, the people who are eventually going to be taking care of the person in the home. Because of the prophylactic program of hands-on care being given to the patient, and taught to all concerned, there is a significant reduction in the complications that occur while in the home. The overall picture has to be of someone who, although seriously disabled, is going to live a life as close to normal as possible outside the confines of the hospital with the prescribed level of care (7).

The high quadriplegic person can have a better quality of life, a more productive lifestyle, and a significantly longer lifespan than in the past. A collaborative study of 216 high quadriplegic persons conducted by three spinal-cord-injury centers reported that 64% of the respirator-dependent quadriplegic patients (n = 128) rated their own quality of life as good or excellent (1).

This optimistic picture, however, is predicated on one critical factor—money. The questions that continue to haunt those that care for the high quadriplegic individual are: What will happen to this person after rehabilitation discharge? Will the family have the necessary attendant assistance, or will they be responsible for the care of this person for the rest of their lives? How will the considerable financial burden be met? We take extreme measures to save them, only to realize that many will not be able to receive basic services, equipment, and placement to provide a reasonable quality of life (8). If we are determined to save a life, we must be willing to also support the consequences of that decision, a responsibility that our society must bear once survival is assured.

REFERENCES

1. Whiteneck GG, Carter RE, Charlifue SW, Hall KM, Menter RR, Wilkerson MA, Wilmot CB (1985): *A Collaborative Study of High Quadriplegia* (Rocky

Mountain Regional Spinal Cord Injury System, Northern California Regional Spinal Injury System, Texas Regional Spinal Cord Injury System). Englewood, CO: Craig Hospital.

2. Wicks AB, Menter RR (1986): Long-term outlook in quadriplegic patients with initial ventilator dependency. *Chest* 90:406–410.
3. Lerman RM, Weiss MS (1987): Progressive resistive exercise in weaning high quadriplegics from the ventilator. *Paraplegia* 25:130–135.
4. Miller HJ, Thomas E, Wilmot CB (1988): Pneumobelt use among the high quadriplegic population. *Arch Phys Med Rehabil* 69:369–372.
5. Fuhrer MJ, Carter RE, Donovan WH, Rossi CD, Wilkerson MA (1987): Postdischarge outcomes for ventilator-dependent quadriplegics. *Arch Phys Med Rehabil* 68:353–356.
6. Perkash I, Leifer L, Hall K, Glass K, Herrera E, Van Der Loos M (1986): Evaluation of robotic aids for the severely physically disabled. In: *Rehabilitation Research and Development Center,* Palo Alto, CA: Veterans Administration Medical Center, Section 2.3.6.10.
7. Lamid S, Ragalie GF, Welter K (1985): Respirator-dependent quadriplegics: problems during the weaning period. *J Am Paraplegia Soc* 8:33–37.
8. Gardner BP, Theocleous F, Watt JW, Krishnan KR (1985): Ventilation or dignified death for patients with high tetraplegia. *Br Med J [Clin Res]* 29:1620–1622.

9

Preadmission Screening and Secondary Transport

Suzanne Nyre and Virginia McKay

Craig Hospital, Englewood, Colorado, U.S.A.

The prescreening and secondary transport options for the high quadriplegic patient are dependent on the admission criteria of the rehabilitation facility receiving the patient, the patient's medical stability, and the type of admission referral.

The emergency admission, which allows for little or no preadmission screening, seldom takes place unless the rehabilitation facility is attached to the receiving trauma center. More often, a rehabilitation facility may have an agreement with one or more trauma centers to accept the transfer of ventilator-dependent patients. This agreement may not allow for denial of the patient, but may allow for implementation of at least some of the preadmission screening and goal-setting processes described below.

The third type of referral is perhaps the most common with today's hazardous funding and consequent admission controls. This referral can be accepted or denied within the established admitting criteria and offers the greatest opportunity to use all possible tools for achieving successful rehabilitation in the most cost-effective way.

Although many of the screening processes and criteria are necessarily financially based, it is important to understand that the focus is less to assure the financial solvency of the rehabilitation facility than to allow the patient's successful rehabilitation outcome. The entire rehabilitation program is and should be designed around the discharge setting that is available to the patient. The setting is determined by the available family and financial support.

For a patient to be discharged to a nonacute medical setting after rehabilitation, he or she must have family/hired nursing home health care available, financial resources for a wheelchair-accessible environment, and durable medical equipment for life support and mobility. It is the height of cruelty to introduce the patient and family to these options and freedoms in the rehabilitation program, to provide that temporary life style of increased mobility and independence, only to take it away when lack of resources demands a discharge back to an acute hospital setting or to an institution that cannot allow the patient out of bed, his or her room, or the facility. Not only is this a difficult reversal for the patient and family to accept, but it often channels whatever finances are available for future care into a rehabilitation program where goals cannot be met. To avoid the emotional and financial drain on the patient and family, the optimal admission process is one that allows for thorough prescreening, family and financial evaluations, and goal setting described in the following pages.

Although we understand the first two referral types do not allow for this thorough process, we believe that any portion of the preadmission screening procedure that can be used will be helpful in producing a positive rehabilitation outcome. Even in cases in which the information cannot be gathered during preadmission, it is helpful to obtain this information as soon as possible after admission.

Not only does this process allow for identification of existing resources, but it is also a helpful tool in developing financial sponsorships. A thoroughly prepared consultation report describing in detail the recommended program, probable outcomes, time, and financial frameworks can be used to establish the cost-effectiveness of the rehabilitation program. In many cases, the eventual discharge plan of having the patient cared for in a nonacute medical setting can offset the initial costs of air ambulance transportation and acute rehabilitation expenditures. When this cost-effectiveness can be demonstrated, it provides the medical review board of the insurance company with facts and figures that may allow flexibility of the strict benefit guidelines. When this flexibility takes place, it ultimately benefits the patient and the family by providing the most appropriate medical and rehabilitation care, the highest quality of life on discharge from the program, and reduces costs to the insurance company. Savings are achieved not only in the long run by providing a noninstitutional discharge program, but often in immediate cost reduction because the rehabilitation program is generally less expensive per day than the acute medical setting from which the patient will be transferred.

This prescreening process is helpful in establishing mutual goals for the treating team, patient, and family. It also establishes the concept of teamwork that will be used throughout the rehabilitation program. By discussing and agreeing on mutual goals for the eventual discharge before commencing the program, all efforts can be directed in a time- and cost-effective manner. As financial sponsorship and benefits are determined early on, they can reduce or eliminate those nonproductive periods when the patient and team must wait for financial approvals for an equipment item and other discharge arrangements.

A thorough screening of basic funding and placement issues should be undertaken before the on-site consultation to avoid needless expense charged to the insurance or family.

INITIAL INVESTIGATION

The referring physician should be directed to call and speak with a receiving physician to establish the basic medical information. Important items to include are the level of injury, any associated injuries, mental status, previous medical history, and current medical treatment, including any postinjury surgical procedures, traction, halo, or bracing devices. At this time, the receiving physician can explain the admission process and get direction from the referring physician as to timing for transfer, how the patient could be most safely transferred, and what prognosis the referring physician has given the patient and family regarding his or her condition. The next step is for the coordinator of high-risk admissions to establish contact with the social worker, financial sponsors, and family to provide them with appropriate information. A call to the social worker at the referring hospital will allow identification of possible funding sources and establish a central information point that will be used throughout the prescreening process.

The financial sponsor should be contacted and an introduction to the rehabilitation program provided both verbally and by sending written information. At this time, eligibility and benefits can be established with emphasis on benefits for rehabilitation, medical transport, durable medical equipment for discharge, home modifications, family or attendant training, home health care, and a skilled nursing facility. Many of these items will not be regularly scheduled benefits, but will require medical review. It is important at this time to establish who will be the contact person for the review process, what information that review board will require, and the length of time they require to review the recommendations they will receive.

Contact should then be made with the family and other support people. They also require a verbal introduction to the rehabilitation program being offered, and this too should be followed up in written form. It is important at this time to identify their areas of concern and provide some counseling and guidance that will help them prepare for the rehabilitation program. It is not necessary for families to make decisions in the area of discharge options, community resources, and finances at this time, but they should be brought up and discussed as options they can begin to consider. Discussions should identify the architectural style of the home the family is currently living in and whether the family desires to stay in that home after the patient's discharge. A brief explanation of accessibility should be given the family at this time. The family should be directed to begin looking for skilled nursing facilities, home health care agencies, and transitional living units available in their home area. These may be used to provide care for the patient on an ongoing basis or for family respite if they are providing most of the care at home. The family should also be directed to investigate possible financial resources in the form of veterans benefits, auto and homeowners policies, step-parent's family coverage, and medical assistance programs, handicapped children's agencies, and vocational rehabilitation programs.

Information should be given to the family about their financial sponsorship and any areas that are perceived to be trouble spots for them. Although this information is not complete at this time, they need to start considering any other sources of assistance. This may include such things as sale of property, community fund-raising efforts, and loans. This is also a time to help the family understand any paperwork process, such as claim forms that need to be filed, applications for extension or conversion of benefits, and need to self-pay premiums to continue coverages.

When any of the factors listed above fail to produce a probability of successful outcome, it is not appropriate to proceed with the on-site consultation and the associated costs.

At this point, assistance can be offered in referring the patient to alternative programs that can be funded within the limitations of the financial resources and to offer telephone consultations from various disciplines to assist the referring facility with direct discharge planning.

ON-SITE CONSULTATION BY PHYSICIAN AND PROGRAM REPRESENTATIVE

When the initial information gathered above indicates that basic funding parameters exist to complete a program and that there is sufficient family support to work towards a discharge to a nonacute medical environment, then an on-site consultation should take place to pin down the details. The consultation team should consist of a physician and a program representative who, regardless of education and background, is prepared to discuss the general rehabilitation program and the financial and discharge issues that are pertinent to this high level of injury. Because of the amount of information to be shared in a brief period of time, it is extremely helpful to split total responsibilities between two team members. Two perspectives also help in reaching a consensus on specific program recommendations.

Areas that will be covered during the consultation include medical issues, such as review of complete medical record and x-ray films, thorough history and physical, a home checkout for wheelchair accessibility, patient/family information, and a summation conference.

This is the time to start establishing the rapport with patient and family that will carry over throughout the rehabilitation program. Not only is this a fact-finding mission for both the evaluator and the patient and family, but it is also when the patient and family begin to feel the support of the rehabilitation team. Up until this time, they have been fighting for survival and have had little time to look into the future. When they have, they have been frightened of the unknown and unable to identify any realistic goals for future independence. This should be a time of free interchange of information between the evaluator and patient/family, and sufficient time should be allowed for all of their questions. Whenever possible, this discussion should be held at the bedside in the presence of both patient and family. This is a reassurance that they are all hearing the same information and that there are no hidden agendas. And because so much information is shared at this highly emotional time, it is helpful for them to use each other as sounding boards when they discuss this information over the next few days.

A layman's explanation of spinal cord injury and the effects it has on future planning should be given as well as treatment options available, such as general versus specialized rehabilitation programs, local versus regional centers, patient population, and the importance of peer interaction. Helping the family to identify other programs they can investigate for comparison helps them to feel they have looked into all options and allows them to feel more comfortable with making their eventual program choice. A thorough explanation should be made of the program represented, including team makeup, length of stay, typical day's schedule, patient population, i.e., age, description of physical environment (pictures help), and any other special programs available to the patient and family.

A discussion should be held regarding discharge options, not only what is available within the community for support, but also helping the family and patient identify their desired discharge outcomes. Playing a large part in these discharge outcomes are the financial concerns. An explanation of the existing benefits should be given to the patient and family, and any limitations or problem areas should be identified so the family can begin budgeting their available resources.

When the physician has completed the review of medical records and physical examination and the program representative has completed the discussions listed above, it is important that the two meet to share information and observations. When they have compared notes, compiled information, shared perceptions as to the patient and family's acceptance of the information presented, then they can reach a consensus on the recommendations and goals to present at a summation conference.

It is important to present "probable recovery" patterns without destroying "hope." Ironclad prognoses are not only discouraging, but if inaccurate, they destroy the credibility of the entire program. It is important to let the patient/family know that although you, as a professional, cannot predict recovery, you are on their side in hoping for it.

This summation conference should again include the patient, if possible, his or her family, hospital staff, and any representatives from funding sources. Areas to be covered include an explanation of past and current medical findings and recommendations for future medical treatment, the projected program goals and limitations, and the cost and time guidelines. A brief program explanation recapping the information shared previously with the patient and family should be presented to the hospital staff and funding sources.

An explanation as to what happens next should include the steps to be taken toward decision to accept or deny the admission and the criteria used to make that decision. If the decision is to accept the patient into the program, an explanation should be given as to what the family can expect regarding transportation and recommended family involvement during the program.

POST-ON-SITE CONSULTATION

A detailed report should be dictated by both the physician and program representative covering all pertinent medical information, detailed cost analysis of the recommended program, and other areas covered in the summation conference. This dictation should be sent to the referring physician and facility, all funding sources, and any other participants in the decision-making process. Patient/family should sign a "Release of Information" for these parties.

Within the receiving facility's established guidelines, the appropriate administrative personnel should meet and review the consultation report and recommendations of the consulting team. Acceptance or denial is determined at this time, and all parties are appropriately notified.

In spite of the careful screening that takes place before the on-site consult, there will still be occasions when the criteria cannot be met and the admission may be denied. At this point, and after expenditure of consult fees and expenses, what can be considered benefits of having received this evaluation?

1. Patient/family have received a number of hours of detailed information regarding medical and financial issues as well as future goals,

outcomes, discharge planning and home modification recommendations.

2. The program recommendations and the financial projections can be used by any facility the family may choose.

3. Funding sources can also use the medical/financial predictions for their account planning.

4. Patient/family can be assured that they have explored possibilities, even if they are not the answer. This is particularly comforting to families if the reason for denial is "no realistic rehabilitation goals."

If proper prescreening takes place, denials after a consultation will be the exception. However, if admission is denied, it is imperative that assistance be given regarding alternative programs, discharge placement, etc. A consultation should never take place without an absolute commitment by the consulting team to assist patient/family/referring facility in every possible manner, regardless of outcome.

Contact is then made with the funding sources to establish the covered benefits and limitations based on the detailed cost information that was included in the written report. Written authorization should be required and any noncovered items must be communicated to the family with a plan formulated for payment of those items. If the discharge placement will not be to the family home, then a written commitment from the facility providing discharge placement should be required before transfer to the rehabilitation program. This document is not legally binding but it does acknowledge the need for commitment and makes the potential receiving facility really think through their decision while there is still time for alternative planning.

SCHEDULE FOR ADMISSION

Information should then be shared with the receiving team, establishing bed availability in the appropriate unit and designating receiving physician and team. The social worker, referring physician, and family members are then contacted regarding date for transfer, determining which family members will accompany the patient and whether they need housing ordered.

SECONDARY TRANSPORT

The ambulance service will be scheduled and funding information will be provided to the transport company. The transport team is then notified of the transfer date and destination and they should receive the consultation report and medical information to initiate the transport process.

Primary transportation of patients with traumatic injuries is often managed by local established emergency medical systems. These patients are then taken to designated hospitals in the area. The transportation of patients from an acute hospital setting to another specialized hospital, or from one area to another requiring the use of medically staffed ambulances, is considered secondary transportation. This type of transport is conducted after planning and preadmittance communication with the receiving hospital or facility, such as secondary transportation to a rehabilitation hospital specializing in the care of patients with high quadriplegia.

The actual mode of transportation and type of transporting team should be discussed and a decision should be made by the discharging physician/facility. The financially responsible party, patient, and family should be included in this decision. It is imperative to engage a qualified air or land ambulance service with experienced personnel to transport the patient. This service should include a medical team knowledgeable in the transportation of patients with high quadriplegia and proficient with the transportation and treatment of patients who are spinal-cord-injured and in need of ventilator support. Some receiving hospitals and rehabilitation centers specializing in the care of patients with spinal cord injuries may have experience with transportation services they believe meet these qualifications and may be of help with the decision on the mode of transportation and the team.

New federal regulations describe the responsibilities of referring/receiving facilities when transferring patients. Details are contained in statute 9121 of the Consolidated Omnibus Budget Reconciliation Act (COBRA) Public Law 99-272 signed into law April 7, 1986. Essentially this law states it is the responsibility of the referring physicians and facility to determine the qualifications of the transfer team, equipment, and receiving facility. Physicians/facilities are subject to a fine for failure to evaluate these and/or for allowing transfer by inappropriate teams to facilities without means to provide the patient with proper care. Additionally, the receiving physician/facility must ensure that space is available and that appropriate services are provided for the transferred patient.

TRANSFER

The transport service receives notice of an impending need, then confirms the date and the medical team needed for the transportation of the patient. Logistical concerns and decisions are made, such as the type of transportation to the admitting facility. Among these considerations would be the following.

1. A Lear jet charter plane that would allow a controlled environment. The jet can be cost-effective and is the fastest method of transportation and can accommodate at least one family member.

2. A fixed-wing aircraft also has a controllable environment, is less costly than a jet, but travels approximately one-half the speed and can take two or three family members. Weather could be a concern with this type of aircraft.

3. A helicopter can be used for short trips, but cannot be pressure controlled and no family can come. This would be an alternative to a long land transport.

4. Commercial airline is considered, but has less controlled environment and limited equipment would be allowed. Oxygen would need to be prearranged at extra cost and the patient would need to sit in a regular airline seat, because domestic aero stretchers are not allowed at this time.

5. Land travel could be used for short distances or in conjunction with air transport.

Our discussion will include specifics for jet or fixed-wing transportation equipped with a stretcher rack and extra oxygen bottles with pressure hose, and for a ventilator-dependent patient with quadriplegia. This can also be adapted to any other lower-level spinal-cord-injured patient and to any mode of transportation decided on.

Total time of transportation should be considered, that is, hospital-to-hospital time, including need for fuel stops, weather and special altitude and pressurization concerns. Routine equipment needs to be arranged by the Advanced Cardiac Life Support (ACLS) certified registered nurse and respiratory therapist. All ACLS and Basic Life Support equipment should be carried on board (1).

All equipment should be portable, battery-operated, or self-contained. Suction, cardiac monitor, defibrillator, first- and second-line drugs for emergency and intravenous (i.v.) insertion, plus i.v. line maintenance equipment should be included. The pack with urinary catheters and supplies, nasal gastric tubes, rectal tubes, and bowel program supplies should also be included. A respiratory pack is necessary, containing equipment needed for intubation, monitoring, establishing and maintaining airway and breathing, a resuscitation bag, and enough oxygen in pressurized tanks to supply 100% oxygen, if needed, for the duration of the trip. Always have a minimum of two tanks of oxygen with pressurized hoses on board the airplane.

Portable equipment to monitor the patient's medical status should be carried on board. An adequate folding stretcher (traction stretcher, if needed), foam positioning pads, a full-length sheepskin, and linen for patient warmth should also be carried to the bedside. The patient should be positioned on the stretcher with sheepskin and pads and secured to the ambulance pram for ground transportation or to the airport.

Special medical considerations and equipment should include a small portable ventilator, one or two 9-h gel cell batteries, all tubing and circuitry, and also an oxygen analyzer for the ventilator-dependent patient. The routine ventilator pack should contain all needed equipment for the ventilator or ventilator-dependent patient to be ready at all times including extra trachs, saline, suction catheters, medications for respiratory treatments, treating tubing and equipment, variable peep valves and equipment, connectors, extra tubing, etc. A 30° stretcher wedge for those with gastrostomy or nasal gastric tubes should be aboard the plane or ambulance.

After reviewing the completed consultation report, updated referral information, and the information from the discharging hospital, the medical team should gather any other specific supplies as needed. The team should keep in mind the family needing to come and who can be accommodated in the specific designated plane or ambulance. The medical team should contact discharging hospital and patient representatives and arrange airport transportation, if needed, and see that medical records and x-ray films are sent with the patient.

The medical team should notify the discharging physician of the team's plans and times, confirm the patient's stability for transport, receive recommendations for adjustments (pre- and in-transit), and answer any questions. These transfer plans should also be left with the rehabilitation person and insurance person. The team should coordinate transport plans with the family and establish luggage space, confirm who is accompanying the patient, and answer any of their concerns. Phone numbers of where the medical transport team members can be reached should be left with the physician, family, contact nurse at the patient's unit, the rehabilitation nurse, and the insurance persons. If any changes or adjustments need to be made, they can be addressed pretransport.

A review of all medical systems should be communicated with the nurse in charge of the patient's direct care. This should supplement the information already obtained. Pretransfer recommendations should be stated by the transport team to allow the transfer to run as smoothly as possible. This information can be used to improve and/or maintain the patient's stability and comfort throughout the transfer process. A pretransfer form should be completed with instructions, information, and considerations as follows.

1. Confirm the consultation and referral report, present condition, and listen to any concerns.

2. Confirm the stated neurological deficit and level of injury, noting any increase or decrease in function or sensation of the incomplete or complete injury site.

3. Inquire about the type of stabilization of bony injury, i.e., surgeries and dates, halo and vest, rods, fusion, braces, etc. Are there any concerns? Is the patient in tongs and traction? Is a traction stretcher or a regular stretcher needed?

4. Inquire about mentation, confusion, or contributing injuries, and whether these are resolving or are a problem.

5. Note bladder management to determine whether there is neurogenic bladder; does he or she use intermittent catheter program, Foley drainage, is he or she reflex voiding, and if so, with or without postvoid residuals? Are there any urinary tract infections in the past or at present with fever and what treatment is being used? A Foley catheter draining system should be requested for transport to prevent acute bladder problems or possible autonomic hyperreflexia in flight. (In systems review, keep in mind the systems or conditions that can be stabilized days ahead to prevent acute problems in flight.)

6. What are the vital signs, i.e., blood pressure, temperature, respirations? Are these abnormal, what could be the cause, are there preexisting acute problems? Consider new problems with a fever, an increased pulse rate, question a urinary-tract infection, an upper-respiratory infection, septicemia, deep venous thrombosis, and heterotopic ossification. Have any cultures and sensitivities shown the source of an infection? Do these problems need to be treated pretransfer or do we need special considerations for these problems in-transit?

7. What type of nutrition and diet is the patient getting? How is his or her appetite? If not all feeding is by mouth, what type of feeding regime is the patient on? Does the patient have a nasal gastric tube? If so, what type? Or, does he or she have a gastrostomy tube? Does he or she have hyperalimentation? If so, what solutions are being used through these tubes and how are they administered? If the patient is being tube-fed, request that the solution be held for at least 4 h pretransfer from the hospital to avoid complications in-transit. Be sure that medications and water are continued to maintain hydration.

8. What is the type of bowel management? Is there need for suppositories, does the patient have involuntary stools, obstruction, or diarrhea? Are there bowel sounds present, nausea and vomiting, other gastrointestinal (GI) disturbances, GI bleeding, is the abdomen soft? Do any of these problems need to be addressed pretransfer?

9. What is the patient's skin condition: are there open sores, decubitus pressure areas, and if so, how are they being treated and are they improving or getting worse? What type of bed is being used? Is the patient being put up in a wheelchair? Does he or she use any special cush-

ion in the chair? How high is the patient tolerating sitting up: 30, 60, or 90°, and how long at a time?

10. Are there any complications existing, such as deep venous thrombosis, present or past? Are the legs of equal circumference, does the patient use elasticthrombo embolitic stockings, is he or she taking deep venous thrombosis prophylactic medications, are there preexisting, resolved, or new cardiac problems? Ask for a description and the treatment. Is the patient being monitored, is there any ectopy or edema? Has the patient had cardiac arrest, anoxia, respiratory arrest? What treatment was given?

11. Inquire in depth about the respiratory system. Were there any preexisting asthmas, etc.? Was the patient a smoker? Does he or she have resolved or present problems, such as atelectasis, pneumonias, infiltrates, effusions, hemopneumothorax? (Update the information since the respiratory consult was written.) Request the latest chest x-ray film result; what type of ventilator the patient is on now, the settings, the type of tracheostomy, the date it was inserted, the size and when it was last changed, or if the patient has an endotracheal tube. Does he or she tolerate the tracheostomy cuff deflated, and if so, how long? Is the patient weaning, and also how long? The date of the last forced vital capacity and results should be noted as well as the current arterial blood gases and the percentage of oxygen the patient is receiving. The team should request any pertinent test to be updated 24–48 h pretransport for a good baseline in-transport and in preparation for the altitude changes the patient may experience.

12. The laboratory results should be reviewed for any abnormal values. If there is deviation from normal, consider what could be the cause and what plans for pretransport stabilization measures could be taken if necessary. If seizure precaution medications are being given, note the blood level and whether the medication needs adjusting pretransport. (Air transport can trigger seizure activity and this could be lessened if the levels are on the higher range.)

13. A list of the patient's medications should be written in the transfer papers. Ask what these are and list on the pretransport form. Include any antibiotics and why they are being used. Are there any allergies? Are any i.v. lines in, if so where and what type of line, what solution is being infused and at what rate? If there is no i.v. line in, would a keep-open rate of i.v. solution for hydration be appropriate, or a heparin-lock i.v. could be requested for transfer in preparation for the transfer. (Better to prepare ahead in the full facility and save the medical team's hands in-transit for emergency situations if they arise.)

14. Request any other pertinent information from the nurse, family, and doctors that would help facilitate a safe and comfortable transfer.

After all the information is obtained and provided for the pretransfer form, the medical team should then recall anyone necessary for a closer update or for any concerns they might have. Discuss real concerns with the receiving physician pretransport. Consider any changes that might alter expectations of medical status, bed plans, or unit placement, and convey these to the proper parties. Check the equipment list and communicate with the transport company of the medical team's needs. Also communicate and present a short written summary of information to the receiving unit, so preparation can be made for admittance, such as proper bed, ventilator prepared and ready, settings, oxygen available, etc. Estimate the time of arrival with the patient and convey this to the admissions department, the receiving unit, and the physician accepting the patient. Leave an itinerary with the receiving hospital personnel where the medical team can be reached, then keep the receiving hospital informed if pertinent changes occur or logistical changes are necessary.

The medical team may request additional adjustments and more information to prepare the patient for the transport, and should explain that they will come to the hospital early with all transport equipment. They will do a pretransport assessment and place the patient on their portable ventilator according to the settings required for adequate arterial blood gases, to transport successfully and within the guidelines of the attending physician. This also allows the patient time to become accustomed and comfortable with the new medical team in attendance. Quite often, this will be a period of 2–3 h.

The transport team should then follow through with the transfer from hospital to hospital until full report is given to the receiving team, and the patient and family are settled in their new surroundings. Before, during, and after the transfer, the team should continuously reassure the patient and family about ongoing and upcoming events, and orient and familiarize them with this new rehabilitation process.

The ACLS medical team should administer to and provide care for the patient in-transit, including proper padding and positioning until the new admission begins. This care should be given according to the discharging physician's orders and recommendations, ACLS standards, and the medical team's established in-transit protocols under the direction of their consulting in-transport physician. Total responsibility is then assumed by the admitting physician.

In summary, we have formulated and provided a working method for successful preadmission screening and secondary air transport of a ventilator-dependent person with high quadriplegia. We have discussed the referral process from an acute hospital, through the medical/financial concerns and decisions, the transport process, and the follow-through to a rehabilitation facility specializing in the care of patients with high quadriplegia.

Although the procedures described require many staff hours, experience has shown the process to be an ultimate time-saver and helps to ensure a safe transfer and successful outcome: one that provides optimal patient care, reduces total hospitalization time, and reduces costs.

REFERENCE

1. American Heart Association (1986): *Textbook of Advanced Cardiac Life Support*. Dallas, TX.

10

Medical Management in High Quadriplegia

Daniel P. Lammertse

Craig Hospital, Englewood, Colorado, U.S.A.

The area of medical management that is most specifically affected by high levels of quadriplegia is clearly the respiratory system and, as such, these special concerns will be dealt with in other chapters. This chapter will provide an overview of the general medical management of the high quadriplegic patient, whose function is greatly affected by the high level of neurologic injury. Although a thorough review of general medical management in spinal cord injury is beyond the scope of this brief chapter, readers requiring a more detailed discussion can turn to a number of available reference texts on the subject (1–5). At the outset we should be reminded that the overall goal of the rehabilitation process is to achieve a transition from a medically unstable, dependent, and uneducated patient situation to one of sufficient medical stability, independence, and knowledge to enable a successful discharge to home. The achievement of medical stability will require proper management (and hopefully prevention) of complications but at the same time the physician team should not underestimate their responsibility in supervising the rehabilitation team in the overall effort to achieve independence and provide education for the patient and family. The truly successful effort will result, at the time of discharge, in a patient and family who are prepared to take responsibility for simple management decisions in the home, the training of the inevitable succession of attendants, and to be sophisticated consumers of health care services. Their medical and nursing management will hopefully have been successful enough and their rehabilitation program broad enough that once home, attention need not be narrowly focused on medical and nursing issues but rather the pursuit of vocational and avocational goals that are such an important factor in the quality of life. To achieve this transition requires a special flexibility on the part of team members. As a result of the high degree of dependence of spinal-cord-injury patients and their special nursing care needs, the provision of a full program will require more medical sophistication and nursing skills on the part of team members. For example, physical and occupational therapists, if they are to treat patients away from the nursing unit, will need to be skilled at performing suctioning and in the management of tracheostomy and ventilator tubing. Recreation therapists will likewise need to be skilled in these and other areas including bladder management and be knowledgeable in the workings of high-technology wheelchairs for issues that may come up on outings. Thus, the general medical needs resultant from the high level of quadriplegia in this patient population affects all disciplines on the rehabilitation team and must be addressed by the team as a whole to achieve a successful program.

MANAGEMENT OF NEUROLOGIC ISSUES

For the vast majority of patients with high quadriplegia, spasticity is an inevitable accompaniment to their paralysis. Patients with high levels of cervical injury, however, may have more difficulty with spasticity because of their lack of spared upper extremity and shoulder girdle function that would enable them to reposition themselves after or to maintain posture during spasm activity. Upper extremities are also frequently involved in mass spasms and, as such, may require wheelchair arm-trough restraints to maintain positioning. When spasticity becomes severe enough to warrant treatment, the options available are similar to those available to patients with lower levels of injury. Medications such as baclofen, dantrolene sodium, diazepam, and, more recently, clonidine, have been tried singularly or in combination, but often even maximal doses do not provide sufficient relief from spasms (6). When medications are either not tolerated or unsuccessful in controlling problematic spasticity, neurosurgical options such as rhizotomy (7), focal neurectomy, or intramuscular neurolysis can be considered. Other experimental techniques such as direct spinal cord electrical stimulation and intrathecal baclofen or morphine infusion may hold promise for the future. The treatment team should also not overlook the role of range-of-motion exercises in the day-to-day management of spasticity.

Central deafferentation pain is generally thought to be less common in cervical levels of injury than in paraplegia, but when it occurs with severity, it may be a significant management problem (8, 9). The neurophysiological mechanism of such pain is not well understood and although a variety of treatments have been proposed including analgesics, psychotropic drugs, antidepressants, antiseizure medications, nerve blocks, transcutaneous electrical nerve stimulation, and neurosurgical treatments, no long-term follow-up data are available for this patient population that could be used to endorse one treatment modality over another. Most clinicians have been disappointed with the long-term results of the modalities noted, and whereas some degree of efficacy has been claimed for neurosurgical procedures such as the dorsal root entry zone microcoagulation (10), results of this procedure in cervical level patients have been disappointing thus far. Thus, in many cases, the high quadriplegic patient with central deafferentation pain is left with psychological treatment options and enrollment in comprehensive chronic pain management programs, many of which do not adequately integrate issues of profound physical disability into their approach.

Signs or symptoms of late neurologic deterioration should raise the question of progressive posttraumatic cystic myelopathy and warrant prompt investigation with magnetic resonance imaging (MRI) studies. Recognition of this problem is especially critical in C4 level patients who may be in marginal respiratory status and in whom even a minor motor ascent may result in respiratory insufficiency. Although logistically difficult, MRI studies can be performed on ventilator-dependent patients using a nonferromagnetic ventilator such as the Monaghan 225 with a respiratory therapist in attendance. Patients in halo-vest immobilization cannot be studied in MRI scanners unless their halo braces are made from nonferromagnetic alloys or composite materials. Evidence of progressive posttraumatic cystic myelopathy would warrant consideration of the performance of a cyst subarachnoid shunt procedure to halt the progression of cystic cavitation of the spinal cord (11–13).

As in any quadriplegic person, autonomic dysreflexia and other autonomic nervous system complications may occur in the high quadriplegic individual. The management of autonomic dysreflexia is no different than at lower levels of injury and should be first directed at postural management and the elimination of the nociceptive source, followed when necessary by pharmacologic management with agents such as adrenergic blockers (phenoxybenzamine or prazosin), calcium-channel blockers (nifedipine), or in more severe crisis conditions, parenteral drugs such as nitroprusside. In addition to autonomic dysreflexia, the traumatic sympathectomy in the high quadriplegic patient may result in significant reflex bradycardia because of unopposed vagal stimulation. This is most prominently manifest during tracheal suctioning and, on rare occasions, may result in asystole. This vulnerability to pronounce bradycardia is temporary in most cases, resolving within the first several weeks to a month postinjury. Thus, most clinicians do not favor the use of cardiac pacemakers, which are usually unnecessary and preclude the use of MRI studies, preferring to manage the situation pharmacologically while awaiting the resolution of the more severe manifestations of autonomic imbalance. These patients also commonly have orthostatic hypotension that is most pronounced early in the course of the rehabilitation process. The use of abdominal binders and progressive upright mobilization typically enables the patient to be conditioned to tolerate the sitting position, although in more difficult cases medication such as ephedrine may also be required.

GASTROINTESTINAL MANAGEMENT

Although ideally the acute hospital management has been successful in maintaining the patient's nutritional balance, often patients arrive in rehabilitation with some degree of malnutrition, especially when their early course has been complicated by recurrent pulmonary infections and other complications. For this reason, a nutritional assessment and aggressive management of deficiencies is an important part of the overall medical management (13). Significant weight loss from premorbid levels is quite common, and although adequate calorie and protein intake to meet energy expenditure and anabolic needs is important, the nutritional assessment should take into consideration a revised ideal body weight considering the patient's loss of muscle mass and decreased energy expenditure as a high-level quadriplegic patient. Many of these patients run the risk of weight gain posthospitalization related to decreased energy expenditure. Nutritional counseling during the rehabilitation phase therefore needs to concern itself with posthospital ideal weight maintenance. In the transition to the rehabilitation phase, many patients initially cannot maintain sufficient oral intake to avoid the need for supplementation. This is commonly provided in the form of tube feeding supplementation either via nasogastric feeding tube, a temporary gastrostomy, or a jejeunostomy. Patients can hopefully be weaned from these supplements and resume full oral nutritional intake within a short period after beginning rehabilitation. During this phase, consideration should also be given to the possibility of dysphagia, especially in the highest levels of cervical or cervicomedullary injuries in which brainstem dysfunction may be manifest. When there is reason to suspect such dysfunction, a full swallowing evaluation, including barium swallow studies with fluoroscopy and various aspiration tests followed by tracheal suctioning, should be performed to assess the potential for aspiration. Other gastrointestinal complications associated with paraplegia such as peptic ulcer disease, gastroesophageal reflux, and cholelithiasis, although not any more common with the higher level of injury, should be kept in mind when evaluating a suspected gastrointestinal tract dysfunction (14,15). The principles of neurogenic bowel management are similar to that in lower spinal cord injury, with the goal of imposing artificial regulation on the bowels through rectal stimulation. As one would suspect, however, it is typically not feasible to perform the bowel program on a high level patient in the sitting position on a commode chair. Lack of postural control typically requires that the bowel program be performed in bed.

UROLOGIC MANAGEMENT

The management of the neurogenic bladder in high quadriplegia is, in theory, little different than for lower levels of spinal cord injury, but some practical issues may warrant consideration. Autonomic dysreflexia is commonly caused by bladder problems. An overdistended bladder is a potent stimulus for dysreflexia and may occur while the patient is on continent intermittent catheterization when the urine production during the catheterization interval exceeds the bladder's "safe" capacity. In patients with indwelling catheters, dysreflexia is usually the result of a kinked or blocked catheter. In those on reflex voiding programs, dysreflexia is usually an accompaniment of sphincter-detrussor dysynergia and thus may respond to α-adrenergic blocking drugs such as phenoxybenzamine or prazosin, which relax the bladder neck while also treating the dysreflexia. In many cases dysynergia in the voiding patient can only be effectively treated by the performance of a sphincterotomy. The type of bladder management chosen is often influenced by practical considerations. Depending on the patient's access to adequately trained attendant care, performance of intermittent catheterization or the management of external collector appliances may be feasible (16,17). Because high-level patients ideally have attendant care available 24 h a day, however, this becomes an issue only in those less-than-ideal situations in which either the funding is not available to provide full-time trained attendant care or the care providers are not able to perform those urologic management techniques. For these reasons in male patients and for female patients in whom continent intermittent catheterization is not a practical method of management, indwelling catheters may be the most practical method of management. Issues of sexual dysfunction, including neurogenic impotence and infertility, are physiologically little if any different from the experience in lower levels of quadriplegia but because of the patient's dependence on mechanical ventilator and the total lack of upper extremity function, sexuality concerns may present a greater psychological burden to a couple. Treatment options available for erectile dysfunction are the same as for lower levels of injury and include penile implants and, more recently, the use of intracavernosal injections of papaverine, although this technique remains controversial (18,19). In recent years there has been a resurgence of interest in the treatment of infertility after spinal cord injury, and reports of childbirth after artificial insemination after both vibroejaculation and electroejaculation techniques have been published recently (20).

ORTHOPEDIC MANAGEMENT

Because of the high quadriplegic patient's lack of functional control of the shoulder girdle and upper extremities, they are less able to compensate than those with lower-level injuries for a mild degree of functional scoliosis and, as such, are more dependent on properly fitted and adjusted wheelchair seating systems and when necessary, orthotic seating components. High quadriplegia in the child or young adolescent will almost inevitably lead to paralytic scoliosis, which commonly requires spine fusion. Heterotopic ossification at the hips, if significant, can lead to pelvic obliquity and also contribute to scoliosis. It should also be remembered that heterotopic ossification can occur in the upper extremities of high-level quadriplegic patients and should be part of the differential diagnosis when range-of-motion restriction and joint swelling in the arms as well as legs are being evaluated. Development of overt heterotopic ossification warrants aggressive treatment with etidronate disodium. Some authors have advocated the prophylactic use of this drug as a means of reducing the incidence of clinically significant ossification (21). Attention should also be given to maintenance of range of motion through passive range-of-motion exercises. Nonsteroidal antiinflammatory drugs such as indomethacin have also been advocated by some authors and may complement treatment with etidronate disodium. When heterotopic ossification is not controlled and results in significant and asymmetric loss of range of motion at the hips, pelvic obliquity resulting in scoliosis is likely to occur. Although heterotopic ossification is fairly common, occurring in 16–53% of patients with spinal cord injury (22,23), fortunately the majority who receive adequate treatment do not go on to develop additional functional impairment due to joint limitation that results in major postural consequences or abnormal skin pressure areas. In this small percentage of patients, surgical resection of the heterotopic ossification is the only remaining alternative and should be postponed until evidence of bone maturity in the area of ossification can be documented by bone scan and alkaline phosphatase measurement.

CARDIOVASCULAR MANAGEMENT

Deep venous thrombosis is a common complication in spinal cord injury, and it has been estimated to occur in anywhere from 12–100% of spinal-cord-injured individuals depending on the method of detection used, with the highest risk appearing to occur in the first several months after injury (24,25). The incidence of pulmonary emboli, the majority of which presumably originate in the lower extremities, is said to be between 5 and 15%. Controversy persists over the efficacy of various proposed prophylactic measures. Low-dose subcutaneous heparin appears to be the most widely accepted prophylactic regimen, but other methods such as low-dose warfarin (Coumadin), combinations of heparin and dihydroergotamine, external pneumatic compression stockings, and electric stimulation of calf musculature have been proposed. Most of the controlled studies on the prevention of thromboembolic complications have been performed on non–spinal-cord-injured patients and to date there remains a lack of well-designed, adequately controlled studies on this topic in the spinal-cord-injured population. Because the risk of thromboembolism is high compared with the risk of prophylaxis in most regimens and there is reason to believe that the incidence of thromboembolism can be reduced with prophylaxis, it would seem prudent to use some form of prophylactic management for the first 12 weeks postinjury (26–28). Once an overt thromboembolic complication occurs, treatment includes full anticoagulation with heparin converted to warfarin anticoagulation after 7 days and continued for ~12 weeks. It is believed that maintaining the prothrombin times at one-and-a-half times control using the standard reagents commonly used in the United States will adequately prevent recurrence and minimize the risk of bleeding complications. If the occurrence of bleeding complications or unacceptable bleeding risk prevents the use of anticoagulation, an inferior vena cava filter should be considered. It should also be noted that a high quadriplegic patient with a high sensory level and on mechanical ventilatory support may not have the classic signs and symptoms of pulmonary embolism and thus thromboembolic complication should be suspected when investigating occult sources of syncope, fever, pleural effusion, pulmonary infiltrate, and hypoxia. Because many centers cannot perform ventilation lung scans on patients who are on mechanical ventilator support, the clinician may more often have to resort to pulmonary angiography to confirm the diagnosis of pulmonary embolism.

SKIN MANAGEMENT

While skin management issues in general are no different than for lower levels of quadriplegia, there are several areas of special concern related to the tracheostomy that warrant comment. Because the trach tube constitutes a foreign body in the trachea, the ostomy itself is typically colonized with respiratory flora. Daily nursing care to inspect and clean the tracheostomy wound is required to avoid superficial infection that could lead to more serious complications and compromise of the stoma. Likewise, when forced to use a cuffed tracheostomy tube, the clinician needs to be constantly aware of its potential to cause pressure ulceration or, as a complication of scarring, stenosis of the airway. For this reason, the respiratory therapy team should use the lowest cuff inflation pressures necessary to insure an adequate seal. It is recommended that the pulmonary treatment team work toward a cuffless tracheostomy as soon as the condition of the lungs permit, not only to avoid these complications but more importantly, to allow the patient to vocalize, an issue of immense psychological importance to the patient and family. Trunk and extremity pressure sores are managed similarly to those occurring in the general spinal-cord-injury population, but it should be remembered that the high quadriplegic patient may be more at risk for upper extremity and particularly scapular sores because of the lack of motor function in the shoulder girdle and arms. This is especially true in patients immobilized in the halo vest in whom periodic pressure relief over the scapulae may be difficult to achieve.

COMMUNICATION MANAGEMENT

Issues of communication in the high quadriplegic patient are all too often overlooked in the intensive care unit and acute care setting, where more pressing issues of survival and achievement of some medical stability naturally take precedence. The psychological toll on the patient, who has lost nearly all control over bodily function, and on the family cannot be underestimated. It is the role of the rehabilitation team to establish effective communications as soon as possible. Unfortunately, lip speaking is not uniformly successful, with some patients being excellent lip speakers but others being woefully inadequate in this regard. Furthermore, it is estimated that only 30% of the English language is interpretable by lip speaking. Ideally, the patient should be allowed to vocalize as soon as the pulmonary condition permits but in the meantime, the team may have to resort to a variety of communication devices including alphabet boards or communication boards. Other devices that can be used before allowing vocalization include the artificial larynx or electromyogram-controlled oral sound tubes. Tracheostomy tubes have also been developed that permit a flow of air to escape into the airway above the cuffed balloon via a second lumen. Unfortunately, this system typically produces only a faint voice that may be obscured by secretions collecting over the tracheostomy balloon. In addition, it requires the listener to control the auxiliary flow of air to produce vocalization. Nonetheless, this device can produce audible vocalization in many patients and should be considered if a more definitive approach to vocalization cannot be used. Ultimately, some means of allowing a portion of the ventilator tidal volume to escape through the larynx can be used to allow the patient to vocalize with adequate power. This will of course require that the patient is no longer requiring a sealed system to maintain positive end expiratory pressure or to treat atelectasis. When the patient has reached sufficient pulmonary stability to allow ventilator leak vocalization, a number of different options are available. Some form of cuffless tracheostomy tube, either the metal Jackson tracheostomy tube or plastic versions, have the advantage of simplicity, easy replacement, and cleaning. Cuffed fenestrated tubes have the disadvantage of trapping secretions above the balloon and pressure complications of the balloon itself as noted in the previous paragraph. An inevitable tradeoff in allowing vocalization via tracheostomy tube "leak" is the decrease in ventilator alarm sensitivity, requiring that the patient and family be thoroughly educated in alarm adjustment. In summary, the psychological importance of communication to the patient, family, and team cannot be underestimated and efforts should be made to establish adequate vocalization as soon as possible with other means of communication used until vocalization can be achieved.

REFERENCES

1. Ozer MN, Schmitt JK, eds. (1987): Medical complications of spinal cord injury. *Phys Med Rehab State Art Rev* 1(3):339–518.
2. Bloch RF, Basbaum M (1986): *Management of Spinal Cord Injuries.* Baltimore, Williams & Wilkins.
3. Berczeller PH, Bezkor MF (1986): *Medical Complications of Quadriplegia,* Chicago, Year Book Medical Publishers.
4. Bedbrook GM (1981): *The Care and Management of Spinal Cord Injuries.* New York, Springer-Verlag.
5. Zejdlik CM (1983): *Management of Spinal Cord Injury.* Belmont, CA: Wadsworth Health Sciences Division.
6. Young RR, Delwaide PJ (1981): Drug therapy—spasticity. *N Engl J Med* 304:28–33, 96–99.
7. Kasdon DL, Lathi ES (1984): A prospective study of radiofrequuency rhizotomy in the treatment of post traumatic spasticity. *Neurosurgery* 15:526–529.
8. Davis L, Martin J (1947): Studies upon spinal cord injuries: the nature and treatment of pain. *J Neurosurg* 4:483–491.
9. Davis R (1975): Pain and suffering following spinal cord injury. *Clin Orthop* 112:76–80.
10. Nashold BS, Bullitt E (1981): Dorsal root entry zone lesions to control central pain in paraplegics. *J Neurosurg* 55:414–419.
11. Quencer R, Sheldon J, Post M, Diaz R (1986): Magnetic resonance imaging of the chronically injured cervical spinal cord. *Am J Neuroradiol* 7:457.
12. Rossier A, Foo D, Shillito J, Dyro F (1985): Post traumatic cervical syringomyelia. *Brain* 108:439.
13. Pfeiffer SC, Blust P, Leyson JFJ (1981): Nutritional assessment of spinal cord injured patients. *J Am Diet Assoc* 78:501–505.

14. Tanaka M, Uchimaya M, Kitano M (1979): Gastroduodenal disease in chronic spinal cord injury. *Arch Surg* 114:185–187.
15. Apstein MD (1987): Spinal cord injury is a risk factor for gallstone disease. *Gastroenterology* 92:966–968.
16. Lapidis J (1984): Neurogenic bladder: principles of treatment. *Urol Clin North Am* 1:89–90.
17. Perkash I (1980): Problems of decatheterization in long term spinal cord injury patients. *J Urol* 124:249–253.
18. Rossier AB, Fam BA (1984): Indications and results of semi rigid penile prostheses in spinal cord injury patients: long term follow-up. *J Urol* 131:59.
19. Sidi AA, et al. (1987): Vasoactive intracavernous pharmacotherapy for the treatment of erectile impotence in men with spinal cord injury. *J Urol* 138:539–542.
20. VerVoort SM (1987): Ejaculatory stimulation in spinal cord injured men. *Urology* 19:282–289.
21. Stover SL, Hahn HR, Miller JM (1976): Disodium etidronate in the prevention of heterotopic ossification following spinal cord injury (preliminary report). *Paraplegia* 14:146–156.
22. Vernier LH, Ditunno JF (1971): Heterotopic ossification in paraplegic patients. *Arch Phys Med Rehabil* 54:475–479.
23. Kewelramani LS, Ortho MS (1977): Ectopic ossification. *Am J Phys Med* 56:99–120.
24. Perkash A, Prakash V, Perkash I (1978): Experience with the management of thromboembolism in patients with spinal cord injury. Incidence, diagnosis and role of some risk factors. *Paraplegia* 16:322–331.
25. Todd JW, Frisbie JH, Rossier AB, et al. (1976): Deep venous thrombosis in acute spinal cord injury: a comparison of ^{125}I fibrinogen leg scanning, impedance plethysmography and venography. *Paraplegia* 14:50–57.
26. Consensus Conference (1986): Prevention of venous thrombosis and pulmonary embolism. *JAMA* 256:744–749.
27. Hull RD, et al. (1986): Prophylaxis of venous thromboembolism, an overview. *Chest* 89:374S–383S.
28. Watson N (1978): Anti-coagulant therapy in the prevention of venous thrombosis and pulmonary embolism in the spinal cord injury. *Paraplegia* 16:265–269.

11

Ventilator Weaning

Allan B. Wicks

Craig Hospital, Englewood, Colorado, U.S.A.

The question of how and when to consider weaning a high quadriplegic patient from a ventilator involves several considerations. The devastation of the injury and associated ventilator dependence causes significant fear for the patient with any proposed change in the mechanical ventilator. There is a significant depression that the patient works through almost invariably, although the timing of this depression and the length may be a consideration when contemplating changes in treatments that require motivation, such as the weaning process (1). Prior pulmonary history including smoking, asthma, or chronic productive cough is also helpful in assessing wean potential.

WEAN PARAMETERS

It is very helpful to have previously monitored parameters of respiration on the patient. This can be obtained despite ventilator dependence by measuring the spontaneous parameters for 30 s. This gives a rough idea of the ability of the patient to spontaneously generate a forced vital capacity. The forced vital capacity is probably the best single indicator of how well a patient will progress with his or her weaning (2). Vital capacity is monitored regularly, often daily for a while. At some specialized centers, vital capacities are measured before and after a wean. Other centers determine how long a wean will go in relation to the initial forced vital capacity, discontinuing the wean when the vital capacity has dropped off 25%. The wean would then be reinitiated after a rest. Other parameters that can be helpful for the weaning process include respiratory rate, minute ventilation, negative inspiratory pressure, and tidal volume.

WHEN TO BEGIN WEANING

There is no specific amount of time that a patient needs to be on a mechanical ventilator before consideration for weaning is practical. If the patient has no major complications, specifically in the form of atelectasis, secretion retention, fever, depression, or other associated injuries, then the weaning can begin as early as 24–48 h after intubation. It is more common, however, to have several minor complications in the medical course of the acute injury that prevent immediate attempts at weaning (3).

There are certain patients who will not be able to fully wean from the mechanical ventilator due to the level of injury. However, this is no reason to avoid weaning attempts. There may be less urgency to begin these weans, but nonetheless every patient should receive a trial of weans for at least a short time to be certain there is no possibility of total ventilator independence.

For the higher quadriplegic patients who, by the level of their injury, would not be candidates for ventilator independence, there are reasons to wean them other than any expected total ventilator independence (2). Wean efforts are always attempted to prevent further muscle atrophy of the respiratory muscles, and to help build some reserve in case of inadvertent ventilator disconnection when the patient does not have an attendant in the immediate vicinity. In these patients, persistent weaning efforts help to strengthen accessory muscles, thereby helping achieve short periods off the ventilator. When these ventilator-dependent patients are at home, the ability to breathe even for 10–15 min on their own may be the difference between life and death in the case of a ventilator disconnect. This is continually reinforced to the patient, who might otherwise become discouraged with his or her lack of significant progress with the weaning process.

When the weaning is to begin the patient is always started in the supine position because cervical-spinal-injured patients spontaneously breathe much better in a supine position (2,4). Later in the weaning process when the patient does attempt to spontaneously breathe in an upright position, an abdominal binder is used to help stabilize the abdominal musculature. This allows for more efficient diaphragm movement and avoids early fatigue.

TECHNIQUES

As mentioned above, wean parameters including forced vital capacity, minute ventilation, etc., are helpful to decide the length of the initial wean. Certainly this can be as short as 15 s to as long as 5–10 min off the ventilator. Shorter weans are preferred initially to give the patients confidence in their own ability to maintain spontaneous respirations. The most commonly used weaning process involves short periods of total ventilator independence, generally with a T-tube to provide moisture and oxygen. Patients are then placed on the ventilator to allow them to rest. There are reports of intermittent mandatory ventilation (IMV) being used to wean the quadriplegic patient, but there is no series of patients done with IMV and there is no study comparing standard weaning with IMV in similarly matched patients (5,6). This does not seem to be a feasible study given the limited number of ventilator-dependent patients in any one center. The physiology of IMV, in the author's opinion, is less conducive to weaning these patients. The fatigue that can be encountered in the already atrophic respiratory muscles with IMV would seem to precipitate further respiratory insufficiency. With our experience at weaning more than 150 quadriplegic patients from ventilators, we never use IMV for weaning a patient, and would generally discourage this technique in these patients (2).

It is very important during the initial weans that a qualified respiratory therapist stay immediately with the patient for reassurance and to be available if the patient requests to return to the ventilator. In general, unless the patient is able to wean for more than 30 min at a time, the therapist is continually at the patient's bedside throughout the wean. Once the patient is comfortable with 30-min weans or longer, a short time away from the bedside is permissible but there should always be someone available and in the immediate area.

The frequency of the weans generally is four times daily. A high quadriplegic patient, for example, might start the weans at 2 min four times daily, whereas a lower quadriplegic patient might start in the range of 5–10 min four times daily. The frequent weans help build strength of the respiratory muscles as in any rehabilitation process (7,8). The progression of the wean intervals depends on several factors with the patient. At times use of the incentive spirometer can help to strengthen the respiratory muscles either during the wean or separate from the wean. Certainly the amount of time between the intubation and the beginning of the weaning process is of major significance. Atrophy of the respiratory musculature progressively occurs with time, and the longer the patient has been on the ventilator, the weaker the muscles will be. In addition, there is variability in the progress of the weans depending on the level of injury (9,10). Chest muscle spasticity occurs in the process of acclimating to the injury. As this spasticity becomes more prevalent, the diaphragmatic motion might become more efficient (4,6,11–15). This may be a contributing factor to the improvement in the spontaneous vital capacity that occurs with almost every patient as the weaning progresses. Of course, the improved performance of the respiratory muscles with the repeated weans would also be a factor in improved vital capacity.

As patients gain confidence in their weans, they often will look forward to longer times off the mechanical ventilator. There is a need to prioritize weans in conjunction with other disciplines. Physical therapy, occupational therapy, educational classes, and conferences demand some use of time. It is important to be sure that the three to four weans per day are arranged among the other activities in the rehabilitation process. This is perhaps best accomplished by scheduling the weaning sessions a bit more frequently during the evening hours.

A wean may progress from 5 min four times a day to 10 min four times a day and even then jump to 15, 20, and 30 min four times a day over a period of 2–3 weeks. The patient can be the best guide to the increased duration of weans. If they have confidence at the present level they are usually amenable to a suggestion from the physician that the duration be increased by 5, 10, or 15 min every 2–3 days. As the wean time increases, the patient must be weaning while participating in other rehabilitation activities. This might even include weaning while sitting in a wheelchair, while in the rehabilitation gymnasium, or while having x-ray tests performed. Vital capacity should be checked with the patient in the sitting position. In cervical spinal injuries, the vital capacity will be lower in the upright position. If the vital capacity drops by 50% or more from the supine to the upright position, the weaning may not be easily accomplished with the patient upright.

From 1 h three times a day, it is relatively easy to go to 2 h three times a day, 4 h three times a day or twice a day, etc. The patient commonly prefers being off the ventilator to being on it by the time the weans are 6 h or more per day (2). Arterial blood gases are occasionally checked during the progression of weans, although not necessarily with every wean increase.

TRACHEOSTOMY MANAGEMENT

Management of the tracheostomy is a separate but equally important aspect of the care of the ventilator-dependent quadriplegic. Soft cuffed tracheostomies are universal at the present time and certainly are important in these long-term ventilator patients. The tracheostomy tube should be changed occasionally. Frequency may depend on secretions, infection, or physician preference, but usually is every 2–3 weeks.

The patient may be allowed to vocalize by having the tracheostomy cuff deflated for short times. This can occasionally work effectively provided that good suctioning is done when the cuff is deflated. If a patient has significant secretions, there may be some difficulty vocalizing, but it works fairly effectively in most patients. There can be a problem with ventilator alarms when the cuff is deflated because there is a loss of volume. Pressure alarms are more efficient in this situation than volume alarms. Occasionally the tidal volume will need to be increased if there is a significant air leak with each ventilator-generated volume. When the respiratory status is relatively stable and often when patients have made a certain amount of progress with their weans, the tracheostomy tube is frequently changed to a metal cuffless tracheostomy, usually a Jackson tracheostomy. With the change, there is usually a significant ventilator air leak and adjustments of the tidal volume and respiratory rate may be necessary to maintain a normal pH. Nonetheless, most patients are extremely happy to get to a Jackson tracheostomy, which allows them to vocalize at will by timing speech with the ventilator cycle (2). An occasional patient does better with a cuffed tracheostomy tube, which is deflated most of the day and then inflated during the sleep hours.

The patient may also vocalize while weaning provided that the cuffed tracheostomy has been deflated. This requires a device that can fit onto the tracheostomy called a Trach-Talk (Olympic) and is very effective in allowing the patient to verbalize during the weaning process.

Generally a Jackson tracheostomy is in the size range of no. 5, 6, or 7 when the patient is primarily connected to the ventilator. When the patient has been weaned off the mechanical ventilator for 24 h, the tracheostomy is decreased immediately to a no. 4 Jackson and the orifice is plugged. This allows the patient to inhale spontaneously and exhale through the mouth and nose. It avoids the tubing over the tracheostomy, while allowing access for suctioning with a normal-size suction catheter (no. 14 French). Any tracheostomy smaller than a size 4 would require a smaller suction catheter than is effective.

Kistner buttons and Olympic buttons can maintain the tracheostomy stoma and allow access for suctioning (11). However, these devices can occasionally fall out. Until the patient can be decannulized and the tracheostomy orifice allowed to heal, the present preference is a no. 4 plugged Jackson tracheostomy.

SUCTIONING

Suctioning is done in the routine way, with sterile suctioning procedure being used when the patients are in the intensive care unit or in the neurotrauma unit where more active medical problems are encountered. In some centers a clean technique is used in the hospital as well as at home. In other centers sterile technique is used in the hospital and clean technique is taught for home use. This clean technique involves a red rubber catheter and good hand-washing technique. Clean gloves may be used electively, although the family would generally use only good hand-washing technique. The catheter is cleared by suctioning sterile saline. It is wiped clear with a 4×4-in. gauze and maintained in a clean, dry container until the next use. A new catheter is used every 8 h. Studies have not been done to confirm the infection rate with this technique as opposed to the sterile technique. However, there are reports in the literature of clean technique being effective under similar conditions (16,17). Clean technique is found to be very practical and less costly than sterile suctioning.

OTHER INFORMATION

During the hospital stay, it is common for fluoroscopy of the diaphragm to be done to evaluate the competency of each of the phrenic nerves (11). The chest x-ray film can give an indication of possible phrenic nerve paralysis with elevation of the hemidiaphragm on the affected side. When done properly, fluoroscopy of the diaphragms can verify the presence of diaphragmatic paralysis. Another option to evaluate the diaphragms is double-exposure chest x-ray films, which can help identify a paralyzed diaphragm.

Phrenic nerve testing has been done on the ventilator-dependent patients to determine whether the phrenic nerve itself has been damaged with the initial cord injury (11). This may be helpful in the consideration of phrenic pacemaker implantation (18,19) (see Chapter 12).

Tracheal stenosis is a significant problem that can be encountered in patients who require long-term ventilation. This can be minimized with a soft-cuffed tracheostomy tube, attention to avoiding overinflation of the cuff, changing to cuffless tracheostomy tubes as soon as practical, keeping the cuff deflated on the usual cuffed tracheostomy tubes, and avoiding malposition of the tracheostomy tube in the patient. Nonetheless, because of the length of time these patients are on ventilators, the problem with tracheal stenosis can be a significant one.

In summary, the weaning process must progress individually depending on numerous factors with each patient. To progress with the weans, patients must have confidence in themselves and in the therapists. It is a mistake to increase weans at too rapid a rate. The patient who becomes overly fatigued with a wean may have setbacks in other rehabilitation and possibly a lack of confidence to progress with the wean schedule. The important point is not the speed of the wean process but the result. The weaning process of a quadriplegic patient can be one of the most gratifying parts of the rehabilitation process, not only for the patient but also for the patient's family as well as the physician.

REFERENCES

1. Lamid S, Ragalie G, Welter K (1985): Respirator-dependent quadriplegics: problems during the weaning period. *J Am Paraplegia Soc* 8:32–37.
2. Wicks A, Menter R (1986): Long-term outlook in quadriplegic patients with initial ventilator dependency. *Chest* 90:406–410.
3. Carter RE (1987): Respiratory aspects of spinal cord injury management. *Paraplegia* 25:262–266.
4. Luce J, Culver B (1982): Respiratory muscle function in health and disease. *Chest* 81:82–90.
5. Downs J, Perkins H, Sutton WW (1974): Successful weaning after five years of mechanical ventilator. *Anesthesiology* 40:602–603.
6. Luce J (1985): Medical management of spinal cord injury. *Crit Care Med* 13:126–131.
7. Lerman R, Weiss M (1987): Progressive resistive exercise in weaning high quadriplegics from the ventilator. *Paraplegia* 25:130–135.
8. Gross D, Ladd H, Riley E, Macklem P, Grassino A (1980): The effect of training on strength and endurance of the diaphragm in quadriplegia. *Am J Med* 68:27–35.
9. Fuhrer M, Carter RE, Donovan W, Rossi C, Wilkerson M (1987): Postdischarge outcomes for ventilator-dependent quadriplegics. *Arch Phys Med Rehabil* 68:353–356.
10. Forner J (1980): Lung volumes and mechanics of breathing in tetraplegics. *Paraplegia* 18:258–266.
11. Berczeller P, Bezkor M (1986): Respiratory care. In: *Medical Complications of Quadraplegia* 1986. Chicago: Year Book Medical Publishers, pp. 25–49.
12. Ledsome J, Sharp J (1981): Pulmonary function in acute cervical cord injury. *Am Rev Respir Dis* 124:41–44.
13. Troyer A, Heilporn A (1980): Respiratory mechanics in quadriplegia. The respiratory function of the intercostal muscles. *Am Rev Respir Dis* 122:591–600.
14. Murciano D, Aubier M, Lecocguic Y, Pariente R (1984): Effects of theophylline on diaphragmatic strength and fatigue in patients with chronic obstructive pulmonary disease. *N Engl J Med* 311:349–353.
15. Cheshire D (1964): Respiratory management in acute traumatic tetraplegia. *Paraplegia* 1:252–261.
16. Jones C (1979): Asepsis in pulmonary care: improving old traditions. *J Neurosurg Nurs* 11:76–82.
17. Harris R, Hyman R (1984): Clean vs. sterile tracheostomy care and level of pulmonary infection. *Nurs Res* 33:80–85.
18. Glenn W, Jogan J, Phelps M (1980): Ventilatory support of the quadriplegic patient with respiratory paralysis by diaphragm pacing. *Surg Clin North Am* 60:1055–1078.
19. Marcy T, Loke J (1987): Diaphragm pacing for ventilatory insufficiency. *J Int Care Med* 2:345–353.

12

Available Respiratory Options*

R. Edward Carter†

with Robert Menter, Marsha Wood, Conal Wilmot, and Karyl Hall

†Institute for Rehabilitation and Research, Houston, Texas, U.S.A.

The major medical difficulty of individuals with high quadriplegia is maintenance of ventilation and prevention of respiratory complications. This chapter begins with a discussion of the importance of initial medical management, and then addresses three major methods of sustaining ventilation at home and in the community, i.e., (a) volume ventilator, (b) pneumobelt, and (c) electrophrenic respiration.

Much of the success of any ventilator-dependent patient program depends on skillful early pulmonary management. In the past, many ventilator-dependent high quadriplegic patients were thought to have no chance of survival on admission to an acute care hospital. They were often maintained by oral feeding despite the known possibility of aspiration, and efforts to keep the lung fields clear were less than vigorous. In addition to aspiration, regurgitation from the stomach or lower esophagus may also occur. Aggressive pulmonary management that takes into account aspiration and regurgitation is now more common as is demonstrated by the increasing number of survivors. Complete swallowing studies should be part of the initial workup for any high quadriplegic

---

*The section on volume ventilators was contributed by Robert Menter and Marsha Wood; the section on pneumobelt use was contributed by Conal Wilmot and Karyl Hall; and the section on electrophrenic respiration was written by R. Edward Carter.

patient. This is in addition to the usual studies of blood count, blood gases, tracheal culture and sensitivity, chest radiography, and fluoroscopy of the respiratory muscles.

Aspiration, unfortunately, is fairly common in the early stages in many of these patients. It is generally thought to occur bilaterally. The right lower lung is more easily cleared than the left by intermittent positive pressure breathing, chest physical therapy, and assistive coughing with suctioning. In nearly all patients, the most severely involved lung area seems to be the left retrocardiac area. The major bronchus to this area is directed more posteriorly and is longer than its corresponding bronchus on the right side. For these reasons, the mucus in the left retrocardiac area is more difficult to clear and effective postural drainage has to be carried out with the patient not only high on their right side but actually three quarters towards the prone and in Trendelenburg's position. Among the first major issues the medical staff must address are the need to clear the chest so that recurrent infections are minimal or preferably absent, to reduce the FIO_2 to 21%, and to begin the patient's progressive sitting program with portable ventilator equipment.

VOLUME VENTILATORS

Volume ventilation is the most common form of respiratory support in spinal cord injury (SCI). The earliest forms of volume ventilation used a negative atmospheric pressure around the outside of the chest to create inspiration and allowed expiration to occur in a passive mode when the negative pressure was discontinued. The negative pressure ventilation was most successfully used in the form of the iron lung and the cuirass chest piece for polio patients. Due to more complex respiratory pathology and needs in SCI, there has been a change in technique from negative to positive pressure ventilation. Today, volume ventilation generally refers to positive pressure in which a prescribed volume of gas is delivered under positive pressure to expand the lungs from within for inspiration. Expiration occurs in a passive mode.

Positive pressure ventilation usually requires a tube (oral tracheal, nasotracheal, or tracheal) to deliver the air into the respiratory system. Under some conditions, a facial mask can be used but the indications are less clear.

Volume ventilators are the most versatile forms of respiratory support available today. Monitors and controls usually include the following: (a) oxygen percentage; (b) respiratory rate; (c) tidal volume; (d) sigh frequency and volume; (e) control/assistance device; (f) humidity; (g) end expiratory pressure; (h) high pressure alarm; (i) low pressure alarm; and (j) volume alarm.

Using the many options available, it is possible to tailor the respiratory support and alarms to the patient's needs with a high degree of

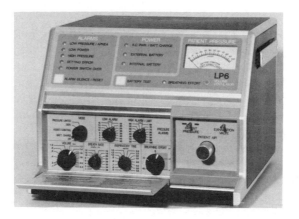

FIG. 12-1. Aequitron LP6 portable ventilator.

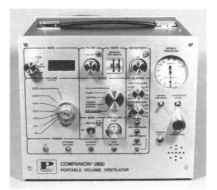

FIG. 12-2. Puritan-Bennett 2800 ventilator.

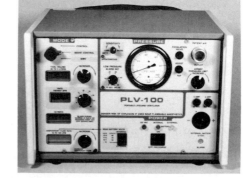

FIG. 12-3. Lifecare PLV-100 ventilator.

accuracy. The control/assist control mode is important once the tracheostomy cuff is down and vocalization has begun. It allows the patient in the assist control mode to trigger extra breaths for talking in addition to the regular rate already set (see Chapters 4, 5, and 11 for information on respiratory management).

There are two general categories of volume ventilators—stationary and portable. The stationary ventilators have many more control features, but they are usually more cumbersome, heavier, and depend on continuous AC current for power. Stationary ventilators are almost never ordered as discharge equipment. Portable ventilators, although having fewer options, are usually smaller, lighter, and have power options of either AC current, external battery, or internal battery power. In response to the increasing need for portable ventilator support, a variety of units are available. Three of the more popular portable ventilators are shown in Figs. 12-1, 12-2, and 12-3. Due to individual patient preferences, and variations in costs and follow-up service, it is desirable to expose patients to more than one choice. Even those patients hoping to go on to electrophrenic diaphragm pacers and/or use a pneumobelt will require a volume ventilator for backup.

We strongly recommend that each person discharged to a home environment receive two ventilators. The concept of two ventilators focuses on the reality that ventilators do break down, require repairs, and that a backup ventilator is needed immediately whenever the ventilator in use malfunctions. Although manual resuscitation is practical for a short period of time, a backup respirator is necessary in nearly all cases to avoid hospitalization and unnecessary disruption in the patient's activities.

Costs should be discussed in terms of the "package" necessary for the ventilators to work. The following represents a typical respiratory equipment package for a first-admission patient in 1988 dollars. Prices will vary by vendor and geography.

(2)	LP6 portable ventilators	@ $7,495.00	$14,990.00
(4)	LP6 circuits	@ 150.00	600.00
(1)	LP6 air filters (5/box)		10.00
(1)	Cascade Humidifier mount for LP6		85.00
(1)	T-0916 Cascade Series Humidifier		741.00
(1)	T-51356 Cascade jar & lid		87.50
(2)	90° connectors with DC battery cable	@45.00	90.00
(1)	Bedside suction		475.00
(1)	Laerdal portable suction		792.00
(1)	PMR or Laerdal ambubag with valve		198.00
(1)	Respirometer		679.00

Table 12-1. *Prices, Maintenance Cost, and Approximate Longevity of Three Popular Portable Ventilator Models*

Ventilator model no.	Manufacturer	Cost	Recommended preventative maintenance	Cost	Estimated life
LP6	Aequitron Medical, Inc., Minneapolis, MN	$7,495	Every 6,000 h	$186	Unlimited, with proper maintenance
PB2800	Puritan-Bennett, Boulder, CO	$7,835	Every 6,000 h or a year, whichever comes first	$350	Unlimited, with proper maintenance
PLV100	Lifecare, Lafayette, CO	$6,600	Every 6 mo; Lifecare sends cards to inform clients that PM is due	Varies	Unlimited, with proper maintenance

(1) Bunn compressor			500.00
(1) Gel cell battery with case			205.00
(2) In-line condensers with cartridge	@ 35.00		70.00
(3) Jackson tracheostomy tubes	@ 64.00		192.00
(1) Ventilarm			230.00

In addition to initial purchase costs, long-term planning needs to include maintenance costs and the possible rental costs of units replacing the unit that is in for repairs. Table 12-1 shows representative costs of purchase and recommended maintenance costs of three popular portable ventilators.

Decisions on purchasing equipment must include patient preference, cost, and local service. We try to establish who is going to be providing respiratory services in the home before making a final decision.

Humidification in portable ventilators can be of two different types depending on the patient's needs and activity pattern. The most common type of humidification is the variable heat moisturizing system such as the Cascade. Cascade style humidification is a standard feature on stationary ventilators and can be attached to a portable ventilator when it is stationary. Unfortunately, the Cascade type of humidifier is very vulnerable to motion such as tipping and is not safe to use on a wheel-

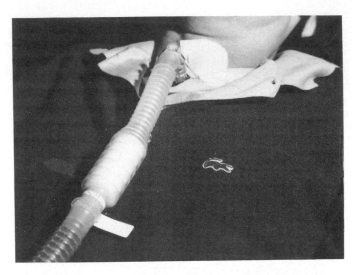

FIG. 12-4. Engstion "Edith" artificial nose.

chair. While the patient is up in the wheelchair, humidification is best provided by an air baffle called an artificial nose (Fig. 12-4). The artificial nose works to trap the moisture during expiration and allows the same moisture to be reused during the next inspiratory phase. The artificial nose most often is used during the day when the patient is up and about, and a Cascade humidifier is used when the patient is in bed. Artificial noses come in both disposable and nondisposable types. The nondisposable type may be cleaned and reused and is most practical for the home environment.

When two ventilators are obtained for a patient's home use, one should be set up as a bedside ventilator with Cascade humidification and the second ventilator should be set up for the wheelchair with an artificial nose. It is very important to note that even those patients going on to electrophrenic pacing and/or pneumobelt use will need a ventilator as backup equipment. No patient or family should ever go on to alternate ventilation program unless they have a solid working knowledge and second nature instinct in the use of a ventilator.

Ventilator use in the acute care setting usually focuses on the more versatile stationary type ventilator. Some specific situations such as air transportation or ground ambulance transportation and transfers to and from diagnostic centers within the hospital are better served by portable ventilators. As soon as the patient begins a program of active mobilization, ventilator support is usually switched to the portable ventilator. A manual resuscitation bag and portable suction must be considered part of both the stationary and portable ventilation programs. If additional oxygen is needed, a portable oxygen cylinder can be used to bleed oxygen into the portable ventilator system. The unique design of portable ventilators allows three options relating to power source: (a) standard AC 110 current; (b) internal battery source; and (c) external 12-V battery source.

The internal battery is charged automatically whenever the ventilator is operating on 110 current. The three options work to give as much flexibility in activities as possible. When in a bedside ventilation location, standard 110 AC current can be used. When not operating on 110-V AC, the ventilator is plugged into the power of the electric wheelchair (reduced to 12 V). When the patient is mobile without the power wheelchair such as to x-ray or other diagnostic centers, the internal battery of the ventilator can be used. For external battery power, a 12-V system created by the power wheelchair, the van, conventional lead acid batteries, or deep cycle sealed gel batteries can be used. In the event that a private or commercial airline is to be used, the external battery must be a sealed gel cell battery approved by the Federal Aviation Administration.

Safety is built into the portable ventilator in several different ways. Power is switched automatically within the ventilator from internal power to external power to AC power depending on whatever power source is available. If the patient is on a standard AC 110 current during the night and there is a power outage, the ventilator will automatically switch to an accessory 12-V battery if it has been hooked up to the ventilator or to the internal batteries of the ventilator. Other ways of dealing with power outages would include a backup electrical generator that would switch on automatically in the event of a power outage or a standard 12-V lead acid battery connected to the vent at night. Typical use time of the ventilator is 45 min on internal batteries, 24 h for standard lead acid battery, and 8 h on a sealed gel battery.

Alarm systems are only as effective as the availability and capability of the person responding to the alarm. Alarm systems fall into two categories: call systems and ventilation monitor systems. Patient call systems are the first line in warning because frequently the patient will sense and/or know of needs before the built-in delay of ventilation monitor alarms. In nearly all cooperative patients, some type of dependable call device can be worked out such as mercury switches in ball, microleaf switch, sip and puff, or eyebrow switch (see Chapter 6 for details regarding patient call systems).

Alarms used in volume ventilation must be discussed with the philosophical prospect that each step down in intensity of care from the intensive care unit introduces additional risk. Alarms are only as effective as there are people to respond to the alarm. Vocalization (deflating of the cuff of the tracheostomy tube in particular) decreases the sensitivity

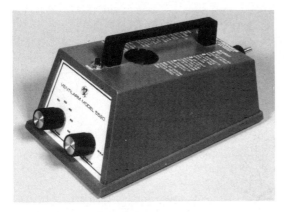

FIG. 12-5. Ventronics low-pressure alarm.

of the ventilator alarm systems. Despite the potential of increased risk, nearly all patients and families want to proceed toward a goal of leaving the hospital.

Ventilator alarms can be categorized as follows: *internal*—high pressure; low pressure; volume; *external*—low pressure; apnea.

All three internal alarms are very accurate when used with inflated tube cuffs. When tracheostomy tube cuffs are deflated or removed, the high-pressure alarm becomes nonapplicable, the low-pressure alarm must be reset, and the volume alarm is of doubtful value. Because of concerns that a power outage or ventilator failure may invalidate all internal alarms simultaneously, we frequently use an independent battery-operated external (not part of the ventilator) low-pressure alarm (Fig. 12-5). Although apnea monitors are widely used in infants, we have limited experience with them in adult SCI.

Despite our best efforts in monitoring and alarm systems, it is recognized that a few patients can become disconnected in terms of effective ventilation without the low-pressure alarms (either internal or external) sounding. The apparent sequence of events centers around the tracheostomy tube coming out partially or completely in such a way that the tip is pushed against the skin or wedged in a way that maintains a low pressure. Although these cases are rare, they have been documented and effectively speak to the need for a philosophical acceptance of risk by the patient and family when leaving the intensive care unit. All alarm systems must be tested regularly and must have a respondent to answer them. Every respondent must be familiar with breathing the patient using a manual resuscitation bag. A manual resuscitation bag must be with the patient at all times. Whenever in doubt as to what is causing the alarm, disconnect the ventilator tubing and breathe for the patient with the manual resuscitation bag.

The connection between patient and ventilator is called the circuit

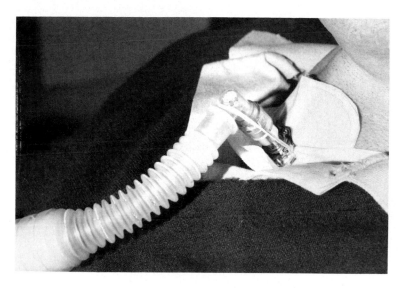

FIG. 12-6. Ventilator tubing can be secured to the trach using a rubber band.

and is comprised of tubing and an exhalation valve. Most ventilator manufacturers make both permanent and disposable circuits for their ventilator. Although disposable circuits are usually used in hospital settings to minimize the risk of infection, permanent reusable circuits are more practical and cost effective for home use.

All ventilator tubing should be supported and immobilized in a way that removes tension or torsion on the tracheostomy tube. To that end we secure all tubes with various types of Velcro chest straps either when the patient is in bed or up in the wheelchair. We also use a 6-in. link of more flexible rubber ventilation tubing between the tracheostomy tube adaptor and harder plastic ventilator tubing. The rubber ventilator tubing bends and twists easily, helping to prevent the tracheostomy tube from being pulled when the patient is turned, transferred, or has spasms.

The connection between tracheostomy tube and circuit is both the most vulnerable and the most critical. Each patient care provider must assume responsibility for that life connection. To assist in preventing disconnection, we use two rubber bands secured around the tracheostomy and looped over the connector (Fig. 12-6).

Suction equipment is the most expensive supportive item in the equipment package. Just as in ventilators, suction equipment falls into categories of bedside (stationary 110-V power) and portable (lighter, smaller, battery power). Stationary suction equipment is very standardized with many models. Portable suction equipment is best represented by the Laerdal unit (Fig. 12-7). It operates off of a battery pack which

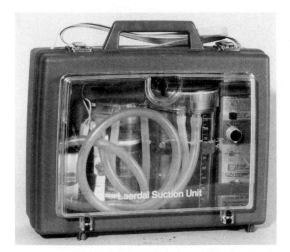

FIG. 12-7. Laerdal porta-
ble suction unit.

is rechargeable by 110 current. By using several battery packs it can be
kept in continuous operation.

This represents an overview of ventilator equipment and its use. All
members of the treating team from nursing to recreation therapy must
have a working knowledge of its use and be responsible for it when the
patient is with them. Everyone must be able to use the manual resuscitation bag without hesitation until additional help arrives to fix or
replace the ventilator.

PNEUMOBELT USE

A review of the development of intermittent negative pressure appa-
ratuses notes the work in 1939 of Sir William Bragg, the Nobel Prize
winning physicist (1). He developed a pneumatic belt made from rubber
football bladders that were strapped around the abdomen and lower chest
and were inflated by a small air pump. Modified to become the Bragg-
Paul "Pulsator," the belt was successfully used with polio cases in England until World War II.

Other published case studies of chronic ventilator use made little
mention of the pneumobelt (PNB) in reporting outcome of ventilating
progressive neuromuscular disease victims. Exceptions are Colbert and
Schock (2), whose survey included ventilator costs and relative use by
the Muscular Dystrophy Association, and Alexander et al. (3), who briefly
describe selected devices and their merits. Splaingard and co-workers
reviewed 20 years of experience with both positive (4) and negative (5)
pressure home ventilators. Almost all SCI cases were confined to the
positive ventilators. They reported that eight died, four had been weaned,

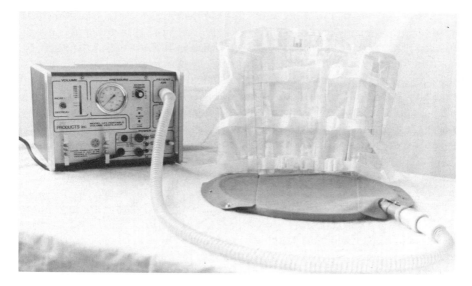

FIG. 12-8. Pneumobelt parts: corset, bladder, tubing, and ventilator.

and four switched to phrenic nerve stimulators (PNS). Survival ranged from 2 weeks in an infant to 11 years using an MA-1 ventilator, but no cases appeared to use the PNB.

The only detailed reported study of the PNB is by Adamson et al., dating from 1959. They failed to give credit to Sir William Bragg for inventing an earlier version of the belt. They outlined trials on 15 poliomyelitis victims with varying degrees of ventilatory paralysis. It was judged "a valuable adjunct to other respiratory aids . . . and for some activities it is the respirator of choice" (6).

Among the available ventilator devices for home use, the PNB appears to have many advantages, yet has received scant attention, particularly for the high quadriplegic population. Because our facility has significant experience with the appliance, we undertook a case review to examine these issues and provide recommendations about its use for the high quadriplegia patient.

Description

The PNB is a corset-type device that is placed around the abdomen and allows for ventilation without a tracheostomy (Fig. 12-8). It was initially called the intermittent abdominal pressure respirator (6) and is also known as an exsufflation belt. It produces artificial ventilation by assisting expiration rather then inspiration. The inflatable flat bladder within the corset fills, compresses the abdominal wall and so causes

the diaphragm to rise and produce active expiration. With bladder deflation, the abdominal contents and diaphragm fall, due to gravitational
pull, and inspiration occurs passively. The bladder is readily replaceable
and the washable corsets are available in three sizes. Together with
adjustable straps and movable buckles, they allow satisfactory fitting to
various abdominal girths and lengths. Increased tidal exchange is
achieved from the semireclining to sitting position and is optimal between 65 and 85°. Cyclic inflation of the PNB is provided by a positive
pressure ventilator pump attached via a single flexible lightweight hose.
A portable pump can be placed between the rear wheels of the wheelchair and is powered by a 12-V battery. It should be capable of providing
up to 18 breaths per minute (BPM) and pressures up to 80 cm of water.
Models used include the LP3 and PVV. The LP3 is no longer made,
which necessitates repair of old LP3s or use of the PVV only. Because
all the patients have had tracheostomies and are on positive pressure
ventilators, the same portable ventilator can be used for the PNB. Most
recently the PLV-100 by Life Care Products can be used satisfactorily
with the PNB as well. Because of the circuitry required, however, it is
noisy on exhale. The PLV-100 is also more complex than the older models.
For these reasons the older models are preferred.

Indications for Use

It is recommended that every respirator-dependent quadriplegic person who meets the following criteria be a candidate for the PNB: (a)
medically stable; (b) lungs are clear clinically and radiologically—that
is, the patient has passed the acute spinal shock phase, any fluid over-
load has been corrected, (s)he demonstrates good volumes and no atelectasis, and the patient is weaned to room air; (c) able to get out of bed
and sit in a wheelchair; (d) without marked abdominal wall obesity or
spasticity; (e) no severe brainstem involvement; and (f) sufficient cognitive ability and motivation to cooperate with the program.

Pneumobelt Fitting

The patient is fitted in the supine position with the corset's horizontal
upper border approximately two finger breadths below the costophrenic
junction. The curved lower border is fitted tighter than the upper part,
which allows a hand to slip without force between the PNB and the
patient's stomach. Once positioned, the patient is placed in the wheelchair for a PNB trial of 20–30 min and is monitored by arterial blood
gases (Fig 12-9). Thereafter, the periods of use are extended according
to the patient's tolerance, exhaled volumes, and serial blood gases.

There are three sizes of PNB: small, medium, and large. The fit has

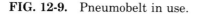

FIG. 12-9.   Pneumobelt in use.

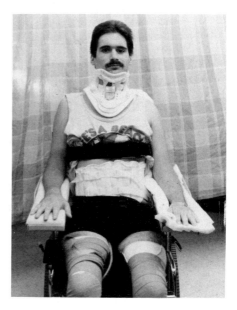

to be tight enough that the belt does not move around in transfers, etc.,
yet allows space between the PNB and the patient's stomach. When fitting, the belt always seems too low when the patient is supine. However, when they sit up in the chair, the belt will rise, but it must not
rise onto the rib cage. If it goes onto the rib cage, it renders the device
totally ineffective (Fig. 12-10). It is interesting to note that in a recent
literature review by Hill on the clinical application of PNBs (7), the
recommendations are not in total agreement with the above. Hill's recommendations are basically those supplied by Adamson in his original
article. These include high placement of the corset, with the upper bor-

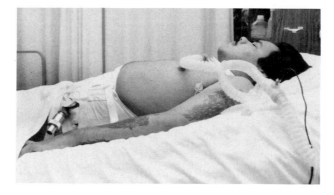

FIG. 12-10.   Proper pneumobelt positioning while patient is supine in bed.

der level with the xiphoid, to ensure enclosure of the lower portion of the rib cage. If this is attempted, the PNB will be ineffective. There will be insufficient air squeezing the abdomen, and therefore exhaled volumes will be too low to be satisfactory. We found other differences with Hill's article. He gives setting rates of 16–28 BPM and +15–+45 cm H_2O pressure. Our average settings were 12–14 BPM with routine pressure attaining +50–+60 cm H_2O pressure. No patient in our experience has been ventilated safely at more than 16 BPM. Hill mentions the limitations about PNB use with the very obese or thin and those with severe respiratory insufficiency. It has been our experience that thin people are difficult to fit but can be fitted, and that women are difficult to fit because of the short abdomen. We also regularly found success in those with a marked degree of respiratory failure. If anything, those with minimal respiratory failure had greater adjustment difficulties.

Psychological Preparation

The psychological preparation for PNB use is of as much importance as the physical/mechanical preparation. Preferably, in the beginning one therapist should be designated for patient training, because this allows the patient to build confidence in the therapist. It is also important to explain the concept to the patient and make sure that the patient understands that this is an external device versus an internal device. The outcome of this understanding will be a successful fitting, which includes the plugging of the tracheostomy. It is important to discuss thoroughly the effect plugging the tracheostomy will have on speech. The patient will have to learn to speak differently and (s)he will only be able to talk on exhalation. Something we have learned from patients is the effect of the use of the PNB on smell and particularly the taste of food. For the first time since being trached, they could smell and taste food, which makes it much more palatable. It should also be noted that there is improvement in hypotension during PNB use. Due to the squeezing of the abdomen and increased venous return, the hypotensive effects are decreased. A minimum of several weeks of supervised PNB use is recommended for adjustment.

We have talked about confidence building. This is important for the patient but it is also important for the staff. The ability of the patient to see and meet other patients using the PNB daily, even before they are ready to be fitted, shows that it is a plausible device. The respiratory therapist, nurse, physiotherapist, and occupational therapist must be totally comfortable with the belt and clearly demonstrate this to the patient. This includes putting on and taking off the belt, and transferring the patient with the PNB on.

Study of Pneumobelt Use

A study conducted at our facility examined use of the PNB among 21 high quadriplegic patients plus two polio cases and provides further valuable understanding.

Method and Materials

The hospital charts and respiratory therapy department records were reviewed from 1976 to 1986 to identify all patients who had used the PNB, however briefly. A survey was also mailed to PNB users. It asked about current usage and patient attitudes toward the device, advantages and disadvantages found, and the quality of life experienced.

Results

Predischarge experience. Most admissions to this acute facility were for initial SCI rehabilitation. Due to their complex spinal and pulmonary management, they were unable to begin early PNB use. The average interval was 3–6 months after the injury. The earliest user was 7 weeks postinjury and two others were late readmissions after 3 and 9 years, respectively. All patients were initially able to use the PNB for at least 15–20 min but tolerance beyond this varied greatly. Three patients adjusted immediately to wearing it for more than 6 h of continuous use and two other patients for up to 2 h at their first trials. Using daily practice, 11 other patients took up to 1 week to achieve 2 h of continuous use. For the remaining five SCI cases to achieve this goal, three of them required 2, 3, and 4 weeks of practice, respectively. A fourth case had an intercurrent infection delaying success until 6 weeks, and for the last case, records were unclear. Twelve of the 21 cases rapidly progressed within days from 2–4 h continuous use of the PNB and generally increased steadily thereafter to 12-h all-day use. Of equal importance are the nine SCI patients who failed to tolerate the PNB, as inpatients, beyond 3 h. Three cases had brainstem involvement with severe communication and swallowing difficulties. Two cases had problems with synchronizing breaths. All 23 cases were able to achieve adequate volumes with corset adjustments and a typical pump rate of 12–14 BPM. Exhaled volumes ranged from an initial 300–700 ml up to 400–900 ml by the time of discharge, all with satisfactory blood gases. The recorded positive airway pressures ranged between 34 and 76 cm H_2O.

The PNB was liberally tried and its overall use was successful. Unsuitable candidates include those with severe brainstem dysfunction (although we found a gastrostomy tube per se need not preclude its use).

It was found that some patients with partial preservation or recovery of diaphragmatic function may have difficulties with its use. Theoretically, serious obesity or spasticity of the abdominal wall may be problematic, although we experienced no such cases. Use of the PNB may be permanent or it may be needed temporarily until diaphragmatic recovery or more typically, patients become adjusted to PNS and no longer require a ventilator.

Survey experience. The survey was sent to 13 of the 23 patients. Three patients were still pending discharge. Of the 20 already discharged, three had died, two had severe brainstem injury along with head injury, and two had recovered diaphragmatic function shortly after admission. Of the 13 surveyed, all but two were regular PNB users at the time of discharge, averaging 12 h continuous use but ranging from 2 to 16 h. Also at discharge, 5 of the 13 were fitted with PNS. Ten of the remaining 13 responded (77%). Patients considered the greatest advantage of the PNB to be cosmetic. In particular, they could avoid the need for tubing around the throat, thus reducing the "invalid" appearance. This in turn allowed tracheostomy plugging and also reduced the fear of accidental disconnection of tubing using chin controls. Further, they highly ranked mobility and independence, and several stated that talking was easier and louder with the PNB. A number considered the PNB to be healthier and to reduce the infection risk, and of the six users residing at home, only one had required readmission for pulmonary infection since initial discharge. For all these cases, comparison was made with portable positive pressure ventilation (PPV). One patient had used the PNB for the whole study period of 10 years, but the other respondents averaged 3 years' use. Survey results also showed users averaged 12–14 h per day on the device. Reported disadvantages of the PNB were few. One complained of pump noise and stomach gas, another that clothing could catch on the corset buckle, while a third still had positioning difficulties. One respondent needed to come off the PNB for large meals. Patients now relying fully on PNS understandably preferred this but even so commented on the comfort, esthetics, improved talking abilities, and lack of problems found with the PNB compared with PPV. Of the 10 respondents, only one had reverted wholly to PPV right after discharge home.

Discussion

A recent collaborative study of high quadriplegia was completed by three regional SCI centers, including our own (Chapter 27)(10). Although restrospective in design and not comparing ventilator types, it was clearly shown that patient self-esteem and quality of life were significantly related to increased mobility and activity. Although costs of follow-up care were extraordinarily high, they were inversely related to time out of bed, mobility, and activity. One obvious conclusion to be drawn is that ventilator devices should be chosen that maximize this lifestyle. The PNB clearly offers just such an advantage. However, patterns of care in facilities aside from our own suggest primary reliance is on PPV for ventilating the high quadriplegic patient (4,8,9).

Experience with the PNB shows the device to offer many advantages. The major limitation of the device is said to be that patients must be sitting. One individual is able to sleep at night while using the PNB. Current sleep monitoring techniques may confirm the PNB's safety for night use, as has been recently demonstrated in a high quadriplegic (C3 complete) using the Rocker bed (9). The latter employs the same principle as the PNB in displacing abdominal contents. Potentially, this may permit tracheostomy closure and thus avoid known complications associated with chronic tracheostomy. We have patients with limited PNS capacity who have already achieved closure using PNS at night and PNB all day. High quadriplegic persons are trained to ensure that daily skin checks are undertaken. We found that abrasions from the corset occurred very infrequently, healed readily, and were generally preventable. Occasionally, patients may need to remove the appliance for a main meal, which is an acknowledged drawback to dining out, but with adequate initial training such problems can be avoided. Other negative pressure devices, e.g., the iron lung, porta lung, body wrap, or cuirass, have not been discussed. For patients requiring only nighttime ventilatory assistance, as in progressive neuromuscular disease, the choice may be different, but for those patients requiring daytime devices, the PNB appears to offer greater cosmesis, mobility, independence, and safety than other ventilator appliances. Findings strongly support use of the PNB, with all but one patient relying on their PNBs in preference to their portable PPVs. Three main conclusions can be drawn from our experience. First, the PNB may well be a leading choice for interim or permanent ventilation of the appropriate high quadriplegic individual. Second, it is underused and its wide acceptance for the high quadriplegic population is strongly recommended. Thirdly, more studies are needed to further evaluate the device.

ELECTROPHRENIC RESPIRATION

Electrophrenic respiration (EPR) was initially developed by Dr. W. W. L. Glenn for patients with Ondine's curse. In this condition, the phrenic nerve to the large volume right lung is implanted with a single electrode and receiver. The transmitter is turned on when the patient desires to sleep. In 1969, Dr. Glenn performed the first bilateral implantation of phrenic stimulators in a patient with traumatic SCI. The second such case was performed in early 1970 at The Institute for Rehabilitation and Research. Both patients are still alive and doing well.

For optimum results, it is extremely important that appropriate guidelines are used in the selection of candidates for this method of ventilation. The suitable candidate is one whose spinal cord is damaged at the first or second cervical level and who has sparing of the third, fourth, and fifth cervical anterior horn cells. These cells contribute fibers to the phrenic nerves bilaterally. A candidate must have both qualitatively and quantitatively viable phrenic nerves to be selected as a candidate for EPR implantation. Benefits of EPR ventilation include its portability, reliability, need for a minimal backup system in case of emergency, and its cosmetic features. The cosmetic features include: an easily disguised transmitter box that can fit on the side of a wheelchair; the lack of any discernible ventilator tubing; and a tracheotomy that can be plugged and/or replaced by a plum button that can easily be camouflaged by a high-necked blouse or scarf.

Breathing maintained by EPRs is similar to normal breathing in that it uses the patient's own diaphragm muscles. It was initially hoped that complication rates would be lower and life expectancy longer in patients using EPRs compared with those of patients maintained by a ventilator machine. However, the small number of cases thus far documented have not demonstrated a statistically significant margin of improvement.

Guidelines for EPR Candidates

The formal guidelines for choosing EPR candidates consist of the following.

1. Family members must be capable of learning and monitoring phrenic stimulator use. In the rehabilitation of SCI patients of any neurological level, the best prognostic sign is that of a stable and supportive family. This factor is of even greater importance in the ventilator-dependent high quadriplegic individual, where family members must be capable of a high degree of psychological support and of technically understanding the use and maintenance of EPR equipment.

2. The patient must be older than 6 years of age. Even then, the phrenic nerves over the anterior scalene muscles in the neck are extremely small. It is very difficult to adequately anchor a large plastic electrode around such a small nerve in the neck without having the electrode slip out of position or having the patient develop a perineural fibrosis. In younger children, it may be best to perform this connection of the electrode to the phrenic nerves in the chest. However, this alternative placement

requires highly sophisticated pediatricians, pediatric pulmonary services, and pediatric surgeons. Teams with this required level of skill are generally found only in major SCI centers.

3. The patient should be at least 4 months and preferably 6 months posttrauma. Traumatically injured quadriplegic patients who have ascending lesions that result in interference with diaphragmatic motion may have a reversal of diaphragm paralysis after a minimum of 60–90 days. Patients with this type of diaphragm paralysis would not become EPR candidates because they would not have the necessary quantitative phrenic nerve viability. Experience reveals that paralyzed diaphragms, unilateral or bilateral, begin to recover after 60 days and some degree of motion usually is seen before 90 days posttrauma. Some injuries to the spinal cord at the second cervical level may have swelling extending inferiorly through the third or fourth cervical level. In this instance, phrenic nerve viability can be permanently compromised or it might return to normal activity after 60–90 days. Waiting an appropriate time after injury allows all chance of normal recovery to take place before committing a patient to surgery.

4. The chest x-ray film should demonstrate clear lung fields with no evidence of pulmonary disease. The patient should be free of recurring atelectasis or pneumonitis. In the absence of pulmonary disease, a minimal amount of suctioning is required.

5. The patient should tolerate room air or an FIO_2 of 21%. EPRs allow a patient a level of wheelchair mobility that would be encumbered by the need for a supplemental oxygen source. Patients with chronic pulmonary disease are not candidates for EPR placement and patients with EPRs must attempt to avoid such conditions. EPR usage is not compatible with chronic endobronchial disease with irreversible bronchiectasis resulting in arteriovenous shunting, or conditions in which collections of mucus leading to recurrent infections require repeated use of major antibiotics.

6. Both a bronchoscopy and laryngoscopy should be performed to ensure the presence of an adequate airway. Meticulous care of the tracheotomy is required to prevent chronic problems that later can impede the closure of the tracheotomy. There must be documentation that indicates the lack of any significant amount of tracheomalacia, tracheostenosis, etc. An adequate airway must be ensured so that once the patient can tolerate bilateral phrenic stimulation, the tracheotomy tube can be plugged or corked.

7. Phrenic nerves must be proven viable, both qualitatively and quantitatively. This should be done with electrodiagnosis under fluoroscopy and will be described in a later section.

8. The patient must have the ability to tolerate the sitting position. It

is extremely important that each patient develop an adequate sitting tolerance, both in angle and duration, to take advantage of the portability and the expansion of mobility that EPRs can facilitate.

9. A surgeon with the skills required for EPR implantation is essential. Ideally, this is a surgeon who has actually seen and/or assisted in an implantation procedure.

10. Bioengineers knowledgeable in EPR equipment and maintenance must be available. Bioengineers perform an integral role preoperatively in the operating room, and postoperatively, documenting response of the phrenic nerves and preservation of viability at all stages of the procedure. They also assist in the calibration of the transmitter after implantation. After discharge, the bioengineer performs periodic checks of the subcutaneous receivers to test for reliability, performance degradation, or failure.

11. Finally, but no less important, a SCI physician knowledgeable in the physiology and pathophysiology of the high quadriplegic patient is essential. The EPR patient must be managed using a preventative program to minimize medical complications and maximize overall health status.

Evaluation of Phrenic Nerve Viability

Phrenic nerve viability is evaluated initially by the absence of voluntary diaphragmatic motion on fluoroscopy. It is important to differentiate a tidal volume emanating from the use of accessory muscles as compared with that resulting from true diaphragmatic motion. The attending and operating physicians should be present during this determination. Under fluoroscopy the dome of the diaphragm, as well as its attachment to the chest wall, is located. Chest surface electrodes are placed opposite and in one space above the insertion of the diaphragm on the lateral chest wall. A ground electrode is placed on the anterior portion of the chest above these electrodes. Then a stimulus using a bipolar electrode is placed medially and slightly posterior to the sternocleidomastoid muscle in the base of the neck. This placement is to stimulate the phrenic nerves as they move from the neck to the chest through the fat pad over the anterior scalene muscles. Initially, a transcutaneous stimulation with a single stimulus (0.2 ms duration at a rate of 1/s) is given to determine the bipolar electrode placement that will result in a maximum twitch of the diaphragm and a diaphragmatic M-wave. At that placement, measurement of phrenic nerve latency is recorded and it should average 6.1–9.2 ms. Next, a train of stimuli (20–30/s for 1 or 2 s) is applied to the same area to measure diaphragmatic excursions and tidal volume. The diaphragmatic excursion should be 4.5–6 cm bilaterally. This level of movement should ensure quantitative viability of the phrenic nerve.

EPR Surgery

Implantation of the EPR equipment consists of making an incision in the base of the neck to isolate the phrenic nerve in the fat pad anterior to the scalene muscles. This must be done without damage to the neurovascular bundle. A curved electrode is inserted and the phrenic nerve is fitted into the curve of the electrode. When there are constraints that do not allow the use of the preferred neck surgery site, an alternative approach is to implant the electrodes about the phrenic nerves in the chest. A subcutaneous tunnel then is formed down over the rib cage and an anterolateral thoracic incision is made just below the rib cage to create a subcutaneous pocket in which the receiver is buried. The subcutaneous wires are attached, via a quick disconnect connector, to wires coming from the receiver so that in the event of receiver failure, there is never a necessity to reexplore the area of electrode attachment. Suitable loops of wire or slack should be allowed because of the potential future growth of the individual. The remaining equipment consists of an external transmitter with bilateral wires attached to a circular antenna.

Postoperative Management

Postoperatively it is desirable to stimulate the patient once daily, including the day of surgery, for one to three breaths to evaluate that the EPR is working adequately. Stimulation continues once a day until the stitches have been removed and the incision is totally healed (~2 weeks). At that point, the patient is scheduled for chest fluoroscopy to evaluate the minimal electrical diaphragmatic response. Then the stimulation is set to afford the maximum tidal volume in the supine position. The initial setting should have a smooth onset of diaphragmatic contraction as opposed to a hiccupping motion. There should also be a slight hold at the end of inspiration to further mimic normal respiration.

The physician should be aware of the possibility of the patient's developing diaphragmatic fatigue syndrome. During the interval from injury to EPR surgery neither the phrenic nerves or diaphragm have actively fired during this time. Thus, a slow, progressive reconditioning program is necessary to rebuild endurance. With several patients who were almost a year postinjury before implant, the initial tolerance to stimulation was only 12–14 min before a significant drop in diaphragmatic motion and tidal volume occurred. Once this tolerance is ascertained, a program of stimulation slightly below that time span is begun twice daily while measuring the tidal volume and response of the patient. The stimulation period should stop when the tidal volume drops more than 25% of the initial tidal volume. This has to be done for each side separately and the stimulation time gradually increased. The increments of increase are apparently highly individualized.

When stimulation approaches 2 h, blood gases are obtained pre- and poststimulation for further checking of the adequacy of ventilation. Then the patient begins a stimulation program while (s)he is up in the wheelchair as well as when supine. Because of the major changes in both vital capacity and tidal volume from supine to sitting, it has been found that simultaneous stimulation of both diaphragms provides adequate ventilation when sitting but results in hyperventilation in the supine position. Therefore, supine patients may use either side alone or use alternate breaths between right and left. During sitting, it is unusual to find stimulation of a single diaphragm adequate to support ventilation. The ultimate goal is adequate tidal volume in all modes with adequate arterial blood gases when the patient is supine on alternating mode and in the wheelchair on simultaneous mode. It may take 2–4 months for the patient to progress to the point of 24-h EPR stimulation with no other ventilatory equipment needed, except as backup. Ultimately the tracheotomy tube is plugged or replaced with a Plum button.

Postoperative Problems

These include loss of viability of the phrenic nerve, either temporarily (with the result of high minimum threshold stimulation) or permanently. Temporary damage subsequently recovers over a period of 6–9 weeks. Permanent damage may also occur in which there is no response to electrical stimulation. This can be the result of damage during surgery to either the nerve or to the nutrient arterial vessels that supply the nerve.

Another possible complication is that of electrode cuff misplacement. As a result of atrophy in the muscles of the neck, it is sometimes difficult to adequately secure the electrode so that the nerve fits in the groove of the electrode. The electrode may, in fact, slip and require increased amounts of current to stimulate the nerve. When there is a large amount of space, either in a circular electrode as was used initially or a semicircular electrode that is in current use, fibrosis tends to occur between the phrenic nerve and the electrode cuff. This makes it extremely difficult to reoperate, if necessary, in the same area. The increasing amount of fibrosis results in a gradual increase in the electrical threshold needed to stimulate the phrenic nerve. Eventually the stimulation required reaches the point where the area finally becomes painful during stimulation and there is a noticeable twitch of the muscles in the neck and shoulder on that side. When this occurs, the patient will generally discontinue the EPR stimulation. Continued viability, qualitatively and quantitatively, is again tested by the previously discussed methods. Reoperation can occur in the neck if there is enough space or the thoracic approach is more commonly used for the second surgery to get adequate placement of the electrode.

Equipment failure may also occur and the most common site is where the wiring attaches to the circular antenna. This is a major area of problems because of bending and pulling. The manufacturer generally supplies an extra set of antennae and wires for just this reason. Another common problem is that of battery failure. Using newer and long-term batteries, a 4–5 weeks' duration can be approached instead of daily changes of batteries. Two complete sets of batteries are recommended with one set being continually in the process of recharging. Another problem is that of receiver failure. This could be caused by the slow leakage of body fluids into the plastic case around the receiver or due to deterioration of the receiver. This has happened in as short a period as 1 year; or, the receiver may last as long as 7–8 years. Both patient and family must be educated and alerted to these potential hazards to manage them at home.

Clinical Results

Results from a series of 37 apneic patients admitted to The Institute for Rehabilitation and Research between 1968 and 1987 revealed 11 females and 26 males. The age at onset varied between 4 and 54 years with a mean of 19 years. There was a total of 35 EPR implants in 18 patients. Onset of injury to time of implant varied from 3 months to 45 months with a mean of 14 months. The status of the 18 patients, as of December 1987, is nine living and nine dead. Of the surviving patients, five are using an EPR full-time and four on a part-time basis. One of the latter four cases could and should be on a full-time basis, but the family physician believes that the nerve may "burn out" and thus the patient sleeps on a mechanical ventilator at night. No evidence of nerve burnout has been found in any cases in this series. In the longest case (20 years from onset) the minimal electrical threshold and amount of electrical stimulation is the same in 1988 as it was initially in 1969. Electrophrenic respiration is a very viable option in carefully selected candidates with apneic quadriplegia on the condition that the guidelines are carefully followed and that the patient and family desire this particular option.

REFERENCES

1. Woollam CHM (1976): The development of apparatus for intermittent negative pressure respiration (2) 1919–1976, with special reference to development and uses of cuirass respiratory. *Anesthesia* 1931:666–685.
2. Colbert AP, Schock NC (1985): Respirator use in progressive neuromuscular diseases. *Arch Phys Med Rehabil* 66:760–762.
3. Alexander MA, Johnson EW, Petty J, Stuach D (1979): Mechanical ventilation of patients with late stage Duchenne muscular dystrophy: management in the home. *Arch Phys Med Rehabil* 60:289–292.
4. Splaingard ML, Frates RC, Harrison GM, Carter RE, Jefferson LS (1983): Home positive-pressure ventilation, twenty years' experience. *Chest* 84:376–382.
5. Splaingard ML, Frates RC, Jefferson LS, Rosen CL, Harrison GM (1985): Home negative pressure ventilation: report of 20 years of experience in patients with neuromuscular disease. *Arch Phys Med Rehabil* 66:239–242.
6. Adamson JP, Lewis L, Stein JD (1959): Application of abdominal pressure for artificial respiration. *JAMA* 169:1613–1617.
7. Hill NS (1986): Clinical applications of body ventilators. *Chest* 90:897–905.
8. Gardner BP, Watt WH, Krishnan K (1986): The artificial ventilation of acute spinal cord damaged patients: a retrospective study of forty-four patients. *Paraplegia* 24:208–220.
9. Miller SL, Sperling KB (1983): Evaluation and respiratory management of a C3 quadriplegic lacking diaphragmatic function. *Arch Phys Med Rehabil* 64:496.
10. Whiteneck GG, Carter RE, Charlifue SW, Hall KM, Menter RR, Wilkerson MA, Wilmot CB (1985): *A Collaborative Study of High Quadriplegia* (Rocky Mountain Regional Spinal Injury System, Northern California Regional Spinal Injury System, and Texas Regional Spinal Cord Injury System). Englewood, CO: Craig Hospital.

13

Rehabilitation Nursing Issues

Barbara R. Vaughn and Phyllis M. Syers*

*Spinal Cord Injury Unit, The Institute for Rehabilitation and Research, Houston, Texas, and *St. Joseph's Medical Center, South Bend, Indiana, U.S.A.*

Rehabilitation for the high quadriplegic patient requires expert medical attention but also demands the interventions from an interdisciplinary team of which the nurse must be a vital part.

Rehabilitation is an ongoing process measured over a period of time. The professional nurse possesses essential qualities in a rehabilitation setting. The nurse serves as the patient's advocate and develops the patient in becoming his or her own advocate. The process of rehabilitation requires a nurse with the innate ability to know when to assist the patient and when to foster or allow independence.

The transition from maintaining life to a focus on stabilization and retraining is at best difficult for the patient and family. It provides the ultimate nursing challenge because of the overwhelming frustration for the patient and family.

The patient may have many reservations about the new staff, and will need to be reassured and given as much background as feasible on the facility's capabilities in working with high-risk quadriplegic patients. Ample time must be given to the patient and the family to express their feelings about the move. It must be explained to the patient that the decision to transfer to a rehabilitation unit is based on the overall improvement in his physical status.

It has been said that "Nurses who practice in rehabilitation possess special knowledge and clinical skills to deal with the profound impact of disability upon individuals, their families, and significant others. Such knowledge and skills are appropriate to the magnitude of disruption to clients' physical, social, emotional, economic, and vocational status throughout their lives" (1).

Within the philosophy of rehabilitation nursing, prevention of complication, restoration of optimal functioning, and maintenance of physical, mental, and spiritual well-being are the keys to the entire process. Special emphasis is focused on the long-term adjustments that would assist individuals and their families in focusing on life after hospitalization.

THE ROLE OF THE REGISTERED NURSE

The registered nurse is generally the first person to greet the patient and the family. She has to make a lasting impression, make the patient comfortable, and introduce the rules and regulations that govern the unit. It is important to the nurse that the patient is motivated and have a general idea of what he would like to accomplish. She will expect the patient to be respectful and cooperative with the rehabilitation program. In return, the nurse will deliver 24-h-a-day skilled nursing care. She will allow the patient choices within limits and will give him the education needed for decision making.

In these changing times when high quadriplegic patients are surviving some of the most severe multitrauma injuries, it is essential that the nursing care be of the highest quality. Certification in the area of rehabilitation nursing has become an important and essential credential for the nurse dictated by the times.

Patients with a high cord injury often view rehabilitation as a means to full recovery no matter what they have been told previously. Once these patients arrive at the rehabilitation center the staff may be viewed unfavorably because this is where a breakdown of natural hopes begins to occur. One of the initial roles of the nurse is the development of trust between the nurse, the patient, and the family.

The family's involvement in the rehabilitation process of the patient with a high cord injury is of the utmost importance. Because of the responsibilities created by respiratory quadriplegia, it is extremely important that the family's needs and reactions to the situation be thoroughly evaluated. One of the major tasks of the team will be to have the adjustment level of the family complement that of the patient. It will be necessary to explain to the family that the main goal during the patient's admission will be that the patient learn to make intelligent decisions about his or her care. However, reassurance must be given that this care will be provided and evaluated to determine when the time is appropriate for others, be it the patient, family, or attendant, to start to take over these responsibilities. Families often need reassurance that it is safe to leave their family member when they have been in constant attendance at the bedside since injury. It becomes the nurse's job to convince them that separation is essential to the success of the program.

The nursing staff is caught in a dilemma of trying to deliver quality care and promoting good public relations. We have to be peacemakers and problem solvers simultaneously. To be proficient caregivers, the nursing staff has to have excellent assessment skills, psychosocial knowledge, and clinical expertise in acute as well as long-term management, coupled with the ability to problem-solve and teach. The nurse not only has to keep abreast of nursing issues, but must also be sensitive to ongoing patient, family, and community needs. Orientation and education of the patient and the family to rehabilitation and rehabilitation nursing turns into a situational priority.

Another goal of the rehabilitation process is to help the patient set obtainable goals. The team will need to work together to provide the patient and family with a clear picture of how the team fits into the accomplishments of these goals. It is vital that the transferring nurse and the receiving nurse have a clear understanding of the long-term goals and the magnitude of potential problems that may surface. If these issues are addressed immediately, a portion of the staff's work with the patient and family will be handled in a more efficient way.

COMMON NURSING DIAGNOSIS OF HIGH QUADRIPLEGIC PATIENTS

The patient entering the rehabilitation center for the first time comes with a variety of ideas related to this injury and to his or her care. Some of these ideas are accurate and others are incorrect. A task of the nurse will be to provide the patient with pertinent data to correct the misinformation. Much of the information from the patient and the family will be based on their interpretation of what was told to them in the acute-care setting.

The high quadriplegic patient may present with several problems during the rehabilitation phase. The nurse in many instances will be responsible for managing or assisting in the management of these problems. In this section of the book we will look at some of these areas and will discuss them in the form of nursing diagnosis. A nursing diagnosis is defined as a "term representing a cluster of signs and symptoms. It can be described as an actual or potential health problem or state of the patient which nurses, by virtue of their education and experience, are licensed and able to treat" (2).

Alteration in Respiratory Status

One of the major threats to the high quadriplegic patient is respiratory insufficiency. The loss of the phrenic nerve's innervation of the diaphragm and loss of intercostal muscles are fairly common occurrences in this population because of the level of their injury. A mechanical ventilator may be used to provide respiratory support or may be necessary to sustain life.

The respiratory involvement with the high quadriplegic patient is one of the major factors that makes them different from other spinal cord injuries. Depending on the level of the injury the respiratory quadriplegic patient will lose sensation and motor control of the head and neck area. The patient with a C1 injury may only be able to control the activities of the face.

The major goal for these patients will be establishing means of maintaining optimal respiratory function. The goal is usually to maintain the patient on some form of portable equipment. Once the patient is on room air, the type of equipment can be determined. The nurse will work closely with the respiratory care department to educate the patient and family on what it means to be "apneic." Inability to breathe without some means of mechanical support can be frightening. They must be taught how to frog breathe, how to care for the equipment, how to suction the patient, and how to determine early that a potential problem may exist. This patient needs to be in view and to have assistance available at all times. Constant assessment of the functioning of the equipment must be maintained.

Tracheal Stenosis of the Apneic Patient

Some factors to consider are long-term ventilation requiring a cuffed tracheostomy tube, the presence of infection, misalignment of the tracheostomy tube such that the tube's tip lies directly against the tracheal wall, incorrect tracheostomy size (e.g., too small a tube not only compromises airway potency but also necessitates high cuff pressures to obtain an adequate seal), the patient's general poor condition, and preexisting disease.

The nurse's intervention will include never adding air to the tracheostomy cuff without measuring cuff pressures, maintaining the tracheostomy tube in midline alignment, securing the tube to prevent unnecessary motion, and arranging ventilatory tubing assembly to prevent traction or pulling on the tube.

Airway Obstruction

The nurse will need to be aware of airway obstruction related to increased secretions or thick secretions or related to inability to pass air through the respiratory passage.

If this problem arises, the patient will produce a large amount of secretions that may be dry from inadequate humidification. There will be an accumulation of secretions around the cuff. The absence of Valsalva maneuver, which limits ability to cough and deep breathe, will also be a contributing factor.

In planning a course of treatment, the nurse must monitor and support respiratory therapy by positioning the patient for the most successful drainage of secretions along with chest physiotherapy, suctioning as frequently as necessary, observing for signs/symptoms of respirations, inspecting the chest for symmetrical expansion, ausculating breath sounds, monitoring vital signs, monitoring blood studies for abnormal gas exchange, and the intended effect of the therapy prescribed for the patient. It may be necessary to liquify secretions by instilling saline into the tracheostomy.

Respiratory Infections

There is always a potential for infection related to dependence on maintenance of an artificial (tracheostomy) airway. The nurse must look for the presence of a moist cough, increased amount of purulent secretions, elevated temperature, and constant need to introduce a foreign object into airway as in suctioning. These make patients more susceptible to infections.

Some simple measures that can be implemented are checking the tracheostomy tube for patency and cleanliness, inspecting for bleeding/irritation around the tracheostomy site, inspecting the chest for symmetrical expansion, monitoring blood studies for abnormal gas exchange, and auscultating breath sounds.

The patient must also be encouraged or assisted with deep breathing and coughing. Ample support should be given to respiratory therapy in the checking of cuff pressure to prevent cuff-related infections. The nurse must monitor and assess the need for tracheostomy tube changes. Sterile technique must be maintained and the patient must be suctioned as needed. The tracheostomy must be shielded from backflow of water in tubes. It is also important to clean and change the tracheostomy dressing as needed. If applicable, the inner cannula must be removed and cleaned daily. The nurse should explain to the patient the reasons for any plans.

Weaning

There may be an inability to remove the patient from mechanical ventilator due to anxiety or fear that they may not be able to breathe.

Before weaning can be accomplished, the patient must build a tolerance of a reduced concentration of inspired oxygen, ideally to room air, have acceptable pulmonary function studies and arterial blood gases, be free from infected secretions, and have stable blood pressure and pulse.

The nurse must explain the weaning process to the patient and to significant others. In planning the process the nurse has to consider and incorporate in the plan reasons for the patient's fear and anxiety. These may include history of previous respiratory arrest, feeling that they need high tidal volumes, history of recurrent infections, and a general fear of being left alone. At this time the nurse should encourage the patient to learn glossopharyngeal breathing. Monitoring arterial blood gases is very crucial at this time to ensure adequate gas exchange. The patient will need to be assessed frequently for distress of ventilation impairment. At the first signs of distress the plug must be removed and the mechanical ventilator restored. The nurse during this phase will be working with the respiratory therapy team to follow and monitor the protocol set by pulmonary physicians.

Alteration in Cardiovascular System

Not all high quadriplegic patients will be affected by the problems identified in this chapter but the nurse must be able to identify the early signs of the problem and help the patient to understand why they may have occurred and what the best management for the problem is. Immobility provides a perfect situation for venous stasis and there are many complications that can exist because of it. Pulmonary embolism is very critical, and the single most common occurrence.

After a spinal cord injury, low blood pressure is often a problem because the size and tone of blood vessels may be altered. Many of the acute situations that arise for these patients are related to the changes in the autonomic nervous system.

Information must be provided on signs and symptoms of dysreflexia, arrhythmias, hypotension, and thrombosis. Dizziness and temporary loss of consciousness is often reported when patients begin a sitting program or are increased to a new position. Abdominal binders and elastic hose are very helpful in the management of these cases. It is absolutely necessary that the patients and their caregivers be aware of the patient's signs and symptoms related to these conditions.

All information that pertains to the patient's circulation must be a part of the care plan and all caregivers must be educated concerning the rationales. The patient's thighs should be measured weekly and any changes should be brought to the attention of the physician because these changes may be the first indicators that thrombophlebitis has occurred.

Advancement to various levels and activities during the rehabilitation stage may be affected by the patient's circulation and time must be allowed for the body to adjust.

Thrombophlebitis

Thrombophlebitis secondary to immobility and decreased circulation is one area that must be addressed with high quadriplegic patients. Often they are immobilized for long periods. The presence of low blood pressure, loss of vasomotor tone, and decreased venous return will provide an atmosphere conducive to the formation of thrombophlebitis.

These patients must be monitored for signs and symptoms of venous thrombosis, i.e., heat, pain, redness, fever, edema, etc. Elevating lower extremities without extreme hip flexion will help decrease chances for thrombus formation. A decrease in the use of constrictive clothing and monitoring closely the use of leg bags will also help. The use of antiembolism stockings when sitting will also help with venous stasis. Range-of-motion exercises should be provided routinely for these patients to promote optimal circulation.

Orthostatic Hypotension

Orthostatic hypotension related to changes in position is often seen in these patients when a sitting program is initiated. It usually occurs during a sudden change from a lying to a sitting position. A history of low blood pressure, tachycardia, and pallor are symptoms that the patient may display. Impaired sympathetic nervous system, especially above T-6, and blood pooling in extremities are contributing factors to orthostatic hypotension.

The patient has to be monitored for dizziness. Avoid turning patients abruptly in bed: progress slowly and smoothly. Elevating the head of bed at least 30° before sitting the patient upright in a chair often is helpful. The use of the abdominal binders and elastic hose when sitting also helps. Elevate the patient's legs when they are sitting until they can tolerate them in a down position. For temporary relief at initial sittings tilt the wheelchair to alleviate symptoms. If not contraindicated encourage the patient to consume foods high in sodium. It is essential also that the patient eat before sitting, especially breakfast.

Alteration in Urinary Status

Urinary complications were once one of the leading causes of death in the high quadriplegic patient. It still accounts for a significant statistic. However, accurate assessment and the prevention of complications has accounted for the reduction of these fatalities. Early recognition of symptomatic signs and appropriate interventions have also contributed to the low incidence of fatalities.

Management of the urinary system is a nursing goal for the high quadriplegic patient. The primary focus in bladder management will be adequate emptying and prevention of urinary-tract infections. The problems with managing the bladder can interrupt the patient's entire day. If patients have to live with the threat of becoming wet they may choose to isolate themselves rather than face this embarrassment.

Instructions must be given to the patient on adequate fluid intake and how it affects the urinary system. They need to understand that taking in too much fluid volume, depending on the type of system used, is just as critical as not taking in enough.

To better prepare patients it is necessary for them to understand the type of bladder they have. The "flaccid" bladder usually occurs immediately after injury but for our patient population we will be looking primarily at managing the "reflex" bladder. This bladder is spastic. A sphincter automatically relaxes when the bladder is full and empties itself. These patients may be permitted to void by external catheter, indwelling Foley (urethral or suprapubic), or artificial sphincter.

Infection-causing organisms can enter the tract in various locations: (a) at the junction of the catheter and urethra; (b) at the catheter connecting to the drainage tubing; or (c) at the end of the drainage set into the collecting bag or bottle.

Special instructions must be given on how and when to change the system, especially if the device is indwelling. Cleanliness of the entire genital area will help the patient to maintain an infection-free tract. Even though the high quadriplegic patient will not be able to physically perform the tasks associated with the bladder, it is essential that they be provided with the information so that they may be able to instruct or direct others in their care.

Problems with the urinary system affect a large portion of high quadriplegic patients. Everything the patient is involved in may be affected by inadequate management of urinary status. The amount of urine excreted is affected by many things, such as the amount of fluid intake and method of urinary drainage.

Urinary Infections

Urinary tract infection related to inadequate fluid intake is a very common occurrence. The presence of an indwelling catheter is one area that must be watched closely. Incomplete bladder emptying, the presence of alkaline urine, and overextension are all factors that must be considered. There also may be an increase in white blood cells that would be indicative of a urinary-tract infection. If the patient has an indwelling catheter or is self voiding, force fluids to dilute urine. Intake should be sufficient to maintain output at ~3,000 ml/day. Maintaining sterile technique for intermittent catherization is a must. The nurse must monitor the urine for changes in color, odor, or presence of sediments. Patients are encouraged to take one-half their daily fluid in water, and must be observed for voiding patterns; fluid intake should be adjusted accordingly.

Choosing the Proper System

In choosing the most appropriate urinary management suited to the needs of the patient's lifestyle one must consider living arrangement for the home, cost and availability of equipment, patient and family's willingness and ability to follow through with the program, and studies that indicate type of bladder, i.e., reflex neurogenic or autonomous neurogenic.

The nurse must provide patients with information on all methods available to them based on the findings of their urologic workup. These are primarily suprapubic, intermittent catherization, self-voiding per external catheter, bladder tapping, and Credé method.

Alteration in Bowel Elimination

The development of an effective bowel program is essential. The nurse must understand the level and completeness of the spinal cord lesion before the type of program can be established. There are two kinds of bowel functions after a spinal cord injury; reflex neurogenic (spastic) and autonomous neurogenic (flaccid). High quadriplegic persons have upper motor neuron lesions and will have reflex bowel function unless two lesions exist. For this population of patients a functioning bowel program is essential or it could cause some compromise of the patient's respiratory status.

Before their spinal cord injury few patients give any thought to their bowel evacuation. This is often the most reluctant part of care for the significant others to learn and assume. The patient must be given information on what alters the bowel program, for example, nutrition, exercise, and emotional stress. The nurse must consider the patient's preinjury habits before establishing a new program. Information must be given on how the program works and why. Explanations need to be detailed but simple. One of the important factors that the patient must be aware of is that eventually, if an adequate program is not maintained, it will affect the patient's other body systems and cause complications that could lead to very serious problems, i.e., paralytic ileus.

The patient must be given information on dysreflexia and how to respond when it relates to the bowels. Information to be included is signs and symptoms of dysreflexia and treatment. The patient must understand that left untreated, dysreflexia can cause death. The symptoms that the patient should be aware of could present as a group or they may appear alone. They include flushed skin, ringing in the ears, shaking, chills, nervousness, splotchiness above the level of injury, elevated blood pressure, and severe pounding like a headache.

Treatment for the problem is based on the cause. If bowel related, an ointment must be used to anesthetize the nerve endings before attempting to evacuate the stool from the rectum. Any restrictive clothing should be removed and the head should be elevated if the patient is lying down.

Paralytic Ileus

Another area of concern is the development of a paralytic ileus related to decreased peristolsis. This usually occurs after 48 h in cervical injury. The patient presents with severe abdominal distention and distress. No bowel sounds will be present. A small amount of flatus and/or stool may be passed. Untreated, this can lead to aspiration, vomitus, and subsequent respiratory arrest. Contributing factors may include prolonged spinal shock, decreased fluid intake, immobility, chronic constipation, and lack of a bowel program.

Some nursing measures include documentation of specific observations to aid in diagnosis. The nurse may need to insert an appropriate size nasogastric tube to low suction. The nurse will need to monitor and assess the need for fluid and electrolyte replacement. The patient has to be monitored daily for the presence of returned bowel sounds.

Increased Flatus

The patient may experience abdominal distention related to increased flatus. The high quadriplegic patient may swallow large amounts of air if the tracheostomy tube cuff is deflated. The supine position adds to the buildup of abdominal distention. Excessive salivation may lead to an excessive swallowing of air. The patient also presents with feeling of fullness, cramping pain, gurgling bowel sounds, and abdominal tympany.

To help alleviate the patient's problem, the nurse must inspect the abdomen for distention, explain to the patient possible causes of the problem, reposition the patient often, discourage iced liquids, discourage use of straws for liquids, restrict intake of gas-forming foods, limit fluids with meals, and assure the patient that the problem is not detrimental to his or her health. Surgery may be necessary for relief of an intestinal obstruction.

Bowel Training

Another major goal for the patient is scheduled bowel movements. The patient may present with recurrent constipation, then diarrhea, then constipation again—the constipation cycle. The nurse has to look at the effects of medications, nutrition, activity, and exercise. The level of injury may also affect the type of program.

To establish the most effective program the nurse must check the bowel program record over several days to have a clear picture of what is actually occurring. Vigorous treatment, i.e., laxatives, enemas, should be implemented if there is no bowel movement for several days. Manual removal may be necessary before the regulated program if there is impaction. The nurse must encourage the patient to eat bulk-forming foods and avoid foods that stimulate diarrhea. The nurse will have to monitor for fluid and electrolyte balance and administer medications as appropriate. Based on patient's needs, an appropriate time for bowel evacuation should be assessed. An ongoing daily assessment of the program will be necessary until the patient becomes regular. The nurse has to evaluate the plan of treatment and adjust as necessary.

Alteration in Integrity of Skin

There are many factors that affect a person's ability to maintain adequate skin integrity. Loss of sensory and voluntary motor ability below the level of the lesion, damage to the autonomic nervous system, and altered circulation are just a few. One of the nurse's major functions will be prevention of skin ulcers. Early detection and constant assessment of the skin is primarily the nurse's responsibility.

General Hygiene

The patient is taught how to take care of the skin. Problems with the skin can delay the patient's entire rehabilitation process and therefore is of utmost importance. Information must be provided to the patient on why the skin breaks so easily and the more successful means of prevention. The nurse should teach the patient to keep the skin clean and dry. The use of extra pads should be avoided. Creams, oils, or lotions may be used to prevent dry, cracked, scaly skin. Changing the patient's position frequently is another key point. Repositioning not only aids in prevention of skin problems, but for the high quadriplegic individual, it is important in the mobility of secretions. The patient's turning schedule may begin at every 2 h and increase to tolerance. The skin should be checked before and after each turn and after sitting until skin tolerance has been established.

Pressure Sores

Protection must be provided for bony prominences by use of cushions or padding. At the first sign of any irritation the most effective treatment is to keep the patient off the area. Overexposure to sunlight can cause burns and skin irritation. Bed rest for a long period, circulatory changes, and dry skin contribute to the possibility of skin breakdown.

Other factors that may relate to this problem are decreased blood flow to skin, excessive capillary pressure, inadequate nutritional status, under- or overweight, contractures, spasms, heat, moisture, cold, and dryness of skin, long periods of bed rest, oversitting in a wheelchair, and sitting with the head of the bed elevated.

Burns

Burns related to decreased skin sensation is one situation that often occurs, but can be easily prevented. Areas to consider in relationship to burns are decreased blood flow to skin, absence of nerve endings regulating sensations to temperature, and lack of sensory warning mechanisms, inability to move freely, and circulatory changes (3).

The nurse has to assess and document any signs of damage to the skin and remove the cause if possible. Instructions should be given to the patient and/or significant other on alteration in sensation of pressure and temperature. The patient should be cautioned about long exposures to sun, avoiding exposure to either extreme hot or cold, using heating pads, and monitoring closely the temperature of water in tub or shower.

Alteration in Sexual Functioning

Sexual functioning remains a priority to those patients with multiple trauma and physical disabilities. Human sexuality becomes a desire that is priceless. Anxiety and fear can be alleviated and sexual gratification can still be achieved with appropriate teaching and interventions.

A firm understanding of sexual potential is as important to high quadriplegic patients and their families as is their respiratory status. Immobility and respiratory compromise cannot interfere with the desire to remain a sexual human being. Nurses can help patients to understand their sexual potential and to identify with their new-found sexual image.

As confirmed elsewhere (4–7), contributors to the patients' sexual inhibitions are role change, changes in body image, lack of privacy, limited communication skills, preinjury dissatisfaction with sexual performance, lack of a willing significant other, values conflict, motor and/or sensory deficits, fear, and anxiety.

Nursing interventions may include but not be limited to: (a) providing education information; (b) listening to the patient's desires and expectations; (c) exploring the patient's feelings regarding his or her sexual image and potential; (d) educating the patient and significant other regarding the effects of sexual activity on the respiratory and cardiovascular systems; (e) offering educational information concerning medications that may affect and/or influence sexual functioning; (f) involving the patient and/or significant other in group sessions, workshops, and/or sexual counseling; (g) involving the significant other in emergency protocols to facilitate pleasurable sexual options and prevent life-threatening crisis; (h) instructing the patient and significant other on ways to optimize sexual relationships; (i) discussing sexual options and alternative means of achieving these options; and (j) discussing fertility and/or the effects of infertility.

Alteration in Nutrition

Chronic disabling conditions often are coupled with nutritional deficiencies. Those deficits often lead to negative nitrogen balance and heterotopic ossification.

Factors that may affect the patient's nutritional status are increased work of breathing, knowledge deficit regarding minimum daily requirements, inability to absorb nutrients, adverse drug reaction, anxiety, depression, and stress ulcers.

Much can affect the patient's appetite. The nurse must work closely with the patient, family, and dietitian to maintain the patient's adequate nutritional status. The high quadriplegic will be unable to feed himself/herself and may find it difficult reverting to being fed. The nurse must recognize this and work it into the patient's plan of care. The patient may also feel fatigued and this also affects the appetite.

Interventions to curtail these problems include assessment of bowel sounds, daily weight, teaching regarding metabolic requirements, monitoring laboratory values: nitrogen balance; albumin; total protein; caloric count monitoring, maintaining adequate oral hygiene, assessment for aspiration, allowing sufficient time for feeding, offering protein supplements as appropriate, minimizing alcohol and caffeine intake, administering fluid intake to prevent dehydration, making appropriate referrals to dietitian or nutritionist, and determining food preferences.

The dietitian should be consulted in assessing a proper diet for the patient. If the patient has to be fed per gastric tube, adequate explanations must be afforded the patient and family. In high quadriplegia, the patient and family must understand that one of the most important factors is to maintain an adequate airway.

The nurse must also evaluate accompanying conditions that may interfere with food intake (i.e., nausea, vomiting, no teeth, poor oral hygiene, loose dentures, etc.).

Alteration in Comfort Level

Because a person has sustained a cervical spinal cord injury does not mean they will not experience pain. The nurse must listen to the patient's complaints of pain and believe that it is real. If patients are to benefit from comfort measures offered by the nurse, they must feel that their pain is being perceived the way they are experiencing it. Treatment of pain in the spinal-cord-injured patient is very difficult to assess, especially if it is below the level of the injury. Routine management becomes more complicated.

Pain

An often misunderstood problem is pain management related to phantom sensations. This problem is difficult to work with because it is hard to understand how pain can exist below the level of the spinal cord injury.

The patient complains of a burning, stinging sensation, often influenced by anxiety, fatigue, and exercise. Phantom sensations are affected by the completeness of the injury. Rarely does total loss of sensation occur below the level of injury. Scarring or nerve-root entrapment causes sensations of numbness, tingling, burning, or stabbing and this is often what causes the patient to have uncomfortable feelings.

The nurse has to reassure the patient that the pain is being taken seriously. It has to be assessed thoroughly and medications administered as ordered. Other measures include positioning extremities and head to allow the most comfortable position, removing any external sources of pain, positioning the body in proper alignment, making the environment as pleasant as possible, allowing the patient to ventilate feelings, and providing the patient with a reasonable explanation as to why pain may exist and recommendations to alleviate it.

Spasticity

Another problem for the patient is compromised comfort level related to spasticity. The patient will have increased muscle tone initiated by emotion and cutaneous stimulation or agitated by environmental changes.

Stimulation of an intact reflex arc below the level of injury is the cause of these uncomfortable spasms. To decrease these spasms the possible cause of the spasm will need to be assessed. Antispasmodic agents should be administered as prescribed, extremities should be arranged as appropriate, and the patient should be provided with information on how spasms may be useful. Additionally, the patient should be positioned to decrease chances for external stimuli, and the environment should be monitored or altered to be more conducive to decreasing the spasm. Lastly, the need for neuroelectric stimulation should be assessed.

REFERENCES

1. American Nurses Association and Association of Rehabilitation Nurses (1986): *Standards of Rehabilitation Nursing Practice.* Kansas City, MO: American Nurses Association, p. 2.
2. Syers P, Ackerman J (1986): *Nursing Care of the "High Risk" Ventilator Dependent Quadriplegic.* Houston, National Institute of Handicapped Research.
3. Zejdik C (1983): *Management of Spinal Cord Injury.* California: Wadsworth Health Science Division.
4. Hogan R (1980): *Human Sexuality: A Nursing Perspective.* New York, Appleton Century Crofts.
5. Masters WH, Johnson VE (1966): *Human Sexual Responses.* London, Churchill Livingstone.
6. Mooney T, Cole RM, Chilgren RA (1975): *Sexual Options for Paraplegics and Quadriplegics.* Boston, Little, Brown.
7. Latimer, AM (1981): Accountability for the sexual awareness of the spinal cord injured patient. *Rehabil Nurs J* 6:8–11.

14

Occupational and Physical Therapy

Gail Gilinsky and Janet McIntyre

Craig Hospital, Englewood, Colorado, U.S.A.

This chapter presents the program and goals of therapy in treating the high quadriplegic patient. From the initial acute care phase and throughout the entire hospitalization, a well-coordinated team effort is required. The focus of this chapter is on the occupational and physical therapy aspects of that team effort. The areas of evaluation, mobilization, program content and progression, some equipment needs, and other special considerations are discussed. Equipment issues will be presented in detail in Chapter 15. The complexities of managing the high quadriplegic patient—such as emergency procedures and dealing with the multitude of equipment—are also addressed in this chapter.

EVALUATION/EARLY MOBILIZATION

As with any therapy program, an initial evaluation is the first step. A comprehensive evaluation should include a detailed sensory test, specific manual muscle test, complete range-of-motion assessment, and functional status evaluation. If evidence of a closed-head injury exists, cognitive-perceptual-motor evaluation is indicated. On completion of evaluation, realistic short-term and long-term goals can be set with an appropriate program and time frame. Goals will vary slightly from the C1 to C4 level of injury and from individual to individual. Some typical objectives for the high quadriplegic patient include the following: (a) to increase or prevent loss of range of motion; (b) to increase strength and coordination of present musculature; (c) to increase endurance; (d) to assess bulbar function and make recommendations for safe diet; (e) to achieve independence in power wheelchair mobility and in weight shifts;

(f) to maximize independence in functional activities—focus on communication skills; (g) to assess home environment and make appropriate recommendations for wheelchair accessibility; (h) to address transportation issues; (i) to train family/attendants in care; and (j) to educate the patient and family regarding spinal cord injury.

Occupational and physical therapy should begin early in the acute care setting (1), even before the patient is mobilized. Most of the evaluation can be accomplished while the patient is still in bed, and this early contact gives the therapist a chance to begin building trust and rapport with the patient.

Some specific therapy activities can also begin during this time. Certainly upper and lower extremity range-of-motion and strengthening exercises could be initiated before the patient is mobilized from bed. Most often the neck is initially immobilized, so neck exercises may be postponed or limited to isometrics. While the patient is restricted to bed, some centers begin a series of tongue and mouth exercises. This will improve strength and coordination of mouth muscles to prepare the patient for mouthstick activities.

Splinting may be considered to prevent foot drop, or resting hand splints may be used to maintain functional position. These may not be necessary if adequate range of motion is maintained by a good passive range-of-motion program. Some centers maintain upper extremities in abduction and external rotation with platform splints to prevent the typical loss of range of motion (2).

Shoulder pain is very prevalent with this population. Early intervention of passive range of motion and mobilization will likely decrease this complication in later stages. If left unattended early on, patients could develop increased pain and joint contractures.

As part of the preparation for mobilizing the high quadriplegic patient, the occupational therapy/physical therapy staff must be thoroughly trained in the respiratory and medical needs of each patient. The therapists are knowledgeable regarding the ventilator alarms, emergency procedures, ambubag use, and suctioning. With the assistance of a well-coordinated team, they are also comfortable in managing possible intravenous lines, oxygen tanks, and supplemental feeding devices during transfers and therapy. This allows for mobilization outside the patient's room to the treatment areas (3). The ability to treat patients away from direct nursing involvement increases the trust and comfort level of both the patient and family in the therapy staff. To help decrease apprehensions, each new procedure is thoroughly explained step-by-step to the patient. Family members are often encouraged to observe.

Successfully mobilizing the high quadriplegic for the first time requires excellent communication between respiratory therapists, nurses, nurses' aides, orderlies, and physical and occupational therapists. To make the transition from bed to wheelchair less threatening and to decrease postural hypotension, a tilt table is often used initially. The tilt table can be used either in the patient's room or preferably in the regular treatment area.

A three-person flat lift, which provides the patient with the most security early on, is used to get the patient onto the tilt table. This process is greatly simplified if a portable ventilator is used. The ventilator and suction machine can be placed on a wheeled cart next to the patient. If enough dead-space tubing is available, the patient can remain on the ventilator throughout the lift. Otherwise, the ambubag may be used until the patient is securely placed on the tilt table.

The tilt table is often used for an hour or for as long as the patient can tolerate. Therapists carefully monitor the patient's blood pressure as the patient slowly progresses to the upright position. High quadriplegic patients are particularly susceptible to hypotension. Abdominal binders and thromboembolic disease hose are often used to help decrease pooling of blood in the lower extremities.

An alternative to using the tilt table for mobilization would be to transfer the patient directly from bed to a reclined wheelchair with elevated legrests, and to gradually raise the back of the wheelchair (4). Raising the head of the bed before transfer from the bed will help alleviate difficulty with hypotension.

When the tilt table is used and the patient manages well in the upright position, the next step is providing the patient with a temporary, full recline, manual wheelchair. Patients use this wheelchair until they receive their own. The wheelchair should have an appropriate headrest, elevating sliding arm troughs or lapboard, elevating legrests, appropriate cushion, and chest and waist belts. It should also have a lapboard or underchair tray to place a portable ventilator, suction machine, and ambubag. The ultimate goal is to get the patient and equipment as compact as possible so that mobility and independence are maximized. Again, a three-person flat lift is used to get patients from tilt table to wheelchair. The wheelchair is generally in the semireclined or tipped-back position for ease of transfer.

The initial transfer into a wheelchair is often a very frightening experience for the patient with new feelings of hypotension, lack of stability, lack of head control, shoulder pain, etc. The body handling and movement often loosen secretions, so additional suctioning may be necessary. The patient must be made to feel as comfortable as possible. Trust in the therapist is crucial.

Education concerning the responsibility for their own skin care is initiated as soon as patients begin using the wheelchair. Tilt-back weight shifts (reclining the back of the wheelchair) are done every 15–20 min. The first time up in a wheelchair is rarely longer than 45–60 min. The patient is then returned to bed so a thorough skin check may be done to make sure there is no redness on ischial tuberosities, greater trochanters, sacrococcygeal or scapular areas. Each day the sitting time is increased slightly, as well as the amount of time between weight shifts. Other options for weight shifts include the dependent forward and side-to-side methods.

The angle toward sitting upright is slowly increased, depending on the patient's comfort level, head and neck control, and overall tolerance. Once a patient develops tolerance for the upright position, the tilt table and/or recline wheelchair with elevated legrests may not be necessary. The patient may be able to go directly from supine in bed to a fairly upright sitting position in the wheelchair. This varies from individual to individual. It may take many sessions to achieve each patient's maximum upright sitting posture. A full 90° upright position may not be feasible for C2 injuries and above, due to decreased neck strength and gravity hindering good trunk and neck alignment.

Throughout the entire early mobilization process, range-of-motion and/ or strengthening and/or relaxation exercises may be done to all extremities and neck. Functional electrical stimulation may be a useful treatment modality. It may be used to strengthen neck extensors and, therefore, improve neck posture. It may also be used to decrease shoulder subluxation (5) either by acting as a type of orthotic device or by strengthening shoulder musculature.

EDUCATION

Early in the patient's program and throughout the course of hospitalization, much effort is directed towards educating the patient regarding spinal cord injury (SCI). The patient should know and understand the aspects of care quite thoroughly. In the beginning, one does not want to overwhelm the patient and/or family with details of SCI. However, certain basic concepts should be taught. For instance, when beginning mobilization on the tilt table, the rationale and benefit of standing should be explained. Likewise, when first up in a wheelchair, the how and why of weight shifts should be detailed. As patients go through the program, they will learn much more and in greater detail, but education starts with day one.

As with any patient, it is better to explain beforehand what you are going to do and why. This is especially important with the high quadriplegic who may be feeling quite vulnerable and helpless. These explanations will help allay fears, as well as increase trust and confidence in the therapist. Families, too, are usually quite involved early on in the hospitalization; they want and need to know what is happening. They should learn a great deal throughout the rehabilitation process, with a final intensive education and, perhaps, trial experience before the patient's discharge home or from the hospital.

PSYCHOSOCIAL ISSUES

The high quadriplegic patient can be an interesting and challenging patient for a therapist. This is an individual who has immense physical losses and may be in a rather depressed or passive state. The therapist's interaction with the patient often highlights this physical loss. It is impossible for patients not to acknowledge this loss. However, the program focus should be on what the patients are able to do—not on what they are unable to do.

It is important for therapists to establish a solid rapport and trust with the patient. The therapist should respond to the patient as a person, not as a "thing" or "freak" with tubes, drains, etc. Although it may be difficult at first, one must see past the machinery. It is helpful if therapists are aware of predictable fears and issues with this type of patient, and are comfortable discussing and acknowledging them. As with any loss, grief may be expected and may have some influence on the therapy program. If uncomfortable or unsure of issues, therapists should refer to other team members such as psychologists or physicians.

Patience is often needed in communicating with the high quadriplegic patient. Lip reading and understanding the choppy, short phrases necessitated by the ventilator are often laborious, but are key in acknowledging the person and establishing some sort of relationship and rapport. Speech therapy may be helpful in the use of communication and alphabet boards and electronic communication devices.

The role of the therapist is one of advisor rather than controller. The therapist has skills and knowledge in the care of high quadriplegic patients but certainly needs the participation and involvement of the patient to be in any way successful. Initial and subsequent goal setting should be mutual between the patient and the therapist. The program is geared to educate patients about resources and techniques available and they should ultimately decide what best fits their lifestyle.

Initially, many patients are quite passive and frightened. They rely on others to give them guidance. Although patients may be passive motorwise, they should be encouraged to be cognitively assertive. Throughout rehabilitation, their participation, involvement, and responsibility should be encouraged. As patients become more mobile, educated, and medically stable, they are encouraged to take increasing responsibility and control for their care and program.

A therapist needs to be flexible and open with goals and plans. The patient must have an investment in the program. When treating any patient, treatment sessions should be planned to provide a positive, successful experience. Providing the patient with graduated successes will encourage the patient's personal investment. In planning treatment sessions, the therapist should be prepared to offer patients choices so that they have control in their program.

The importance of increasing the patient's independence and self-esteem cannot be overemphasized. Each of the specific therapy activities described in this chapter offers opportunities for the therapist to foster these feelings, as well as develop individual patient skills.

WHEELCHAIR EVALUATION

A major aspect of the high quadriplegic program is evaluation and training in a power-drive recline wheelchair. This is initiated as soon as possible. Ideally, these wheelchairs are available for trial. A power wheelchair can increase a patient's self-esteem and attitude by providing independent mobility. Figure 14-1 illustrates a patient in a fully equipped power-recline wheelchair. By giving them the means to do their own weight shifts, patients then become more responsible for their own skin care. Dependence on family members and staff is also decreased. It should be noted that some centers do not use power-recline wheelchairs but rely on a patient's ability to build skin tolerance to avoid the need for frequent weight shifts.

Having trial wheelchairs available serves a twofold purpose. First, it provides the patient independence in mobility and weight shifts on a consistent basis. Second, it allows the therapist to thoroughly evaluate the type of chair appropriate for this patient. (See Chapter 15 for details on ordering wheelchairs.) Patients are thoroughly trained in the use of

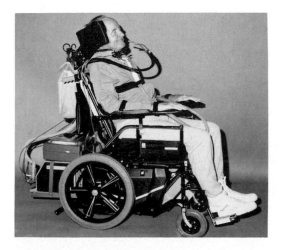

FIG. 14-1. A spastic C2 quadriplegic man with poor neck control is shown in a fully equipped power-recline wheelchair. Note how ventilator, portable suction unit, ambubag, and oxygen tank are compactly attached to the wheelchair.

the wheelchair on smooth and rough terrain before the arrival of their own wheelchair. A manual wheelchair is also ordered as a backup for power failures, or for use in areas where power wheelchairs are not manageable, e.g., stairs and loading into cars.

FUNCTIONAL ACTIVITIES

Another major role in therapy is the pursuit of functional activities for the high quadriplegic patient. For the patient with good head and neck control, the mouthstick will be a valuable tool (4). For training and evaluation, a temporary mouthstick can be made with heavy wire, dowel sticks, and respiratory care mouthpieces. Weighted or suction cup holders or goosenecks with magnets can be used to station mouthsticks when they are not being used.

With the mouthstick, the patient should be able to manage page turning, typing on an electric typewriter, computer, and telephone usage. The patient can also write, draw, and play simple board games (Figs. 14-2 and 14-3). A birdbeak/pincer mouthstick, which is available commercially, is ideal for card playing, as well as other games with small pieces to manipulate. The patient is encouraged to do mouthstick activities, not only for future vocational (4) and/or avocational interests, but also as a method of increasing neck strength, endurance, and range of motion. If the patient does not have adequate head and neck control to manage effectively with a mouthstick, electronic methods of managing telephone, computer, and page turning are explored. Environmental

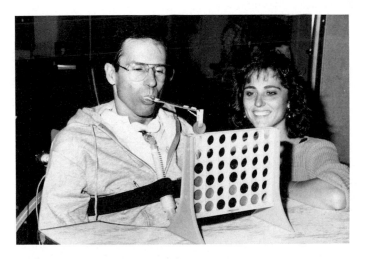

FIG. 14-2. C3 quadriplegic patient using pincer mouthstick to manipulate game pieces.

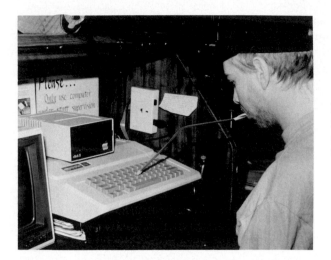

FIG. 14-3. High quadriplegic patient using a computer for prevocational activity.

controls can be interfaced with the telephone and computer, as well as with remote control for most household appliances. Access modes to these devices can be pneumatic; voice activated; head, eyebrow and tongue switches; or powered by laser light sources, to name just a few possibilities (6,7).

Most high quadriplegic patients are educated about general environmental control information, but few pursue anything very elaborate during their first hospitalization. It is generally found that neither patients nor their families are capable of determining what their specific needs will be after discharge.

Alarm and call systems are explored to cover a variety of emergency situations. At times, simple homemade methods of activating a loud noise to get a family member's attention from another room is sufficient. Other times, elaborate intercom or emergency telephone systems may be more appropriate. The individual needs of each patient are considered in this area.

TRANSFER TRAINING

Regarding transfers, the therapist has several options for the high quadriplegic patient (3,8). One must choose a "flat" transfer with the patient supine, a sitting transfer, or use of a mechanical lift. It is recommended that all types be tried with the patient. The decision can then be made by patient and therapist as to which is most appropriate. Very often in the hospital setting, there are enough personnel to do dependent patient "lifts" involving three to four lifters. However, home situations may have only one person available to do the transfer. Some

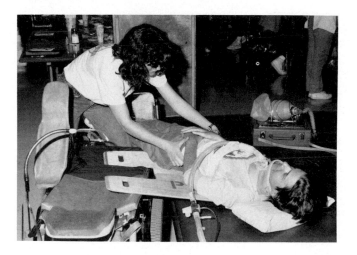

FIG. 14-4. With wheelchair fully reclined, C2 quadriplegic patient is transferred from mat to wheelchair by one person using two sliding boards.

factors that affect the decision about type of transfer include patient safety and comfort, number and size of persons able to assist, patient size, spasticity, and neck strength and stability. An important consideration with these patients is the placement of tubing and ventilators during the transfer. Tracheostomy site irritation must also be considered.

The "flat" transfer method involves the patient being supine throughout the entire transfer. This type of transfer is most often used for patients with compromised head/neck control or problems with hypotension. The size of both patient and attendant also influences this type of transfer. A full-recliner wheelchair with small rear wheels (i.e., 20-in diameter) is needed for this method. One could use either two or three sliding boards or one large board such as the commercially available Buch Board. In Fig. 14-4, the wheelchair is aligned parallel with the mat, boards are placed, and then the patient segmentally is moved (lower extremities, hips, and head and shoulders).

Another transfer method has the patient being moved in the sitting position (Fig. 14-5). For this, the patient should have some head/neck control. In some cases, a hard collar may be worn by the patient to protect an unstable neck or substitute for weak neck muscles. The same factors previously mentioned, such as attendant size, patient size, and spasticity, affect the feasibility of this transfer. If the patient is small or the attendant large, one could do a "butt-pivot" transfer without a board. In this transfer, the patient is brought from supine to sitting and leaned forward. Then, through the use of good body mechanics, the therapist

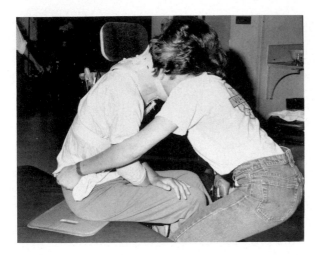

FIG. 14-5. One-person-assist sliding board transfer.

pivots the patient's buttocks from bed to wheelchair seat. This involves an actual lift with the pivot. This transfer also requires the patient to be able to tolerate sitting to at least 90° of trunk flexion and probably more forward than that.

Yet another option involves the use of a mechanical lift. This method is especially good for exceptionally large patients. In selecting this method, one must keep in mind several points. Extra space is needed to store this piece of equipment. The patient must be able to tolerate at least 90° of upright sitting. Ideally, the patient's skin would be able to tolerate sitting on the sling for the same duration as sitting in the wheelchair. However, it is possible to remove and replace the sling while the patient is sitting in the wheelchair.

In summary, when choosing a transfer method, one should bear in mind the principles stated previously and then actually try different transfers with the patient to determine which works best. Of course, the easiest transfer situation to practice is on and off a raised mat. This situation should be used to determine the best transfer method. Once this best system is worked out, other transfers can be taught, such as bed, commode chair, car, couch, airline seat, and possibly floor transfers for emergency purposes.

BODY HANDLING

As a part of a comprehensive treatment program, the high quadriplegic patient can and should be involved in a mat exercise program. The mat is an excellent place to work on range of motion, strengthening, and general body mobility. Also, the vestibular system can be stim-

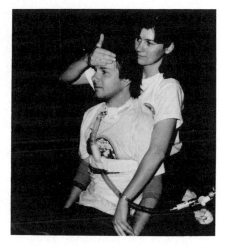

FIG. 14-6. C2 quadriplegic patient working with physical therapist on neck strengthening exercises.

ulated by the variety and type of movement (9). It shows patients that they are not "breakable" and gets them used to being handled, which prepares them for later transfers.

Figure 14-6 demonstrates a typical mat exercise with the patient long-sitting on a mat, supported by the therapist (3,9). A mirror may be placed in front of patients so they can see and control their efforts. Good neck and shoulder posture is almost always a goal. This involves both strengthening and relaxation. The upper trapezius muscles are often overly contracted and the patient must learn to relax them specifically. If any prone positioning is indicated, for instance as a potential sleeping position or to stretch hip flexors, the mat is an ideal place to introduce this activity.

In some centers, physical therapists may be responsible for respiratory evaluation and treatment. The evaluation would assess muscle strength, chest wall compliance, and bronchial hygiene (10). Treatment techniques may consist of muscle strengthening exercises (especially diaphragmatic), providing abdominal support (to help diaphragm function more effectively), increasing chest mobility (by manual chest stretching, deep breathing, glossopharyngeal breathing, etc.). To improve bronchial hygiene, one may use assistive cough techniques, suctioning, and postural drainage.

If the patient does not have a tracheostomy, aquatic exercise might be an appropriate therapy tool. The warmth and buoyancy of the water make it a terrific medium in which to work on both strengthening and relaxation, as well as range of motion. Being in the water gives the patient another sense of mobility and movement, and it can be used as a modality to decrease pain.

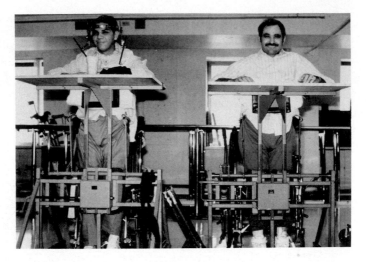

FIG. 14-7. Hydraulic standing tables being used by two high quadriplegic patients.

With some patients, a standing program may also be used. Standing the high quadriplegic patient is generally accomplished by means of a tilt table or standing table (Fig. 14-7). Initially, the tilt table is used to decrease hypotension and it allows graduated increase of upright towards 90°. The standing table is an all or nothing operation—sitting to full standing. The benefits of standing are somewhat controversial (11). Mainly, it helps maintain good range of motion of the lower extremities, particularly in hip and ankle joints. It has debatable benefit in the areas of improving circulation, decreasing spasticity, improving bowel and bladder drainage, and increasing bone density secondary to stress on long bones. Another consideration for standing is that some patients enjoy being at "eye level" once again. If interested, patients may be exposed to the standing program. Experience has shown, however, the high quadriplegic patient who pursues a standing program at home is certainly more the exception than the rule.

TRANSPORTATION

The area of transportation must be examined thoroughly. A properly modified van is the most safe and efficient method to transport a high quadriplegic individual using a power wheelchair. Because van modifications are costly, equipment recommendations made to the insurance companies should be accurate and reflect medical necessity. To help take the guesswork out of writing prescriptions, some centers have a "van clinic." At this clinic, a community vendor provides fully modified vans,

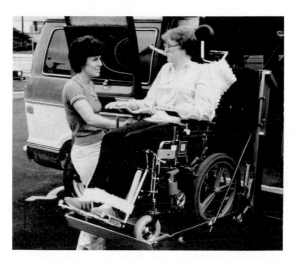

FIG. 14-8. C4 quadriplegic patient and her therapist evaluate the use of a fully automatic lift for a van.

thus making accurate evaluations of maneuverability, visual field, and proper fit of vans and lifts possible. Because of the weight and size of the power wheelchair, a fully automatic lift is most ideal (Fig. 14-8). Safety issues and equipment recommendations should be specifically outlined by a qualified therapist and/or driving instructor.

Some patients do not have the financial capability to purchase a modified van for transportation. In this case, community-based public transportation resources should be investigated. Inquiry as to whether ventilator-dependent persons are allowed to ride on public transportation should be made. If the family must use their car for transportation, positioning issues must be discussed and problem-solved for safety.

HOME ACCESSIBILITY

Another important aspect of the patient's program is the assessment of home accessibility. If the patient lives locally, it may be possible and preferable to do an actual home visit. If the patient is medically stable, he or she may accompany team members on the visit. If not, therapists should take an appropriate-size wheelchair and go through the home to ensure that hallways and doorways can accommodate the wheelchair and turning radius.

A home modifications questionnaire and booklet can be sent to the family or primary caregiver for the nonlocal patient (12,13). The questionnaire asks for pertinent information about the home and strongly encourages the caregiver to return a scale drawing of the house layout and photographs for evaluation. Team members review these plans and write suggestions or recommendations regarding home modifications.

Their recommendations are based on the equipment with which the patient will go home and should reflect the simplest, most cost-efficient modifications.

Typical wheelchair accessibility issues should be considered in evaluating the home. In addition, there are some considerations specific to the high quadriplegic: (a) a work station for communication needs, e.g., wheelchair height table; (b) van accessibility in a garage (height of van, side or back loading lift with van); (c) an auxiliary power source or generator; and (d) a good heating and/or air conditioning system (important because the high quadriplegic individual lacks temperature autoregulation).

GROUP ACTIVITIES

Because spontaneous socialization with others is often difficult for the high quadriplegic person, it is believed that group educational opportunities are extremely beneficial. Many centers have a variety of ways to meet these educational needs. The Re-entry and Exhaler classes will be discussed as examples (14).

The Exhaler Class was developed to better meet the physical, psychosocial, and educational needs specific to the high quadriplegic person. Class instructors are a multidisciplinary group, consisting of occupational and physical therapists, nurses, speech therapists, recreational therapists, respiratory care personnel, and dietitians. The 45-min class is held weekdays for a 6-week rotation. To participate, the patient must be a C4 or above quadriplegic who is deemed ready physically and emotionally by his or her treating team. The patient should be able to sit in a wheelchair, preferably upright, and attend and actively participate in the class. The class begins with passive range-of-motion and simple neck and shoulder exercises. After the warmup, one designated discipline presents a lecture. Topics may include such subjects as skin/bowel/bladder care, recreational options, wheelchair maintenance, transportation needs, care/cleaning of ventilator, airline travel, and nutrition. During this 6-week period, the therapeutic recreation department conducts an outing in the community. This outing is used for socialization, as well as training for patient and family.

Toward the end of the patient's stay, he or she is enrolled in the Re-entry class in which all SCI patients participate. This is a 3-week series of classes held every weekday morning. The various groups are led by family service counselors, recreational therapy, nurses, physicians, and peer counselors. The topics focus on discharge issues and life at home, including areas such as attendant care, sexuality, stress management, SCI research, and drug and alcohol abuse.

DISCHARGE EDUCATION/TRANSITIONAL LIVING

As stressed earlier, much of the therapy program for the high quadriplegic patient is education for the patient, family, and possible attendants. Ideally, this is ongoing throughout hospitalization. However, if the family was not present during a good portion of the patient's admission, an intensive training period is recommended. For example, a 2-week period could be used for general education with a focus on actual "hands-on" care. Even if hired attendant care is planned, a designated family member is usually trained thoroughly in case of inconsistency or illness of attendants. Of course, patients themselves are trained so they can instruct others in their own care. Often audiovisual and written aids are provided to take home. Toward the end of this 2-week period, the patient and family would be encouraged to participate in a transitional living program in an apartment complex nearby (15). If insurance will not cover this outpatient experience or apartments are not available, the patient and family are encouraged to function in an "independent living" capacity within the hospital. This situation calls for the family members to assume full responsibility for the care of the patient while he or she is still in the hospital room. However, the apartment experience itself seems the best way to ease the transition from institutionalization to real life at home.

SPECIAL CONSIDERATIONS

Other issues that complicate the high quadriplegic patient's therapy program are immobilization devices, spasticity, pain, postural problems, and brain-injury involvement. These issues are discussed below in more detail.

Initial halo vest or neck collars for orthopedic stabilization can slow down the functional aspects of the high quadriplegic patient's therapy program. For example, mouthstick activities are quite difficult, but may be possible for simple tasks if the patient is extremely motivated. The halo vest, however, should not restrict wheelchair mobilization or any general education aspect of the program.

Spasticity is often a significant problem for the high quadriplegic patient. Moderate to severe spasticity poses difficulty in their handling and management for obvious reasons. It may also limit functional capability. Range-of-motion and standing programs sometimes help to decrease spasticity. Positioning in bed and wheelchair may also be used to inhibit tone. Physicians often rely on therapists to assess and monitor the effects of drug therapy on the patient's spasticity.

Pain and contracture formation can also be an issue with this population. Most often, these contractures are in the neck and shoulder region. As discussed at the beginning of this chapter, attention and care should be given to prevent contractures. Pain is often addressed with traditional therapy techniques, such as the use of modalities, joint mobilization, relaxation, etc.

Shoulder subluxation is quite common and is best managed by proper support, especially when the patient is up in the wheelchair. Proper support is easily provided by arm troughs or lapboards on the wheelchair. Caution should always be exercised when transferring the patient to avoid pull on the glenohumeral joint.

Proper positioning and posture are quite important in the care and management of the high quadriplegic patient. Because of the significant motor loss, these patients often need stabilizing devices when sitting up in a wheelchair. Specialized headrests and trunk supports give the patient stability needed to perform functional activities. For example, a C2 quadriplegic patient with poor neck strength may need not only good trunk stabilization, but also a headrest that provides good stability to allow use of a puff-and-sip or chin control to drive the wheelchair. Special wheelchair seats and backs, trunk supports, arm troughs, cushions, and headrests are used to properly position and stabilize a patient in the wheelchair. The different devices available and the rationale for their use are discussed in Chapter 15.

A difficult complication to deal with in high quadriplegia is brain injury or brainstem involvement. The extent of the therapy program will depend on the injury site and severity of the head injury. Communication can be severely limited, or may not be present at all. Brainstem injuries can lead to the loss of facial musculature, decreasing the person's ability to express emotion. There can be memory loss and decreased reasoning skills, which can make teaching cumbersome or impractical. Patient involvement in problem solving may be minimal.

Bulbar involvement in the head-injured patient can make swallowing unsafe with certain food substances. Thorough oral-bulbar evaluations, including evaluation of the impact of head position on swallowing, along with video-fluoroscopy, will identify and specify problems. Even very small amounts of aspirated food can lead to chronic respiratory infection.

Therapy goals are usually limited for those patients with significant head injury. The main goals may be to provide the equipment and family training necessary to safely care for the patient after discharge. Because of a patient's brain injury, the therapist may rely on family as a source regarding the patient's likes and dislikes. Families may be necessary to make all decisions. The severity of the patient's injury may make any functional activity virtually impossible. Even with sophisticated pneumatic or myoelectrical switches, the patient with a severe brainstem involvement may not be able to activate electronic devices.

Mobilization may be possible only in a manual wheelchair as opposed to driving a power wheelchair independently. However, getting this patient into an open treatment area can help increase general stimulation and the possibilities for socialization.

CONCLUSIONS

This chapter has shown the scope of the occupational and physical therapy program for high quadriplegic patients. The therapy program is geared toward education, providing equipment and offering resources and techniques. It is up to individuals to choose those that best suit their lifestyle.

Closely coordinated teamwork is required to care for the severe and complex nature of this injury. Occupational and physical therapists are integral parts of this team effort from the initial acute care to discharge, as well as with follow-up needs postdischarge. Reevaluation and follow-up plans will be addressed in a later chapter. Often, therapists believe they have "nothing to offer" this group of patients. On the contrary, there is much therapists have to offer to contribute to a better quality of life for these individuals.

REFERENCES

1. Sargent C, Braun MA (1986): Occupational therapy management of the acute spinal cord injured patient. *Am J Occup Ther* 40:333–337.
2. Donovan WH, Bedbrook G (1982): Comprehensive management of spinal cord injury. *Ciba Clin Symp* 34:23.
3. Dingeman L, Jawn JM (1978–1979): Mobility and equipment for the ventilator-dependent tetraplegic. *Paraplegia* 16:175–183.
4. Lathem P, Gregorio T, Garber Lipton S (1985): High-level quadriplegia: an occupational therapy challenge. *Am J Occup Ther* 39:705–714.
5. Benton L, Baker L, et al. (1981): *Functional Electrical Stimulation—A Practical Guide,* 2nd ed. Downey, CA: Rancho Los Amigos Rehabilitation Engineering Center.
6. Dickey R (1986): Electronic technical aids for persons with high level spinal cord injury. *Centr Nerv Syst Trauma* 3:93–110.
7. Dickey R (1986): *Electronic Technical Aids for Persons with Severe Physical Disabilities.* New York: Mary Ann Liebert, Inc.
8. Alvarez S (1985): Functional Assessment and Training. In: *Spinal Cord Injury* (Adkins HV, ed), New York: Churchill Livingstone, pp 132–137.
9. Gerhart K (1979): Increasing sensory and motor stimulation for the patient with quadriplegia. *Phys Ther* 1518–1520.
10. Wetzel J, (1985): Respiratory evaluation and treatment. In: *Spinal Cord Injury* (Adkins HV, ed). New York: Churchill Livingstone, pp 75–98.
11. Kaplan P (1981): Reduction of hypercalciuria in tetraplegia after weight-

bearing and strengthening exercises. *Intern Med Soc Paraplegia* 19:289–293.

12. Garee B (1986): *Ideas for Making Your Home Accessible.* Bloomington, IN: Cheever Publishing.

13. Erickson G (1981): The accessible home: remodeling concerns for the disabled. *Better Homes and Gardens, Remodeling Ideas,* 65–116.

14. DePasquale P (1986): Exhaler class: a multidisciplinary program for high quadriplegia patients. *Am J Occup Ther* 40:482–485.

15. El-Ghatit A, Melvin J, Poole MA (1980): Training apartment in community for spinal cord injured patients: a model. *Arch Phys Med Rehabil* 61:90–92.

15

Equipment Considerations

Carole Adler

*Department of Occupational Therapy, Santa Clara Valley
Medical Center, San Jose, California, U.S.A.*

The high quadriplegic patient requires highly specialized equipment for all aspects of daily life, from basic life support to driving a wheelchair. Thorough evaluation of equipment recommendations will not only enhance the patient's potential for relative independence but will assist the caregiver in meeting the needs necessary for providing optimum quality of life.

The objectives of this chapter are (a) to identify the complex problems related to evaluating and ordering equipment for the high quadriplegic patient; (b) to identify evaluation considerations when evaluating and ordering wheelchairs, positioning, activities of daily living, and communication equipment; and (c) to highlight some appropriate equipment options. Refer to Chapter 12 for information on portable ventilators, alarm systems, and suction machines.

In reviewing the literature, only two references were found to be pertinent to this topic. Dingemans and Hawn (1) discuss the team-oriented treatment approach in the rehabilitation of the high quadriplegic patient. Mobility equipment, including wheelchair, portable life support, and transfer equipment are discussed. The importance of early mobility and introduction to adaptive equipment is stressed as important to the self-esteem and psychological acceptance of the patient to the disability. Whiteneck et al. (2) briefly discuss the long-term use of equipment by the high quadriplegic population.

Secondary to the limited information available, expertise in this area depends on trial and error and commitment to understanding the realistic and unique needs of this specialized patient population.

Due to the limited number of rehabilitation centers treating high quadriplegic patients and the few numbers seen per year in those centers, therapists may lack clinical experience in assessing their patient's short- and long-term functional potential and thus in determining their specific equipment needs. Recognizing the numerous problems encountered by the professionals responsible for the evaluation, ordering, and training in the use and care of high quadriplegic equipment may assist in expanding one's awareness of areas of expertise to develop.

Medical equipment vendors are a vital resource to the therapist, yet may lack the experience to thoroughly understand the application and realistic capabilities of high quadriplegic equipment. Because most high quadriplegic equipment requires customizing, the vendor must be committed to working with the therapist to create the most efficient system and with the patient postdischarge to ensure continued maintenance and follow-through. Demonstration trials of necessary equipment are extremely important in determining the patient's specific ability and needs. However, most vendors do not have high quadriplegic equipment readily available. Much equipment is ordered without adequate trial by the patient.

Due to the advances in engineering technology and the expanding role of the rehabilitation engineer, equipment for the high quadriplegic is developing beyond the sophistication of most therapists and vendors. Maintaining a working understanding and awareness of this costly and sophisticated technology is difficult. The most experienced resources should be used whenever possible.

Therapists must justify purchase of this costly equipment to either governmental or private payment sources in a way that will increase awareness of the unique needs of this patient population and ultimately facilitate payment authorization. Justifications must be written in a clear and concise manner and reflect that the specific equipment requested will best meet the patient's needs. The therapist must maintain credibility with the insurance company by requesting payment of only absolutely necessary equipment. It is the therapist's responsibility to educate not only themselves as to realistic need and appropriateness of equipment but to educate the vendor, patient, caregivers, and payment sources as well.

Poor patient attitude, compliance, and follow-through can be a result of inappropriate equipment recommendations. Considerations must be made as to the patient's discharge environment and must include support systems available to maintain the good working condition of all equipment and availability of service.

WHEELCHAIRS

A high quadriplegic person depends on the assistance of others in almost every aspect of daily life. The most probable area of freedom and independence is that of mobility via a thoroughly evaluated wheelchair system. All aspects of the patient's needs while in the wheelchair must be considered; the wheelchair must make up an integrated system that will meet these needs. A thorough evaluation must include range of motion, strength, and endurance of functioning musculature, body build, effects of spasticity on positioning, cognitive ability, motivation, accessibility of the discharge environment, and long-term mobility needs.

Transportation options and social and financial support available while an in-patient and long term must also be considered (3).

When determining the type of wheelchair to be ordered, whether it be manual or electric or both, the therapist must choose not only the frame design but weigh the following considerations with the patient's specific needs: (a) What is user's current and potential sitting tolerance? The goal is to be up in the wheelchair all day every day. (b) What type of weight shifts are required and what is their frequency? The goal is to prevent skin breakdown at all times. (c) How will the patient breathe? The goal is to provide a reliable, efficient, and portable life-support system. (d) What are the patient's positioning needs? The goal is to prevent deformity and enhance respiratory function by ensuring proper skeletal alignment while the patient is sitting in the wheelchair. (e) What are the patient's mobility needs? The goal is to permit access to all appropriate environments: home, school, urban, and rural. (f) Will the patient be dependent or independent in wheelchair propulsion? The goal is to maximize independence in wheelchair mobility on all indoor and outdoor surfaces. (g) What is the patient's functional potential? The goal is to optimize patient's functional ability via an efficiently integrated mobility system while meeting the above goals.

MANUAL WHEELCHAIR EVALUATION CONSIDERATIONS

The following questions should be asked before ordering a manual wheelchair: (a) Will the manual wheelchair be the user's full-time wheelchair or used in conjunction with an electric wheelchair? (b) What are the user's positioning and portable life-support needs? (c) Will the user require weight shift and position changes throughout the day?

MANUAL WHEELCHAIR OPTIONS

For optimum skin care, upright tolerance, body alignment, and to facilitate management by caregivers, the patient will most likely require a semi- or full-reclining wheelchair. The patient should be expected, however, to sit upright and not rely on a head support unless available musculature is insufficient for good head alignment and support. If the patient will be using the manual wheelchair full time, then a top-of-the-

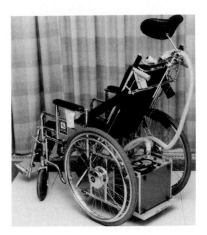

FIG. 15-1. Manual wheelchair with ventilator cart.

line manual recliner should be considered for its durability and ease in use of the recline mechanism and custom frame options, such as Everest and Jennings Premier. Consider the style of the ventilator cart that must fit under the seat and within the dimensions of the wheelbase while still allowing the chair to fully recline if indicated (Fig. 15-1).

ELECTRIC WHEELCHAIR EVALUATION CONSIDERATIONS

The therapist must weigh the subsequent considerations relative to the individual patient before assuming that an electric wheelchair is appropriate: (a) Does user *demonstrate* the motor control and endurance on a consistent basis sufficient to drive a wheelchair independently? (b) Is it the *user's goal* to drive an electric wheelchair independently? Does the user *demonstrate* the cognitive and perceptual ability to safely operate the wheelchair? (c) Can user adequately instruct others in the operation, care, and maintenance of the equipment? (d) Will the user have a van available to transport an electric wheelchair? (e) Does the user have the financial resources available to purchase and maintain this costly item? (f) Are the user's family or caregivers committed to or have the resources available for the care and maintenance of an electric wheelchair?

ELECTRIC WHEELCHAIR OPTIONS

There are basically two frame styles available. The standard folding frame with belt-driven motors can be customized to accommodate commercially available ventilator carts or trays, recline systems, and positioning and drive-control needs of the high quadriplegic patient (Fig.

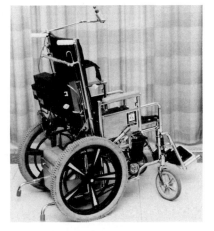

FIG. 15-2. Standard electric wheel-chair frame.

15-2). The frame is stable enough to accommodate most custom seating. This is essential for chin-drive or puff-and-sip control systems due to the patient's inability to compensate for trunk instability.

The solid base frame (e.g., Fortress 655, Invacare Arrow XT) accommodates most custom seat styles, recline systems, and drive controls and uses direct drive motors (Fig. 15-3). Due to the solid base frame, ventilator equipment must be mounted via a custom tray on top of and behind the chair, extending the overall chair length by at least 1 foot. Thought must go into the tray design to efficiently house the ventilator and other needed equipment while still allowing the chair to fully recline. A customized tie-down system is required for safe van transport. Due to the single center post-seat mount the seating surface is more unstable than a standard frame style. This can create postural instabil-

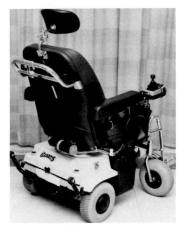

FIG. 15-3. Power-base electric wheelchair frame.

ity for the user when driving on outdoor or uneven surfaces. For a harness-type drive control, or when using a puff-and-sip, a chest-strap mounting should be considered that will compensate for increased vibration and head movement while driving this style of chair. Another option is for an experienced vendor to design extra support struts into the seat frame. Thorough trial by the user should be evaluated on all driving surfaces.

CONSIDERATIONS FOR THE PURCHASE OF TWO WHEELCHAIRS

If it is determined that an electric wheelchair is appropriate, then a manual wheelchair should be ordered as well. The manual wheelchair must meet all the above-mentioned goals in the event of electric wheelchair breakdown or for emergency transport if a van is unavailable. Because the user will only require use of this second chair occasionally, it does not need the durability requirements of a full-time wheelchair. Therefore, a bottom-of-the-line manual wheelchair such as Everest and Jennings Universal or Traveler or Invacare may be sufficient. Custom options are limited for this less expensive style of chair and should be thoroughly considered before ordering. Written justification should be clear as to the purpose for a second wheelchair to ensure reimbursement.

ELECTRIC WHEELCHAIR DRIVE CONTROLS

Once it has been concluded that the patient has the potential of independently propelling an electric wheelchair, then the propulsion system must be carefully evaluated. There are various styles of commercially available high quadriplegia drive systems on the market as well as the availability of designing a custom system. For the purpose of keeping costs down and repair and parts accessible, all commercially available options should be evaluated before considering a custom system. Researching the latest drive systems should be done by the therapist before planning demonstration trials to ensure the most comprehensive and up-to-date evaluation. Vendors can be a valuable resource in providing the necessary information.

Drive systems and their component parts have varying degrees of mechanical sophistication and with that comes inevitable mechanical breakdown. Not only should the patient's physical needs and capabilities be considered but also the financial resources, caregiver skills available, and local vendors who are experienced and committed to maintain the equipment in good working order.

CONSIDERATIONS FOR DETERMINING DRIVE CONTROL SYSTEMS

When determining the appropriate drive control system the following should be considered: (a) Does the user have mouth, jaw, and neck strength, range of motion, and endurance sufficient for independent control of chair? (b) Does spasticity interfere with operation of the drive control, especially on uneven surfaces? (c) Is the user sitting at an angle sufficient for optimum visual field? (d) Does the user have the cognitive and perceptual ability to safely operate the system? (e) Does the user require an independent recline option to be built into the drive control system? (f) Will the user's lifestyle warrant including environmental control interface to be included in the drive system? (g) What brands of drive systems will interface with the brand of electric wheelchair ordered? This should be determined before the chair order. (h) What drive system style (i.e., harness versus boom mount) is most functionally appropriate and cosmetically pleasing for the user? Consider that the drive system will most likely be in front of the user's face at all times. (i) Will the user's mouthstick use and environmental control system use interfere with operation of drive control? (j) Has the user been involved in problem-solving the above considerations?

DRIVE CONTROL OPTIONS

Joystick on Boom Mount

There are several styles available for both the joystick and the boom. The user need not have fully innervated neck musculature to operate this style of drive control. Exertion is minimal using this system and the user can increase strength and endurance in available musculature necessary for neck-accessory breathing and mouthstick use. Experience has shown that even a patient in halo immobilization can successfully operate a chin drive joystick with mouth and jaw if it is precisely positioned and the patient and therapist are motivated to succeed.

The boom should be as unobtrusive as possible while providing the stability and adjustability necessary for optimum positioning of the joystick. The most reliable booms are manually positioned because the power-retractable designs have been found to be mechanically unreliable. They should be easily adjustable because the user's precarious trunk instability may require daily repositioning by caregivers.

The most successful type of joystick is the short-throw proportional style (Fig. 15-4). The user will master a smoother ride with less exertion. Nonproportional microswitch controls create a "jerky" ride that can compromise the user's trunk stability, especially on outdoor surfaces.

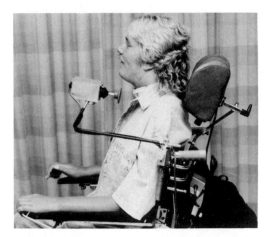

FIG. 15-4. Short-throw joystick on boom mount.

If user-operated recline or environmental control system interface is
required, then the need for a separate switch should be investigated.

Harness-Mounted Joystick

The "DU-IT" joystick by Control System Group, Inc., is attached to a
harness that is secured around the patient's neck (Fig. 15-5). This may
be preferable to the boom mount if the user is relying on only jaw or
very little neck control because it can be mounted very close to the patient's face while remaining cosmetically pleasing and not obstructing
the tracheostomy or ventilator hose. The user requires only jaw muscu-

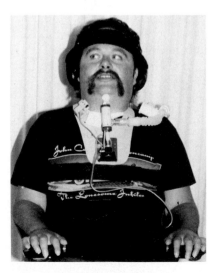

FIG. 15-5. "Du-It" harness-mounted
joystick.

lature to successfully operate this type of control. If the patient's trunk alignment changes due to spasticity or rough driving surfaces, the joystick remains in place, because it is attached to the user's body. The independent recline and environmental control system operation can be integrated into this style of joystick, affording the patient one control center for many functions. This type of drive control is technologically more sophisticated than the conventional boom mount, and thus requires an experienced dealer to repair the system in case of mechanical breakdown. The user and the caregiver's ability to care for the equipment, as well as the availability of vendor and manufacturer support, is essential for the therapist to consider when recommending this style of drive control system.

Pneumatic "Puff-and-Sip" Drive Control

This style of drive control requires only mouth musculature to operate. There is very little exertion on the part of the user and, although initially challenging to operate, it can be mastered by most patients. The puff-and-sip drive control is cosmetically pleasing because only a small tube is placed near the user's face (Fig. 15-6). An advantage to using this system is that it is less sensitive to movement from spasticity or uneven surfaces than a boom mounted joystick is. The control is usually mounted via gooseneck onto the back frame of the chair and is easily adjusted. Drawbacks to this style of drive control are that the electronics are extremely sensitive and may require frequent maintenance if caregivers or vendors are not familiar with the system. Also, users are not required to use the jaw and neck musculature that they may have available.

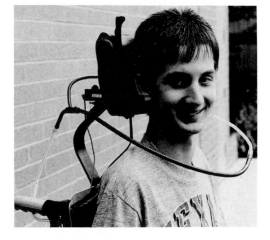

FIG. 15-6. "Puff-and-sip" drive control.

Custom Drive Controls

Currently there is much innovation in the area of custom wheelchair drive control such as voice- or eye-activated systems. These are still in the development phase and not recommended. To ensure reliable and safe propulsion of the chair the drive control must have been thoroughly evaluated on the specific user, and be affordable and repairable.

RECLINE MECHANISMS

The reclining option is a necessary addition to a high quadriplegic wheelchair system. An adjustable back angle will enable the patient to find a seat angle that will best accommodate the trunk alignment against gravity. It also provides an effective weight shift for pressure relief, reduces the need for transfers to bed required for catheterizations and rest, and provides for independent position change. There are problems, however, with skin shearing and system breakdown that may dissuade from its use.

There are several types of electric recline systems available. The standard power recline is a rigid seat with a reclining back and a hinged system with the pivot point below the hip joint. After reclining, manual repositioning is usually required due to the patient's sliding forward in the seat. This can contribute to poor sitting position in relation to the drive control and potential for skin breakdown.

The "zero-shear" recline system by La Bac and "rug seat" system by Falcon are two schools of thought addressing the same problem of the need for repositioning after the recline process. The "zero-shear" recline system (La Bac) is preferable not only for providing the minimal amount of skin shearing during the reclining process but in allowing the patient to resume an upright position with the least amount of forward sliding in the seat (Fig. 15-7). It is also optimal for patients with positioning problems due to spasticity. The standard recline may be appropriate for an individual in whom skin shearing or sensory loss is not a problem.

When considering the brand of recline system, take into consideration how the components will fit with the rest of the wheelchair and ventilator components. Everything must be mounted so that the chair can be reclined fully. Careful consideration must be given as to location of recline switch for independent access by the patient or easy access by a caregiver.

Currently there is no complete system available. The electric wheelchair manufacturers make electric wheelchairs and the power recline manufacturers make recline systems. It is up to the therapist and the expertise of the equipment vendor to aesthetically interface these products along with the drive control into an efficient system. The user's

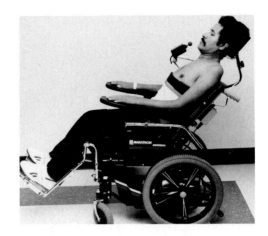

FIG. 15-7. "La Bac zero-shear" recline system.

entire lifestyle must be considered including needs at home, vocationally, and during leisure activities (see Chapter 20).

VENTILATOR CARTS OR TRAYS

The ventilator cart houses the portable ventilator equipment including battery and charger as well as the electric wheelchair batteries. It must carry all components under the wheelchair frame, while protruding as little as possible behind the chair (Fig. 15-8). It is important to be aware of the specific ventilator and battery dimensions when ordering the cart so all parts will fit as efficiently as possible while allowing the chair to recline fully. Different systems of breathing require different-size batteries. Using a pneumobelt requires a larger battery than breathing trach-positive (see Chapter 12). All of the wheelchair and

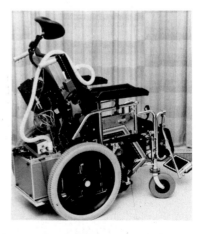

FIG. 15-8. Ventilator cart on standard electric wheelchair frame.

ventilator components must be readily accessible for ease of adjustment and repair.

WHEELCHAIR POSITIONING DEVICES

Careful assessment and application of wheelchair positioning devices will greatly enhance appearance, mobility, and functional skills of the high quadriplegic patient. Also, early consideration must be given to long-term skeletal alignment, skin care, and respiratory needs.

When assessing the patient's positioning equipment, the therapist must keep the following outcomes in mind: (a) to prevent pressure sores by recommending appropriate wheelchair cushioning; (b) to prevent deformity and enhance respiratory function by maintaining appropriate skeletal alignment throughout the *entire* body; and (c) to maximize function, comfort, and cosmesis at all times.

An understanding of the anatomical position desired as well as an awareness of technological advances and available trial equipment to meet those needs will assist the therapist in providing the most optimal system (4).

WHEELCHAIR CUSHIONS

A precursor to good total body positioning while in the wheelchair is an accurately positioned pelvis. The most desirable position places the pelvis in slight anterior tilt, which facilitates a normal lumbar curve and good head positioning. The cushion that is recommended should achieve this position and contribute to maintaining skeletal alignment throughout the rest of the body. The cushion should provide optimal pressure relief from buttocks to distal thigh and facilitate good lower extremity positioning while affording maximal pelvic stability.

When evaluating the cushion it should be placed on a *rigid,* flush-to-the-frame wheelchair seat to provide a stable base of support (e.g., Everest and Jennings 941 hl) (Fig. 15-9). The cushion measurements should match that of the wheelchair seat and fit snugly so as not to slide when the patient is transferred or repositioned. The patient should be placed on each cushion being considered and observed in a variety of recline angles to evaluate how well pressure relief and stability are preserved. Pressure evaluators such as the Texas Interface Pressure Evaluator or Sciamedics Pressure Gauge may be used to determine objective pressure measurements but should not be the only information considered. Total body positioning and direct skin observation and quality of cushion maintenance by caregivers should also be carefully assessed.

A dry floatation or ROHO cushion, although providing excellent pressure relief for most patients, may not provide enough pelvic stability in patients with pelvic obliquity or considerable trunk and hip spasticity.

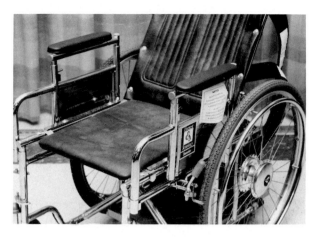

FIG.   15-9. Flush-to-the-frame   wheelchair seat.

For the high quadriplegic individual, it has shown to be an excellent cushion, however, since the patient can be well stabilized in the trunk to maintain position as opposed to the lower level quadriplegic patient, who may not require as much trunk fixation. The cushion requires regular attention by the patient and caregivers to maintain adequate internal air pressure and for that reason may not be appropriate for the patient who demonstrates poor follow-through of care.

The high-density foam base with Flolite top pad (JAY, JAY ACTIVE) provides a very stable base and has been shown to assist in maintaining symmetrical pelvic support. This low-maintenance cushion can be ordered with overfill "Flolite" pads and extra gel inserts. Also available is a "recliner" model to maintain position of gel at various recline angles. Necessary pressure relief over a long period should be watched closely by performing "skin checks" on a regular basis.

High-density foam cushions are rarely ordered for the high quadriplegic patient because they have not been shown to provide the long-term pressure relief and durability required in cushions for this patient population.

For most patients, commercially available cushions afford optimal support. However, when severe spinal deformity or chronic skin breakdown is present, a custom-contoured seating system may be indicated. There are several systems available and the therapist should be aware of all aspects of cost, fabrication, and how they integrate with the wheelchair frame before ordering.

TRUNK SUPPORTS

Trunk supports are necessary to maintain stability in the trunk after the pelvis has been accurately positioned. The high quadriplegic individual will almost always need some form of trunk stabilization added

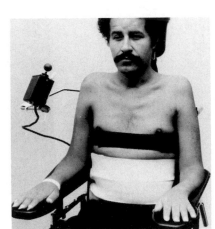

FIG. 15-10. Velcro seat belts for trunk support.

on to the wheelchair frame. The long-term benefits of good skeletal alignment due to an efficient trunk support system are now being seen in patients, not only in growing children, but in adults several years postinjury. Before determining the style of trunk support, place the patient on his or her own cushion and wheelchair with appropriate arm support, and at their optimum upright sitting tolerance observe the effects of gravity on their alignment. Seat belts placed both at the hip and just below the axillary level of the chest provide very good trunk support if the patient's chair fits properly and if the patient has no functional or structural trunk deformity (Fig. 15-10). Velcro cinch type seat belts are preferred because they do not cause pressure as do car-type seat belts and are unobtrusive and easy to adjust. If more rigid support is required then mounted rigid supports may be required. The daily, precise positioning of rigid lateral trunk supports is critical to the benefit they have on the patient's total body positioning. The supports can be placed symmetrically or obliquely in the case of excessive scoliosis or pelvic obliquity. Otto Bock manufactures a lateral trunk support that is easy to manage during transfers, maintains its position once adjusted,

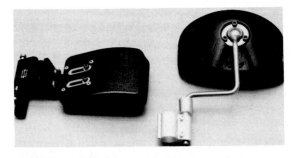

FIG. 15-11. "La Bac" and "Otto Bock" lateral trunk supports.

and is not bulky (Fig. 15-1). The trunk support must remain properly adjusted no matter at what angle the patient is sitting. A trunk support attached to the back frame of a "Zero-shear" recliner will change position as the patient reclines (Fig. 15-11). The therapist must be aware of this and the options available to accommodate for it. "La Bac" manufactures a trunk support mount that will accommodate this style of back. The trunk supports stay in a fixed position to the chest and do not require repositioning after position changes.

HEAD AND NECK SUPPORT

Some style of head and neck support will be necessary either to maintain head position due to muscle weakness or to provide comfort and support while in the reclined position. There are many styles available and the therapist should be aware of options available for the headpiece and wheelchair mount. How the head support integrates with the other positioning devices is important in that it should look streamlined and "clean," enhance function of the head and neck, and be easily adjustable. The more support the patient requires, the more surface area and contour will be necessary for alignment and comfort. If neck extension is weak or absent, resulting in head instability when sitting upright or driving on rough terrain, a simple athletic headband has been found to securely and comfortably hold the head in place.

Wheelchair and recline system manufacturers design their own head supports, some with built-in strip switches to control recline or emergency functions. Some bracket designs are bulky and difficult to adjust. Otto Bock manufactures several styles of headrests and a simple streamlined mounting bracket. La Bac manufactures a head support and bracket that is less costly and works well for a patient requiring inter-

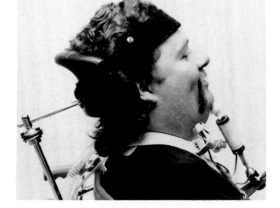

FIG. 15-12. "Otto Bock" headrest with headband for additional support.

mittent support, because the headpiece is easily removed. Rehabilitation engineers and vendors design head supports as well. The therapist should be aware of the various options available and that the systems can be interchanged to meet the individual needs of the patient. Cosmesis should always be a high priority when considering head and neck supports (Fig. 15-12).

UPPER-EXTREMITY POSITIONING IN THE WHEELCHAIR

Accurate upper-extremity positioning will assist in maintaining total body alignment and stability while sitting. It will inhibit shoulder subluxation, pain, and range-of-motion limitations, as well as improve overall appearance. Properly supported upper extremities will also assist in maintaining positioning of the head and trunk.

Arm troughs provide the support and adjustability necessary to maintain upper-extremity alignment. There are several styles of arm troughs that, when attached to reclining brackets on the back of the wheelchair, will adequately support the arms and shoulders in any angle of sitting. The therapist should take note of the length of the arm trough in relation to the patient's arm, its width in relation to the rest of the wheelchair, and the complexity and durability of the mounting bracket (Fig. 15-13). It is important to be aware of the options and how they integrate into the entire system. Some mounting brackets are difficult to operate and maladjustment is often a problem. The material used in fabricating arm troughs is important to note. If the trough is made out of vinyl it will tend to rip easily and require frequent repair. La Bac and Otto Bock manufacture arm troughs that meet most patients' needs, including du-

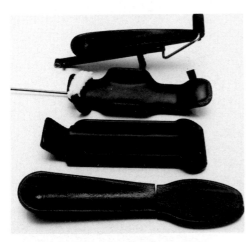

FIG. 15-13. Various arm trough styles.

rability and appearance. Some are contoured and bolstered to provide necessary elbow stops and hand positioning.

Lapboards can support the upper extremities and provide a portable functional surface for functional activities and carrying items. Commercially available lapboards come in many materials, the most preferable being clear Plexiglas or Lexan because they do not obscure the patient's view of his/her own body. The therapist should consider mounts that are durable and easy to manage by the patient's caregivers. Disadvantages to a lapboard are that it may appear to create a barrier, making the patient look less accessible to people. It can also be difficult to apply and remove when the patient requires repositioning. If the patient is using the lapboard for arm positioning then some type of padding will most likely be required at the elbow to prevent skin breakdown.

When considering all of the positioning devices that are required to meet the patient's needs, it is essential that they all be considered in relation to one another and integrated well with the rest of the wheelchair, drive, recline, and ventilator systems. Optimal total body positioning, function, and durability of component parts, integrated into an attractive and space-efficient system, should be primary goals of the ordering therapist.

ACTIVITIES OF DAILY LIVING

Beds

The hospital bed that is ordered for the high quadriplegic patient should have the features necessary to meet the primary needs of the patient, such as daily respiratory care and activities of daily living. Because the patient will require maximal assistance for all self-care and positioning needs, the bed must be easily adjustable in high–low, head, and feet positioning. Brakes on the bed must be freely adjustable, safe, and durable for stability during transfers. Bed rails should be easy to operate.

The patient's respiratory needs may vary. A treatment of choice in assisting in the prevention of respiratory complications is prophylactic daily chest percussion in the Trendelenburg position (head lower than feet) to promote drainage of chest secretions. A bed that will easily assume this position will assist in consistent follow-through of this procedure by caregivers.

Standard "three-motor" hospital beds will assume the varied positions necessary. However, they require manual positioning of Trendelenburg placement. The HILL-ROM and JOERNS beds, although more costly than standard hospital beds, will mechanically assume the Trendelenburg position. A head-operated bed control is also available with the

HILL-ROM bed. It is important that manual controls be accessible to the caregiver as a backup in case of power failure. Substantial justification to payer sources is necessary to educate and to justify the increased cost of this type of bed.

Bathroom Equipment

Bathing in a tub or shower while requiring mechanical ventilation must be thoroughly evaluated to determine its appropriateness. It is advisable that the therapist, patient, and caregivers participate in an actual wet shower on a commode or gurney, while the patient is in the hospital, to fully comprehend the task. Once this has been done, the following considerations should be weighed before making equipment recommendations: (a) How much attendant care will be available during the bathing process? (b) What financial resources are available for the costly bathroom modifications if the bathroom is currently inaccessible? (c) What type of ventilator support will be required during the bathing process? (d) What is the experience of the rehabilitation team in providing training to the patient and caregivers?

The timely and energy-consuming task of bathing in a shower may not be an efficient use of time for someone who will require physical assist throughout a 24-h period. The time it takes to perform a bath in an actual shower may interfere with other important daily activities such as going to school or work or socializing. It can be more taxing on caregivers (several additional transfers may be required) whose extent of daily physical exertion should be minimized to promote a positive and safe working environment.

Most residential homes do not afford the luxury of wheel-in showers or a bathroom large enough to manage large reclining commodes and gurneys. The cost of recommending such modifications is high. Shower gurneys such as those found in hospitals are extremely expensive and difficult to store when not in use.

It is not recommended that ventilator-dependent quadriplegic individuals use a shower due to the possibility of aspirating water and the electrical precautions necessary to consider. If, however, the patient and family can accommodate the above issues then a reclining commode (ACTIVE-AID) is recommended over a shower gurney due to its adjustable position and decreased cost and space requirement.

In many cases minimal bathing equipment and no bathroom modifications are required. Caregivers are taught to give a very sufficient bed bath, which usually can be given on a more frequent basis than a shower due to time and energy conservation. An inexpensive inflatable hair-washing tray (SHAMPEZE) has been found to enable frequent hair washing while the patient remains in bed (Fig. 15-14). Inflatable bath-

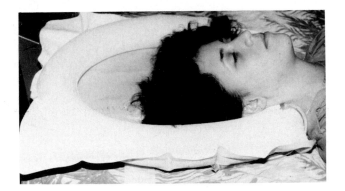

FIG. 15-14. Inflatable hair-washing tray for use in bed.

tubs are available but are extremely time and energy consuming and are rarely used. The high quadriplegic patient's bowel program as well as oral and other hygiene activities may also be conducted in bed. It is preferable that a sink be located close by for the caregiver's convenience and that an accessible mirror be available for the patient to see him or herself while sitting in the wheelchair.

TRANSFER DEVICES

There are varied methods of transferring a high quadriplegic patient that may require equipment (see Chapter 14). If manually transferring the individual, a slideboard is indicated for safety. Flat sliding transfers can be performed by using a larger slideboard, extending the length of the patient's torso.

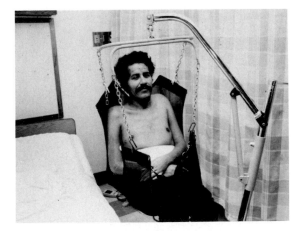

FIG. 15-15. Sling design is important for good total body support.

If a mechanical lift is being used then a lift should be ordered for the home that has a safe and reliable boom and sling design. The TRANS-AID LAT II with no. 309 full body sling securely positions the patient during the lift and can also assist in positioning in the wheelchair (Fig. 15-15). The C-base design is stable and facilitates turning tight corners if necessary. The sling design allows easy placement and removal by one person while the patient is sitting in the wheelchair. The U-shape base may be necessary if the patient is extremely heavy.

COMMUNICATION DEVICES

Mouthsticks

A mouthstick is a relatively inexpensive, nonelectronic piece of equipment that will prove functional for the high quadriplegic patient. By using intact or weak neck musculature and good mouth strength and coordination, the motivated patient can successfully turn pages, use a standard keyboard, and participate in table-top avocational activities such as drawing, writing, painting, playing cards, or board games (see Chapter 14). This is significant in that an essentially dependent person has the ability to actively perform an activity by using available musculature and uncomplicated, easily fabricated, and repairable equipment.

It is important that the therapist look beyond traditional expectations when evaluating a patient's potential mouthstick use. Commonly, only a patient with fully innervated neck control is considered appropriate to use a mouthstick. Experience has shown, however, that a person with very little to no active neck musculature or an immobilized head, such as in a halo, still has the ability to independently read or use a keyboard if the proper mouthpiece and stick configuration is considered.

Mouthsticks and their docking systems can be ordered commercially or can be custom fabricated. There are many styles and lightweight materials that are used. The most commonly used mouthstick is simply for turning pages or pushing buttons. This can be easily fabricated in the clinic using materials such as Plexiglas drinking straws (ordered from adaptive equipment catalogues), wooden dowels, or fiberglass arrow shafts. Others have the ability to pinch for picking up papers or cards, such as Ad-Lib, and have changeable tips for writing and painting (Fig. 15-16). The patient's specific needs will determine the appropriate mouthstick style. The therapist should thoroughly investigate both commercially available and custom options.

Commercially available mouthsticks may have simple nonmolded mouthpieces usually, in a V shape or paddle shape. The V-shape mouthpiece (e.g., "Ad-Lib" or "Extensions for Independence") allow for tongue

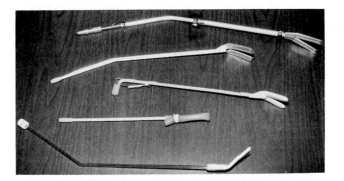

FIG. 15-16. Various commercially available and custom-made mouthsticks.

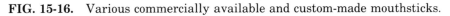

movement, talking, and swallowing and are comfortable for many patients, especially those with little head control, because the mouthpiece is easy to manipulate with lips and tongue. Custom-molded dental-impression mouthpieces can be more expensive and less versatile because they are difficult to comfortably manipulate in the mouth, especially if mouth control must compensate for weak neck musculature. There continue to be questions as to the long-term effect of noncustom mouthpieces on teeth and jaw; however, experienced long-term mouthstick users have not appeared to have ill effects from the nonmolded style.

Mouthsticks vary in functional design. Some have changeable tips and telescoping features such as "Extensions for Independence." The style should depend on how avid and creative a user the patient is and will be. A mouthstick that is too sophisticated or heavy for the user will not be used.

FIG. 15-17. Mouthstick docking system should be space-efficient on work surface.

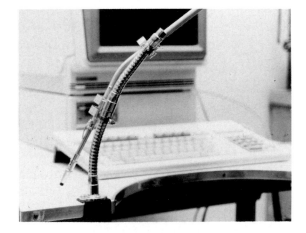

Various docking systems should be experimented with that enable the user to work for longer periods by independently changing tips, docking, and retrieving the mouthstick. The docking system should take up as little space as possible on the work surface to provide room for books, computer, and other necessary items. Docking systems such as a simple gooseneck with broom clamps attached to table or wheelchair by a small clamp have been simple to fabricate and successful (Fig. 15-17).

The therapist's experience and creativity will enhance the patient's motivation and thus the success of long-term mouthstick use.

ENVIRONMENTAL CONTROL SYSTEMS

There have been many technological advances in the field of specialized electronic equipment for the high quadriplegic patient. A wide range of equipment is commercially available such as remote-control door openers and telephone systems. There is also a considerable amount of research and development in process using microcomputers and robotics.

It is an area that is extremely specialized and challenging for the occupational therapist. Not only must there be an expertise regarding the patient's long-term functional needs, but the therapist must have a general understanding of current electronics, programming abilities, interface and upgrade capabilities, and how the equipment will integrate into the patient's lifestyle and other equipment. Due to the complexity of the situation, including the desire to provide as much as possible to a patient population almost totally dependent on equipment, the occupational therapist and patient must remain realistic regarding their expectations of what function environmental control systems will reliably perform. In many cases, sophisticated, expensive, highly customized systems may be an overuse of technology for the high quadriplegic individual. Staying simple is preferred. Creative use of mouthsticks and well-managed attendant care may be more than adequate to consistently meet the patient's needs as well as remaining within financial constraints.

Relatively simple, commercially available technical aids may be appropriate after thorough evaluation of the patient's functional and lifestyle needs. The technology continues to change and the therapist should be aware of currently available options by contacting experienced resources and local agencies. In California, for example, the various telephone companies offer a variety of modified telephone options, including the only state-wide free loan program of voice-operated wireless telephones, allowing independent and private placing and receiving of phone calls. Electronics stores provide a variety of remote-control switches to the general public that may be appropriate.

Not only is the task of determining the specific environmental control equipment complex, but mounting and operational switches definitely pose a challenge. The therapist must be aware of options available and have access to trial equipment. Ideally, affiliation with a rehabilitation engineering department that can assist in the setup of devices will assist in successful long-term use. The occupational therapist should interface with the engineer to ensure *realistic* and appropriate application of the equipment to the unique needs of the individual.

Financial considerations are a major issue because this equipment is extremely expensive at this point in development, requiring considerable customizing and constant maintenance. Funding sources very likely will be unwilling to pay for what they consider luxury items. Few patients benefit from the current development in sophisticated environmental control systems other than in vocational or research settings.

Rather than discuss specific brand names and options in this text, it will be the therapist's responsibility to become informed by contacting appropriate experienced resources familiar with this equipment such as Rehabilitation Engineering Research and Development at the Veteran's Administration Hospital, Palo Alto, California. There are other excellent resources for commercially available environmental control systems (1,4,5).

TRANSPORTATION

Equipment recommendations for attendant-driven vans should be left to experienced adaptive driver evaluation programs. The extensive evaluation will ensure that all equipment recommendations will be proven safe and appropriate for the high quadriplegic individual and necessary caregivers.

There are some general medical and technical concerns necessary to recognize with high quadriplegic patients. Before the evaluation, patients must be in their own purchased wheelchair with all positioning equipment in place. This is essential, because the overall dimensions of the patient in the wheelchair, including ventilator equipment, will affect the type of lift, placement of tie-downs, and the need for a lowered floor. Ample headroom is necessary, not only to maximize the patient's visual field, but for caregiver safety and comfort. When living in climates where extremes of heat and cold are experienced, rear-mount air conditioning and heater vents are recommended because the high quadriplegic patient will always be in the middle to the back of the vehicle as a passenger. This is necessary to ensure adequate temperature control. Auxilliary suction and ventilator equipment including a power source compatible with the ventilator plugs is essential for the person dependent on a ventilator.

The therapist must assure that the vendor responsible for making the van modifications does not make changes in the van setup without specific authorization, because any change will have a great impact on the safety of the patient.

If a personal van is not an option and public transportation is available, assisting the patient and family in reliable options in the community is required.

DISCUSSION AND SUMMARY

The therapist has considerable responsibility in assessing an array of equipment, from simple to extremely sophisticated, that can be a major factor in enhancing the quality of life for a high quadriplegic patient. Experience in working with this level of spinal cord injury, medical equipment vendors, engineering and manufacturing personnel, and thoughtful equipment justification will support making equipment recommendations that will best meet the short- and long-term needs of the patient.

The therapist must be able to realistically appreciate the needs of their patient, especially long-term physical and functional potential. Experience is limited, yet growing, in this area and spinal cord centers experienced with this level of injury should be used as resources that can offer a comprehensive perspective.

The therapist should apply the skills of durable medical equipment vendors, manufacturers, and rehabilitation engineers in fabricating and customizing equipment. Coupled with the knowledge of the patient's needs, lifestyle, and support systems, the therapist can evaluate, recommend, and train in the use of the most appropriate equipment.

Technology is advancing and efforts to remain aware of recent developments should be pursued. At the same time, consideration of simplicity and practicality will ensure compliance and follow-through by both patient and caregivers.

In today's changing reimbursement climate, equipment justification is becoming increasingly important. Recommendations should be based on a thorough evaluation of clinical, functional, and financial issues that will best serve the interests of the patient and payment source as well. It is the responsibility of the therapist to maintain credibility with payer source and to consider the absolute necessity and appropriateness of all equipment ordered.

REFERENCES

1. Dingemans L, Hawn M (1978): Mobility and equipment for the ventilator-dependent tetraplegic. *Paraplegia* 16(2):175–183.

2. Whiteneck, GG, Carter RE, Charlifue SW, Hall KM, Menter RR, Wilkerson MA, Wilmot CB (1985): *A Collaborative Study of High Quadriplegia* (Rocky Mountain Regional Spinal Injury System, Northern California Regional Spinal Injury System, and Texas Regional Spinal Cord Injury System). Englewood, CO: Craig Hospital.
3. Adler C, ed. (1987): *Wheelchairs and Cushions; A Comprehensive Guide to Evaluation and Ordering.* San Jose, CA: Santa Clara Valley Medical Center.
4. Dickey, R (1986): *Electronic Technical Aids for Persons With Severe Disabilities.* Washington, D.C.: National Rehabilitation Information Center (NARIC).
5. Hill JP, ed. (1986): *Spinal Cord Injury, A Guide to Functional Outcomes in Occupational Therapy.* Rockville, MD: Aspen Publishers.

16

Counseling During the Rehabilitation Phase

Patricia Tracy

Craig Hospital, Englewood, Colorado, U.S.A.

Counseling the patient who has a high-level spinal cord injury in the rehabilitation setting addresses many aspects of the patient's self and his or her life. The counselor's role is varied and ranges from therapeutic to concrete issues. The counselor can be cheerleader, confidant, organizer, case manager, and liaison for the family, patient, staff, and outside resources. Although the counseling functions described in this chapter presume that one individual is fulfilling the role, some centers use a variety of social workers, psychologists, and other rehabilitation team members to perform these functions.

Counseling begins with a positive initial contact, then a thorough psychosocial history. A preliminary plan for services mutually determined with the patient provides a basis for ongoing counsel. The goal of discharge from the rehabilitation setting to a safe and caring environment hopefully will provide the patient with the security and courage needed to lay groundwork for a fulfilling life ahead.

REHABILITATION COUNSELING

Meeting the Patient

Shortly after the patient's admission to the rehabilitation floor or facility the counselor meets with the patient and available family members for an introduction. The family members who are absent can be telephoned and/or mailed a letter of introduction. It is essential that this initial contact bear with it the message that the nuclear family and those who have a significant relationship with the patient are an important part of the rehabilitation process.

At the time of the introduction the counselor presents clear information including the counselor's name, title, and function, telephone number and location of office, working hours, and availability. The counselor needs to clarify the patient's name (including pronunciation, spelling, and preferred name for addressing the patient), and the names and relationships of those in attendance at the time of the introduction. An orientation to the rehabilitation floor or facility can be confirmed or arranged at this time. The length of time or planned visits by the relatives can be clarified so future time with them can be scheduled. Information on local community resources can be provided to out-of-town relatives. A general understanding of how the hospital system works, the team concept, schedules, conferences, and expectations can be reviewed with the patient and the family.

The initial meeting is also a time to evaluate, by observation and after reviewing the chart information, the physical condition and communication status of the patient with high quadriplegia. If the patient cannot speak it will be important to identify the most efficient means of communicating with him or her. Family members or attendants who have accompanied the patient to the unit are often helpful in providing this information. Counselor consultation with occupational therapy or speech therapy might be needed to further establish the most effective communication techniques. Eye contact and touching the patient in sensory present areas on the shoulder, head, or face can also be an important reassuring means of initial communication.

At the end of the introductory meeting, a time can be arranged to meet with the patient and family again. After the patient is settled, and orientation and initial tests are completed, a session to secure a more detailed psychosocial history is scheduled.

Psychosocial History

The psychosocial history involves the patient and any appropriate family members he or she invites to attend. This interview can be a means of obtaining helpful background information to guide the counselor in identifying needed services, to assist in establishing rapport and understanding of the patient's past life, and in aiding in evaluating the patient's knowledge, processing, and communication skills.

The psychosocial history includes the patient's report of the injury, the details of its occurrence, and the patient's understanding of the implications of the disability. This report can also shed light on such things as the relationship of alcohol to the accident and possibly be a guide for future referral for drug or alcohol treatment. It is also an opportunity to check for the presence of amnesia or unconsciousness after the injury because this information, combined with behavioral and response patterns, could possibly indicate the need for a neuropsychological evaluation. An overview of the patient's hospital course, surgeries, and information about the injury provided to the patient before admission to the rehabilitation facility is helpful in guiding the counselor in understanding the patient's present level of anxiety, understanding, or confusion about the disability. The presence of problems such as persistent pain can also be revealed during this interview and can be a guide for referral for pain management.

Encouraging the patient to share concrete, nonthreatening background information about his or her family system can then be helpful as a means of identifying members of the family, relationships, and residences. A family genogram can be a helpful tool and quick reference in organizing this information. Intermingled with this information can be more sensitive topics such as sexual history, substance use history, and mental health history.

In the history, the type of housing and transportation available to the patient should be noted as well as the size and type of community in which the patient lives. These are important pieces of information in planning for the patient's eventual discharge from the rehabilitation setting. Recreational activities enjoyed before the injury can be noted for use in encouraging recreational involvement at the rehabilitation facility. Coping strategies can be explored with the patient for feedback on how he or she sees themselves managing the disability. This information can be used as a guideline for encouraging family support systems and contacting support systems beyond the family (for example, religious leaders or specific cultural organizations). Also, the patient's notation of severe depression or reaction problems to the disability could indicate the need for further psychological counseling. The psychosocial history should also include a review of the patient's financial status, including insurance and income. This is essential in beginning to understand the resources available in planning for the patient's future needs. This information also serves as an indicator for the counselor to make the necessary referrals for benefits.

Information about the patient's vocational background is important for future planning and referrals to outside vocational agencies. The last year of school completed, job history, and history of military service is helpful information to the counselor and patient in sorting out the patient's future employment potential.

The concluding part of the psychosocial history includes the counselor's impression of the interview and of the patient and family responses. This is professional interpretation of the facts provided and the manner in which they were provided. This information is the counselor's opportunity to note significant communication patterns or behaviors that can be important in pinpointing areas of sensitivity or difficulty for the patient. This can also serve to indicate who is important in the patient's life and the quality of those relationships. These areas could denote need for particular awareness or specific counseling. It is important that the counselor listen throughout the psychosocial history with eyes, ears, and heart open.

Finally, the history concludes with a plan for services mutually agreed on with the patient. The plan is based on the background information provided and how this spinal cord injury will affect that. This is often the patient and family's first clear permission to openly discuss discharge plans—what it will be like to leave the hospital in a wheelchair and what it will take to do that. For the counselor, a list (Table 16-1) can help in organization and efficiency with the discharge plan.

Patient/Team Communication

As a part of the planning, the counselor will make the patient more aware of the services that the rehabilitation facility has to offer. To keep the counseling plan coordinated with the patient goals of the other multidisciplinary team members, ongoing communication with all is essential. After the initial history, regular conferences with the patient, family members, and all team members (physician, physical therapist, occupational therapist, counselor, psychologist, nurse, recreation therapist, respiratory therapist, speech therapist, flight nurse, etc.) are scheduled. Others invited by the patient (for example, friends, lawyers, insurance representatives) can also attend these conferences. This conference, held approximately once a month, is a chance for reviewing of tests and of progress toward rehabilitation goals. It is also a time for the patient and family to ask questions and for all team members to coordinate goals and plans for discharge.

Weekly chart rounds with the physician and the rehabilitation team is another opportunity to stay in tune with the changes occurring and to alter goals or approaches accordingly. In addition, there are occasionally specific team meetings held usually involving the psychologist, team members, and the patient. These are an attempt to resolve, often by contract or schedule, behavioral issues that present difficulty to the staff or patient in progressing toward discharge goals. The counselor's role in these meetings is to coordinate plans and schedules and to be supportive to both patient and staff in reaching goals.

Individual counseling sessions can be regular and scheduled or consistent but unscheduled contacts and are a means of addressing the specific needs of the patient on an ongoing basis.

Documentation of progress in the medical chart is another way of sharing information with the team. The counselor has an obligation to share essential information while protecting the privacy of the patient.

Table 16-1. *Discharge Planning Checklist for Family Service*[a]

Task	Target date	Completion date/initial
Attendants		
Communicating who will be attendants	2 mo. pre d/c	
Communicating no. of h/day	1 mo. pre d/c	
Letter on funding for attendants	2 mo. pre d/c	
Inform family and team of training schedule	1 mo. pre d/c	
Arrange with family for nursing agency/private attendant back home	1 mo. pre d/c	
Communicate contact person at agency to flight nurse	2 wk. pre d/c	
Mail medical records and/or doctors' orders to agency (fl. nurse will do if involved)	1 wk. pre d/c	
Counseling family		
Stress management related to trip home and possible problems re: equipment delivery, etc.	1 mo. pre d/c	
Equipment		
Funding letters to insurance	2 mo. pre d/c	
Free-care and other forms	6 wk. pre d/c	
Communicate to all team if *no* funding for any item	1 mo. pre d/c or ASAP	
Notify floor nurse of conference *before* d/c conf.	6 wk. pre d/c	
Home modifications		
Letter to insurance	6 wk. pre d/c	
Home checkout form received and meeting held with OT and PT	2 mo. pre d/c	
For local patients, home checkout with OT/PT	6 wk. pre d/c	
Bring up checklists at rounds	ASAP	
Follow-up checklists	At weekly chart rounds	

[a]d/c, discharge; OT, occupational therapy; PT, physical therapy.

Confidentiality can be more difficult when family and team members are also closely involved in interpreting patient behavior and needs.

Educational classes are a way to provide information and support to the patient and families. Classes can offer sessions on topics such as social skills, sexuality, stress management, and financial benefits. Patients can also profit from the thorough review of the current research on spinal cord injury. A list of periodicals and journals related to spinal cord injury can be provided as well as the spinal cord injury hotline telephone number and numbers for local related community resources.

Emotional Support

Support groups within the rehabilitation facility or in the community can be helpful to patients and to their family members. Some rehabilitation facilities offer specific groups for spinal cord injured patients with high quadriplegia, for family members, or for women with spinal cord injuries. The opportunity to share with and learn from others in similar circumstances is often a means of support not able to be duplicated in any other kind of support system.

Elsewhere, emotional support for the patient with high quadriplegia and his or her family often comes from extended family members, friends, church, community groups, and rehabilitation staff. Other patients on a one-to-one basis can provide the most intimate awareness of the patient's suffering and through this be the most supportive and encouraging.

While being supportive, the counselor can help to identify the patient and families' coping styles and resources. Sharing this with other staff can enlist the best sensitivity and understanding of how the team can be helpful to the patient. Hearing the patient's fears, comprehending his/her bravado, or trying to imagine what it is like for the patient to be paralyzed can help each team member appreciate the position of the patient. This appreciation is basic to using the patient's strengths while recognizing but strengthening the weaknesses. This approach, facilitated by the counselor, combined with the patient's exposure to other patients with high-level quadriplegia and the allowance for the passage of time, are often the basis for the patient's beginning to understand and adjust to the disability. Those patients or family members who struggle excessively with the grief process will warrant a referral for more intensive therapy with the counselor, psychologist, or psychiatrist.

Financial Counseling

This continual emotional support related to the patient's adjustment to disability is part of the counseling effort that goes into other counseling issues as well. After injury, personal and family finances become even more essential to survival and quality of life. The counselor's evaluation of available assets includes exploring insurance, salary, disability income, and other income or assets. This information is a guide to planning benefit referrals and funding for discharge needs. An initial contact with the insurance claims adjustor and/or the contracted rehabilitation case manager begins the process of outlining the patient's needs to the insurance company. This contact also assists the counselor in learning the limits and process of securing funding through the insurance company to meet these needs. Financial coverage for such things as equipment, attendant care, or home modifications can vary depending on the individual insurance policy or company (see Chapter 26). Often a combination of insurance is involved and sorting out the primary insurance and method for working cooperatively with secondary insurance can be clarified. Health and accident insurance, worker's compensation, car insurance, and government insurance (for example, Medicare, Medicaid, Champus) are examples of the varieties of insurance of which the counselor needs to be knowledgeable. Ongoing telephone contacts, letters of justification, and feedback from conferences (written summaries or tape recordings) can assist in keeping the insurance company informed and involved. Hopefully, in this way a hospital stay will not be prolonged because of a need to wait for funding decisions related to discharge needs.

Eligibility for specific resources and gaps in funding resources are identified with the counselor, patient, and family. Subsequent referrals are made to appropriate agencies to explore eligibility for income (e.g., Social Security), insurance (e.g., Medicaid), or other services (e.g., churches, civic organizations). Some agencies, such as the Department of Vocational Rehabilitation or Handicapped Children's Program, can provide funding for specialized services if the patient is eligible. Some states now have federally funded model waivers for the heavy care needs of the severely disabled (1). Some state Medicaid programs can apply the "Katie Beckett" waiver to help fund care needs at home for the disabled child (2). Creative ways of securing needed funding are continually researched by the counselor in trying to meet the discharge needs of the patient with high quadriplegia (see Chapter 26).

Discharge Planning

The patient and family financial resources are a primary basis on which the patient's discharge plans are made. After being in the rehabilitation setting, discharge to the patient's or family's home is often the patient's preference. Available housing, personal care, transportation, supplies, equipment, and financing are essential to make this plan workable. An adult with high quadriplegia with no family could have more difficulty using this home discharge plan, especially without financing that could fund adequate attendant care.

The counselor can help the patient find attendants in several ways. People can be selected and trained by the patient or they can be hired professionals from a home health agency (see Chapter 17 for details). Trained, willing, dependable family or friends can provide personal care but with the caution that this responsibility on a continual basis can lead to stresses in the relationship with the patient. For the person with high quadriplegia who needs many hours of hired attendant care, the continual presence in the home of an attendant can also be a stress on the family's privacy. Some patients have found more creative ways to find attendants through organizing volunteers from specific service groups.

In addition to helping find attendants, the counselor can ascertain that the patient is aware of durable medical equipment vendors and local or mail-order pharmacies and medical supply providers.

The counselor, with the patient and family, must locate or identify appropriate housing for discharge. Once the house has been identified, the team members (counselor, physical therapist, occupational therapist) and the patient can make a home visit. If the house is not in a nearby location, floor plans, measurements, and snapshots of the house can be reviewed by the family, patient, and team. Appropriate suggestions for modifications to the house are made by the team and the patient. Accessibility to the main entrance, bedroom, bathroom (and its fixtures), and main living quarters are usually considered as minimal modifications needed for long-term residency. Some suggestions are based on specific needs of the patient with high quadriplegia and could also entail alarm systems, air conditioning, and environmental controls. A summary of the recommendations is submitted by the counselor to the funding sources and contractors. The counselor can provide the patient and family with literature showing modification designs for such things as ramps and bathrooms.

As with home modifications, the patient will work with the occupational therapist to evaluate transportation. The counselor can assist with assessing funding for the patient's special transportation needs such as attendant-operated van modifications. The counselor can also help the patient and family identify and contact their local emergency services for transportation or care should those be needed after discharge home.

The counselor arranges with the family for their coming to the rehabilitation facility for intensive predischarge training. Before the patient leaves, a transitional living arrangement close to the hospital or an opportunity for the family to assume all care of the patient while he or she is still in the hospital is helpful. The counselor can assist with organizing this and support the family and patient in this process.

Other options besides going home are sometimes selected by the patient with high quadriplegia (see Chapter 17). Transitional or independent living centers or group homes are options in certain communities. Some patients choose to return to college or boarding school with hired attendant care whereas others will go to a nursing home or extended-care facility. The counselor can assist in locating and evaluating appropriate placement that can serve the physical and social needs of the patient with high quadriplegia.

Although the person with a high-level spinal cord injury can be quite physically dependent, it is important for the counselor to advocate the patient's intellectual and social input into his or her family and social systems. In planning discharge it is crucial to keep the patient involved in the decisions to be made. If the patient, however, chooses to have a legal conservator to manage his financial affairs, the counselor can assist with appropriate guidance and referral regarding this.

Who Am I Now? Counseling for Role Adjustments

For the patient with high quadriplegia, reviewing, seeking, and maintaining identity is a struggle that often begins to surface during the rehabilitation phase of treatment (3). The counselor can assist the patient in looking at the personnel, social, sexual, spiritual, and productive parts of himself/herself. In these, the basic needs for human affirmation, diversion, and personal contribution can be confirmed and encouraged. Social and recreational activities can be promoted as can vocational pursuits. Concrete information, counseling, and guidance to resources can be the counselor's role with the patient. For school-age students, tutoring can be arranged by the counselor so that the patient can continue studies.

The counselor can also arrange for injured patients who did not complete high school to earn their general equivalency diploma. This can be a boost for vocational goals after discharge. Joint contacts with schools, employers, or vocational counselors are often indicated to initiate the process of reentering this aspect of the patient's life. Counseling related to peer acceptance, dating, and meeting others can be incorporated into the socialization aspect of returning to school, work, and outside activities.

In more personal relationships the patient's sexual role is frequently a primary concern. The need for physical closeness, gender confirmation, and acceptance are often experienced by the patient with spinal cord injury. Struggling with a changed body image and roles (for example, as husband, father, or bread earner) is an ongoing process that warrants counseling of supportive, educational, and psychotherapeutic natures.

Exploring with the patient and his or her partner their sexual history, including roles and expectations, is a helpful beginning for the counselor. The basic information about sexual anatomy and physiology and changes in sexual functioning after spinal cord injury can be provided by the counselor. The patient's level of physical functioning and areas of bodily sensation need to be taken into consideration as part of the counseling process. For the patient with high quadriplegia, movement and sensation can be notably restricted for sexual activity. It is therefore important for the counselor to supportively encourage the partner's participation in counseling. Special concerns of the partner's role in sexual activity can be identified during counsel. It is the counselor's role to openly and comfortably discuss the options, whether it be penile implants, positions during intercourse, techniques, devices, or alternative means of sexual satisfaction, because this provides the patient and partner permission to thoroughly evaluate this topic. Often patients with a high-level spinal cord injury are not as interested in the details during their first rehabilitation stay as they might be at a later time. Nevertheless, the counselor can provide the basic background information for the patient's reference.

The sexual history also includes the patient's plans for having children. The counselor then, if appropriate, must incorporate information regarding fertility into the sexual counseling. To men with high-level quadriplegia, fertility techniques and options should be made available to him and his partner. The female patient with spinal cord injury might need specific information and counseling related to birth control, pregnancy, and delivery. Parenting and child care issues might be present or future concerns that could warrant discussion with the counselor. Sexual counsel can be provided in individual sessions or in group classes. Educational literature and films can assist the process as can visual aids such as vibrators or samples of implants used for penile erection. For young patients parental permission is needed for counseling using explicit materials.

As part of counseling related to intimate relationships, it is not uncommon for patients with a high-level spinal cord injury to express concern about not only their physical attractiveness but also their overall value as people. Fears related to being able to contribute to a relationship are often reflected in the sexual expectation of the patient but are readily seen to go beyond that role. The questioning of the meaning of life, exploring and calling on resources of faith, courage, and hope are part of this reckoning process. The counselor can get assistance from other resources in this area of counseling such as through the hospital chaplain, clergy, the patient's friends, and from other patients with spinal cord injury. Whether a spiritual exploration to find meaning and courage to get through the here and now or an educational awareness of what is being done to try to change, treat, or cure spinal cord injury to identify hope for the future, the counselor will find these questions as underlying themes in the rehabilitation counseling process.

While helping the patient adjust to body changes and role alterations brought about by the disability, the counselor leads the course of rehabilitation counseling toward the goal of discharge. The counselor works to finalize discharge plans with the patient, family, and outside resources. Assistance with transportation from the rehabilitation unit to the discharge destination can be arranged. The counselor is careful to verify reservations with cabs, ambulance, or airlines. Also important is the confirmation of trained attendant care accompanying the patient. A termination interview is held with the patient and family to again review the discharge plan and to offer support for the transition from the rehabilitation setting (see Chapter 19). A dictated discharge summary will include the patient's progress through the rehabilitation program, the discharge plan, and recommendations for services for follow-up after discharge.

CONCLUSIONS

In the rehabilitation unit the counselor's role consists of helping the patient adjust to the here and now while preparing the patient with a high-level spinal cord injury for life after the hospital. Counseling means thorough evaluation and planning of concrete needs, mixed with appreciation for the emotional and psychosocial needs and values of the patient and family. Finding or instilling a sense of belief in oneself, the meaning of one's life, and a searching for what gives life quality is part of the motivation toward specific discharge plans. It is not surprising that findings in a survey by Menter et al. (4) shows long-term survival rates of patients with high-level spinal cord injury are significantly more positive in those patients who are discharged to their homes after rehabilitation. It also appears from these findings that the home setting is more conducive to living out one's life roles in a personal, social, sexual, vocational, and spiritual capacity. Rehabilitation counseling promotes the value of the patient's living out his or her own life roles in a caring, supportive environment after discharge.

REFERENCES

1. Loyer S (1987): *Ventilator Dependent Funding.* Ann Arbor, MI: University of Michigan.
2. *Brook Lodge Invitational Symposium on the Ventilator Dependent Child.* Augusta, MI: 1983.
3. Ginsburg M (1986): *Ventilator Dependent Quadriplegia.* Englewood, CO: Craig Hospital.
4. Menter R, et al. (1983): *Outcome: Ventilator Dependent Quadriplegia: 42 Cases, 1974–1982.* Englewood, CO: Craig Hospital.

III

Discharge Planning

Overview

Daniel P. Lammertse

Craig Hospital, Englewood, Colorado, U.S.A.

The following chapters review various aspects of discharge planning for the high quadriplegic patient, including patient and family education, equipment, arranging for attendant care, and preparing for the psychological impact of the return home. Although these issues are not unique to the high quadriplegic patient, the magnitude of these problems often appears much greater than for patients with a lower level of injury. The complete physical dependence and the amount of high technology equipment required for a successful discharge from the hospital create requirements for successful home placement that in terms of both hours of care and financial costs are far greater than for other patients. Because of the need to respond at a moment's notice to the inevitable ventilator equipment malfunction, high quadriplegic patients require 24 h of attendant care per day, and although their direct care needs for activities of daily living, self care, and hygiene may not be significantly different from other dependent quadriplegic individuals, this issue of attendant availability in the event of equipment malfunction has a profound effect on the real costs of community placement for these individuals. In situations in which third-party funding for such help (either in the home setting or in a nursing home) is not available, the "cost" burden is borne by family members if available and willing. When these resources are not available, the patient can oftentimes not be discharged.

Another issue that sets this group of patients apart when planning for discharge is the cost of equipment. It can be said that the rehabilitation of the high quadriplegic patient is primarily the evaluation, prescription, and fitting of equipment and the training of patients and their caregivers to use equipment. To be sure there are other issues of education, training of nursing skills, and maintenance therapy programs,

247

but because this group of patients exhibits such profound physical dependence, any achievement of independent mobility and control of the environment requires the use of sophisticated high technology and expensive equipment. The cost of two portable ventilators, one primary and one backup in case of failure, plus related respiratory equipment can easily cost between $20,000 and $25,000. Mouth-controlled power-recline electric wheelchairs can cost between $10,000 and $15,000. When van modifications and other equipment are added to this list, one can readily see that the equipment expense alone is very high.

Because of these unique factors, the successful rehabilitation and community placement of the high quadriplegic patient is not always feasible. The discharge planning process must therefore take into account the availability of resources to achieve a community discharge and such an exploration of resources should ideally begin before accepting a patient into the rehabilitation program. Thus, for this group of patients more than any other, the discharge planning process must begin before admission. It does the patient and family little good to have the carrot of rehabilitation held out only to be out of reach when it is learned that insufficient funding support exists for equipment, attendant care, or nursing home placement. Having accepted such a patient prematurely, the rehabilitation facility (which is usually in the best position to advocate for what are novel but farsighted and discharge-enabling expenditures on the part of the insurance company), will potentially have lost some of its leverage to lobby with third-party payers on the patient's behalf.

Once the patient is admitted and involved in the program, the discharge planning effort requires a great deal of coordination between the team members. The prescription, delivery time, setup, and troubleshooting of sophisticated equipment are often the determining factors in length of stay and must be carefully coordinated with the required home modifications and the hiring and training of attendants. Patient and family education, because it involves not only nursing and maintenance therapy issues but also the use and maintenance of sophisticated electronic equipment, is of such magnitude that it cannot be put off for the last week of hospitalization but must continue apace throughout the admission.

Finally, because most high quadriplegia rehabilitation by necessity occurs at tertiary centers, careful preparation for transition to local resources must be made. Follow-up medical specialists in rehabilitation medicine, pulmonary, urology, and other relevant specialties should be identified and contacted before discharge. Local equipment vendors for respiratory equipment as well as wheelchairs and van modifications should be identified to assist the patient and family in arranging for maintenance. Along these lines, it is critically important that the patient and family be fully educated in the maintenance schedules of life-support ventilator equipment and to strictly adhere to the manufacturer's recommended maintenance schedule.

In summary, because of the extraordinary financial and attendant care requirements of high quadriplegic patients, the discharge planning process must be thoroughly integrated into the rehabilitation effort and ideally begun before admission to the rehabilitation unit. All disciplines on the team have a role to play in the discharge planning process which, because of this complexity, requires careful coordination of the individual efforts of the team members. Most importantly, the patient and family must be thoroughly involved in the process of goal setting and in ensuring that the community placement is both realistic and achievable.

17

Personal Care Attendants: The Alternative to Institutionalization

Scott Manley

Craig Hospital, Englewood, Colorado, U.S.A.

OVERVIEW

Personal care attendants can be the key to successful independent living for individuals with severe disabilities (1–5). A person who has survived a high cervical spinal injury cannot live independently without the assistance of attendant care services. Independent living requires the disabled individual to be responsible for directing his or her own life: choosing where to live, addressing community and social responsibilities, and managing personal and financial affairs. Individual choice allows each person to direct his life even if it involves taking risks and making mistakes (2,3,5,6).

Attendant care is a major issue of the independent living movement because it allows severely disabled individuals the freedom of choice in making decisions affecting personal independence (2,6). The attendant care model incorporates many of the values and concepts advocated by the independent living movement, including civil rights, institutionalization, freedom of choice, and independence (2,6). "Attendant care is more important to a person with severe physical disabilities than accessible housing, special parking, or affirmative action programs" (6).

SCOPE OF SERVICES PROVIDED

Attendant care services may be performed by either a paid or nonpaid person and may occur on a full or part-time basis. It also can be categorized according to the type of assistance provided. Personal care is the most common type of attendant care. It is medically oriented and prevents inpatient hospitalization or institutionalization. The services are directed at long-term care or maintenance as opposed to short-term skilled care for an acute illness. Specific tasks performed by personal care providers include assisting the patient with personal hygiene, dressing, feeding, and transferring. Assistance with household chores or housekeeping would not be allowed under personal care services unless they were essential to the individual's health and comfort or incidental to medical need. Changing bed linens, providing transportation for medical treatment, or preparing meals for special diets, for example, would be considered incidental to medical care or essential to the patient's individual health.

Personal care services are usually supervised by a registered nurse who periodically evaluates the ongoing need for services and the quality of services being provided. Services are generally recognized as a reimbursable expense by Medicaid, but usually not paid for by private insurance plans. Medicare may also pay for personal care services, but only if they are provided in conjunction with skilled medical home health services.

The second general classification of attendant care is medical home health service. This assistance involves giving injections, inserting of catheters, irrigating with sterile procedures, changing sterile dressings, caring for decubitus ulcers, administering medications, or giving physical and occupational therapy. These services require a physician's order and are performed by a registered nurse, licensed practical nurse, occupational therapist, or physical therapist. The insurance industry generally recognizes reimbursement for these services, but may impose a frequency or financial limit.

Home health services are also more expensive because of the involvement of trained medical personnel and are viewed as less desirable by advocates of the independent living movement because they are medically directed as opposed to being self directed (2). The home health care model is closely related to the medical model in which consumers become more like patients rather than becoming independent and taking responsibility for directing the services they deem necessary. The independent living movement, however, has increased the sensitivity of home health care agencies to the concerns of the disabled and, as a result, are allowing the disabled individual more control in directing the activities of agency personnel.

Attendant assistance may also be classified as chore services, including housecleaning, washing clothes, or shopping for the disabled individual. Chore services are not usually considered to be a reimbursable expense by private health insurance plans.

Individuals with high-level quadriplegia may use several types of attendants to assist with personal care or activities of daily living. Patterns of care and service may vary widely. A personal care attendant may provide assistance with activities of daily living on a full-time basis, whereas part-time attendants are used to provide assistance with housekeeping chores, meal preparation, equipment maintenance, shopping, or providing transportation. Attendants may also assist those enrolled in educational programs by providing transportation to school and assistance with note taking or school work. High-level quadriplegic individuals will be heavily dependent on attendant care services that must be coordinated to assure ongoing independence. Unfortunately, all attendant care services are not recognized as reimbursable expenses by the insurance industry and services frequently overlap, creating a complex process that only adds to the frustrations of the disabled individual.

Due to funding inadequacies, family or friends generally assume a major role in the provision of personal care services. Family members should not be expected to provide long-term attendant care without deterioration of the family unit and ultimately higher medical costs when the family unit reaches a point of not being able to provide adequate care and support. Enlightened insurance carriers recognize the cost benefits of providing financial support to family members providing attendant care and recognize the benefits of providing additional attendant care services.

The medical profession and insurance industry need to work together in providing the high quadriplegic person with medically indicated attendant care, while assuring the cost effectiveness of the services provided. When the two professions do not work together, an adversarial relationship usually develops. In this case, the insurance carrier insists on paying only for services provided by an RN or LPN. The physician, recognizing that 24-h supervision is required, orders 24-h RN or LPN services. These services can be supported medically based on the medical needs and life support equipment involved in managing a high quadriplegic person. If both parties are willing to work together, a compromise can be reached that still provides the medical care and supervision required, but at a significantly reduced cost. In lieu of providing 24-h RN or LPN attendant care, a combination of RNs, LPNs, and aides can be employed as a team to assure that proper care is provided and adequately supervised. The result is a reduction in the hours of direct care provided by a RN or LPN. Costs are significantly reduced and proper medical care can be safely monitored. Costly medical complications are avoided and long-term medical management costs are significantly reduced.

The author has observed too many cases in which the family and insurance company end up in an adversary relationship. Ultimately, no one wins. The family unit deteriorates, the patient develops medical complications, and the insurance company ends up paying for hospitalization costs or related medical treatment. All parties involved need to work together to develop a cost-effective model based on the 24-h medical care and supervision required for high quadriplegic individuals.

SERVICE DELIVERY MODELS

Attendant care services can be provided in a variety of ways. A high-level quadriplegic person who lives in an urban area may be able to use shared attendant care services with other disabled individuals within the community. Under this model, an attendant may be hired full-time to assist several individuals, allowing several persons to combine their financial resources. Because high-level quadriplegia is associated with significant dependence, many individuals will use a combination of both models: using a full-time attendant for primary care while using other attendants for supplemental care to several individuals.

Another adaptation of this model is frequently used by college students who find it cheaper to live together and share attendant resources. Although the clustering of disabled individuals is not always desirable, the savings may outweigh the preference for living alone instead of in a group living arrangement. The group model may involve as few as two individuals living together or as many as four to eight individuals living in specialized college housing adapted for the severely disabled individual.

Numerous colleges, universities, and communities have established special housing arrangements that provide for attendant care services, transportation, meals, and recreational opportunities. Although the individuals may not be fully integrated into the able-bodied community, this model has received strong support because of the financial benefits of providing accessible housing, transportation, and attendant care services within a centralized location. There may be lower financial costs and the ability to provide backup services may be easier to arrange when attendants are ill or absent.

As the U.S. population shifts to an increasing number of elderly individuals who may require the assistance of personal care attendants, our society must recognize the need to develop a better model of providing transportation, accessible housing, and attendant services. Unfortunately, until our society recognizes this need plus the financial benefits of planned attendant care services, accessible transportation, and accessible communities, our current models will remain fairly limited.

PROVIDERS OF ATTENDANT CARE

There are a number of resources that provide attendant care services. High-level quadriplegic individuals commonly combine available attendant care resources with family members to provide personal care assistance.

The newspaper ad is the most common means of obtaining attendant care. Ads provide a variety of responses, from those who have had previous attendant care experience and enjoy assisting others in achieving independence, to those who have had no experience or formalized training. Individuals providing attendant care may not have to be previously trained or licensed if they are supervised by competent medical personnel. Needs and systems of care may vary from individual to individual. College students can be used on a part- or full-time basis, but they may not be able to provide for continuity of care due to school schedules.

Vocational school students specializing in the health care field may also be a good resource. Some vocational schools offer specific training programs in attendant care services and students completing the program may seek positions in hospitals, nursing homes, or institutional settings. Placing an ad in a nursing home or hospital may secure health care professionals who are looking for part-time employment. As mentioned earlier, home health care agencies also provide professionals and paraprofessionals who can provide attendant care services. The agency cost is generally higher, however, and the disabled individual will not have the control they might have over an attendant they have hired and trained themselves.

Using a developmentally disabled individual has also been successful depending on the complexity and skill involved in the attendant care services. The author is aware of several situations in which developmentally disabled individuals have been used. They have provided excellent, reliable care over an extended period. Some community agencies or organizations may also maintain an attendant registry that can be accessed by individuals with a disability. Volunteer organizations or churches may also be a source of attendants. Although Social Security recipients have been used to provide personal care attendant services, individuals requiring total assistance in transfers, turning, or positioning should determine if the elderly individual has the physical strength and stamina required to assist safely. Assistance with housework, shopping, meal preparation, or transportation, however, can be provided by elderly persons interested in supplementing their income.

FINANCING OF ATTENDANT CARE

The cost of attendant care varies, depending on the location, previous training, specific duties, and qualifications of the attendant. The cost may range from minimum wage to $25–30 an hour for home health care agency personnel with specialized training. The payment source of attendant care services can also vary. Some insurance policies (such as

Worker's Compensation and no-fault or liability insurance) may provide for full coverage of attendant care services that are prescribed as medically necessary by a physician. The majority of individuals needing attendant care are not covered by insurance policies that provide comprehensive coverage for attendant care. Although some health care indemnity plans will provide coverage for registered nurses if medically indicated, some of the attendant care provided does not require the professional training of a registered nurse or therapist.

The federal government also provides funding for attendant care for those individuals who meet specific eligibility guidelines. Under Medicaid regulations, personal care services can be provided in a person's home by a qualified individual. The services must be prescribed by a physician in accordance with a plan of treatment that is supervised by a nurse. Medicare patients can also receive home health aide services but only if the individual is also receiving skilled nursing or therapy services. The Medicare program focuses on short-term skilled care and not on long-term personal care services for disabled individuals. Fortunately, Medicaid does not require a test for skilled services, allowing eligible recipients to receive the services of a home health aide if home health services are part of the state Medicaid plan. In most state Medicaid programs, home health care is perceived as an appropriate alternative to unnecessary institutionalization or hospitalization. Medicaid's requirements address long-term care and do not have any statutory basis for requiring skilled care.

The Rehabilitation Act also provides a funding source for attendant care services. Under Section 110, funds may be used to pay for attendant care services if the disabled individual is a client of vocational rehabilitation. Unfortunately, the services available are usually of limited duration and available only to vocational rehabilitation clients. Social Service Block Grants (SSBG) may provide another source for attendant care if the services provided prevent or reduce the need for institutionalization. California's In-Home Supportive System is an excellent example of using SSBG funds to pay for attendant care (7). The major problem with the SSBG program is the lack of appropriated funds. Some states also provide for credits or refunds to disabled individuals who are employed and pay for personalized attendant care services (7). Tax deductions have also been allowed for the portion of attendant care expenses related to groceries, rent, and utilities (8).

Some of the major disadvantages of government-supported programs include the limitation of available funds, the focus on service for poor people only, and the low rate of reimbursement for providers of attendant care services. The majority of disabled individuals are not eligible for government-supported attendant care services and have to rely on family members or friends for attendant care services. Although the availability of attendant care services for the severely disabled is limited because of the lack of financial support, the need for attendant care on a national basis continues to increase. As our population grows older, the number of individuals with physical disabilities will continue to rise. Many of these persons will require assistance with activities of daily living. As Findley and Findley state, "Between 1966 and 1976, the number of persons with limitations in any of their activities rose by 37% at a time when the general population increased by only 10%" (9).

The increased medical technology available in our society has also resulted in increasing the number of individuals with severe disabilities. These individuals will also require services of personal care attendants if they are to remain independent outside of an institutional setting. If our society continues to support the deinstitutionalization of the disabled and the aged, then there will be an increasing need to support the personal care services for these individuals. As the make-up of the family unit changes with an increasing number of women entering the work force, a greater demand will take place to provide outside assistance in providing for the personal care needs of disabled or elderly individuals.

All of these changes will increase demands on our society to find a more effective model for providing personal care assistance for the disabled or elderly. The model must also be financially sound, taking into account what is appropriate to spend while still being affordable to the increasing number of individuals who will require attendant care services.

COST–BENEFIT ANALYSIS

There has been very little written that examines the cost of providing funds for attendant care in the home as opposed to the costs of institutionalization. The benefits of Section 2176 of the Omnibus Budget Reconciliation Act of 1981 provide some basic data. This section of the Act granted the Secretary of Health and Human Services the authority to waive existing Medicaid statutory requirements and permit states to finance noninstitutionalized long-term care services for Medicaid-eligible individuals (1).

The 2176 Waiver Program is designed to provide home and community-based services (HCBS) for the disabled, the developmentally disabled, or the elderly who would remain in or would be placed in institutions without HCBS services (10). The Medicaid Waiver Program was passed by Congress as a cost-containment measure with the stipulation that the level of expenditure for all long-term care services would not be greater under the Waiver than the level of expenditures would have been in the absence of the Waiver (1). It was estimated that the Medicaid Waiver Program would save $250 million dollars in its first year of operation for the 26 states with approved programs as of February 1983 (1).

These costs are only estimates and reflect cost savings for a wide spectrum of disabled individuals. Attendant care requirements for the general population of disabled individuals is 2–6 h of attendant care per day (2). For the individual with a high cervical injury, the average direct medical care requirement per day is closer to 10–12 h, with most ventilator patients requiring 24-h medical supervision initially when discharged (11). The cost–benefit analysis used by the government to determine the costs for maintaining an individual in a hospital or institution rather than at home does not provide an accurate indication of the actual cost associated with a ventilator-dependent individual in the home. The rate of reimbursement allowable for an institution or hospital is based on a formula that does not take into account all of the expenses of providing care to a ventilator-dependent individual. Nursing homes or hospitals, therefore, may be reticent to accept ventilator-dependent quadriplegic patients because of lower reimbursement when compared with private pay or insurance sponsored patients. Home health care providers also believe the allowable Medicaid reimbursement rate for providing attendant care to ventilator-dependent individuals is significantly below rates paid by the private insurance industry.

The current cost–benefit model also does not take into account the hidden costs associated with placing a young disabled person in an institution. Most nursing homes take care of the elderly who have significantly different needs and interests than a young, disabled individual. A nursing home or hospital environment is not designed to provide the psychological and social support necessary for the normal growth and development of a young individual over a prolonged period of time. In this sense, the cost formula does not recognize the potential hidden costs that can be associated with ongoing medically related complications due to a passive existence in a nursing home, or the physical deterioration that can result from psychological factors associated with confinement. Further research is needed to determine the long-term effects of institutionalization on a young individual and the effects of institutionalization on long-term medical costs. It is unreasonable to expect a young disabled individual to develop his or her full potential if placed in a restrictive environment that is not conducive to normal maturational growth socially and psychologically.

PROBLEMS IN THE PROVISION OF ATTENDANT CARE

Individuals with high-level quadriplegia have been greatly concerned with the difficulty of obtaining and training individuals for attendant care services (3). Thornock and colleagues conducted a survey involving 131 agencies and found that only 42% of the agencies provided organized programs to teach necessary attendant skills, and only 18% provided ongoing evaluation of attendant performance (4). Even though 90% of the respondents reported that their client populations included persons who would require attendant care to live independently, the majority of the programs were not providing specific training programs or any type of follow-up services to evaluate the attendant care services being provided (4). Whether it is the responsibility of the rehabilitation facility to provide attendant care, or whether the community is responsible, is a question yet to be resolved.

The funding available to pay for training programs or attendant care services has always been a low priority. The majority of individuals rely on their own resources, both financially and otherwise, to obtain attendant care services. As a result of the independent living movement, there have been some excellent manuals and resource guides developed that help the disabled learn about hiring and maintaining an attendant. Once the problem of locating an attendant has been solved, obtaining funding support for attendant care services presents ongoing problems. If funding is available from a government agency, periodic adjustments in wages are limited because of the difficulty in obtaining cost adjustments once reimbursement rates are established. One of the major reasons for turnover of attendants that has been cited is low pay (2,4,6,12).

In some states, licensing requirements may be an additional concern. If personal care services require the changing of catheters, suctioning, or administering of medications, state licensing requirements may be strict in the required credentialing of individuals providing these services. Because most high-level quadriplegic persons will need some assistance with suctioning, catheter care, and medications, an individual with a severe physical disability is left with the choice of obtaining a qualified attendant who is licensed to provide these specific services, or using someone who is not licensed to provide these services under state requirements. This situation can become difficult for attendants if they are in a state that requires licensing for specific personal care services. If attendants provide these services, even though they may have been authorized to do so by the disabled individual, they may be at risk legally and financially if medical complications develop or if they are reported for being in violation of state law.

Attendant care services provided by family members is another major issue. Families usually provide some of the attendant care services for the high-level quadriplegic individual. The amount of care provided usually depends on the availability of financial resources and/or the availability of attendant care services within the community. In a follow-up survey of 30 ventilator-dependent quadriplegic persons, Charlifue (13) indicated 25% of the required attendant care services were being provided by a family member. The impact on the family has not been studied due to lack of available data. There have been numerous reports, however, about the stress that providing attendant care has on the family over a long period (4,14,15).

Family dynamics may be altered significantly when family members assume the major responsibility for attendant care. The established family role of being a spouse or parent is changed to one of being a nurse or attendant. This can have a significant impact on the normal interaction of the family and the role each has assumed in the past. The provision of attendant care services for a high-level quadriplegic person can also be very demanding (4,14,15). Unfortunately, there are few data available on the long-term effects psychologically, socially, financially, or physically when family members provide the major portion of attendant care services day after day. Although the literature may lack information related to specific impact of family members providing attendant care services, a review of literature indicates that articles are beginning to appear that address the need for providing support to family members responsible for long-term care to elderly or disabled family members. Two organizations that provide supportive services and assistance for caregivers are the Association of Carers and the National Council for Carers and Their Elderly Dependents.

CONCLUSIONS

According to Dejong, "Attendant care is viewed (in our society) as a survival right, a benefit necessary to the survival of the individual, since a severely physically disabled person cannot participate in school, work, recreation or the political life of the community without it. Because of its indispensable nature, attendant care takes on the character of an inalienable right with status compared to a civil right" (16). Although the need for and importance of attendant care services for the disabled is easily understood and relatively simple to provide in its basic form, our society has chosen to make it complex. This dilemma continues to have a significant impact on the ventilator-dependent quadriplegic individual who must rely on these services to remain independently at home.

Individuals who are ventilator-dependent need to align with other disabled individuals who are advocating an increase in governmental support for attendant care services. Our society needs to recognize that attendant care is important not only to the disabled poor but to all individuals with disabilities who cannot function independently without attendant care services. Rehabilitation professionals need to become involved in research efforts that will analyze the effects of placing young disabled individuals in institutions intended for the care of the elderly.

What impact does long-term institutionalization have on long-term outcomes and costs? The increasing number of the elderly and the disabled provides an opportunity to address more effective ways of treating these individuals whom society has chosen to save through improved medical care. Our society, unfortunately, has been unwilling to take responsibility for assisting these individuals in maintaining independence after the individual has survived the initial trauma.

REFERENCES

1. Lakin KC, Greenberg JN, Schmitz MP, Hill BK (1984): A comparison of medicaid waiver applications for populations that are mentally retarded and elderly/disabled. *Ment Retard* 22:182–192.
2. DeJong G, Wenker T (1979): Attendant care as a prototype independent living service. *Arch Phys Med Rehabil* 60.477–482.
3. Hutchins TK, Thornock M, Lindgre B, Parks J (1978): Profile of in-home attendant care workers. *Am Rehabil* 4(2):19–22.
4. Thornock M, Hutchins TK, Meyer S, Kenyon A, Williams M (1978): Attendant care needs of the physically disabled: institutional perspectives. *Rehabil Lit* 39(5):147–153.
5. Litvak S, Zukas H, Heumann J (1986): Attending to America: personal assistance for independent living. *Executive Summary of the National Survey of Attendant Services Programs in the United States.* Berkeley, CA: World Institute on Disability.
6. Smith NK, Meyer AB (1981): Personal care attendants: key to living independently. *Rehabil Lit* 42:258–265.
7. Zukas H (1986): *Summary of Federal Funding Sources for Attendant Care.* Berkeley, CA: World Institute on Disability.
8. Watson S (1979): IRS deductions for attendants. *Rehabil Gaz* 22:20.
9. Findley TW, Findley SE (1987): Rehabilitation needs in the 1990s: effects of an aging population. *Med Care* 25(8):753–763.
10. *Medicare and Medicaid Guide,* vol 1 (1987): Chicago: Commerce Clearing House.
11. Staff presentation (1980): Care of high quads C-4 and up, multi-center conference. Englewood, Colorado, Craig Hospital.
12. Atkins BJ, Meyer AB, Smith NK (1982): Personal care attendants: attitudes and factors contributing to job satisfaction. *J Rehabil* July–September:20–24.
13. Charlifue S (1987): Ventilator-dependent spinal cord injured adults: long-term outcome data on quality of life. Paper presented at American Congress of Rehabilitation Medicine Conference, Orlando, Florida.
14. Gloag D (1985): Severe disability: 2—residential care and living in the community. *Br Med J* 290:368–372.
15. Hollinghurst V (1984): Supporting the carers: in at the deep end. *Nurs Times Commun Outlook* December:445–446.
16. Dejong G (1984): Monograph on issues related to independent living. *Holistic Approaches to Independent Living (HAIL).* Prepared for U.S. Department of Education/Office of Special Education and Rehabilitation Services/Special Need Section. Contract RF300-81-0366.

18

Reflections on the Process of Education for the Patient with High Quadriplegia

Kevin McVeigh

Craig Hospital, Englewood, Colorado, U.S.A.

The process of teaching and learning is complicated, especially in the health care setting. Why? Because many professionals have never been taught how to teach. The patient educator has to overcome many barriers to teaching and learning—barriers that lead to statements of frustration such as, "We tried to teach them, but they didn't learn."

High quadriplegia is so complex that it presents an enormous challenge to team members whose goal is effective patient education. There are many reasons for this difficulty—the resistance of the patient to accepting the situation, the staggering amount of information the patient needs to learn, and the possibility of the concomitant head injury, to name but a few.

Because educating this patient is so challenging, staff members need to approach teaching the high quadriplegic patient with special thoughtfulness and energy. It is particularly important for staff members to recognize that a patient needs to come to grips with the problem before he or she will engage in learning to solve that problem.

In the book, *Living, Loving and Learning* (1), author Leo Buscaglia quotes Carl Rogers as saying, " 'You know that I don't believe that anyone has ever taught anything to anyone. I question the efficacy of teaching. The only thing that I know is that anyone who wants to learn will learn. And maybe a teacher is a facilitator, a person who puts things down and shows people how exciting and wonderful it is and asks them to eat.' "

If the outcome of patient education is to be successful, the patient and the patient educator must develop a joint venture from the early planning stages to the final evaluation, each making individual contributions.

Unfortunately, in many situations teachers or educators teach as they were taught. Health care professionals have been involved in the formal education process for many years, first obtaining one degree and then continuing on to graduate work. In these academic settings, the teacher knows in advance what the learner needs to be taught. For example: in the primary grades—reading, writing, arithmetic; in the later grades—science, history, calculus. In patient education there is a different situation. Staff members know little or nothing about the patient's previous knowledge level or abilities. Some patients will be quite sophisticated, whereas others may be examples of the demise of the public education system and why Johnny can't read. Before any plans for teaching can be made, the patient's learning experiences must be determined.

In addition to the normal range of intelligence to be expected among patients, staff members must be prepared to deal with a significant number of high quadriplegic patients who have concomitant head injuries. In this case, educational material must be vastly simplified or presented to family members rather than the patient.

INCREASING INDEPENDENCE

A major goal in patient education is to increase competency, confidence, and independence. This is especially important for patients with high quadriplegia for several reasons. First, they have suffered a severe change in body image that can leave them depressed and hopeless. Second, the success of their rehabilitation and future life depends on their ability to learn about their physical needs and effectively direct others in their own care to become teachers themselves.

It is clear that to accomplish the goal of increased independence, a relationship of trust between staff and patient must be established. Trusting relationships take time, yet time is of the essence in the daily routine of team members. This "time crunch" forces the assessment of patient readiness to learn to be determined by the discharge date.

If patient education efforts on the part of the health care staff are to be effective, psychosocial factors must be taken into account. Spending time disseminating information about what to do and what not to do without considering the psychosocial factors is a waste of time; it also leads to poor outcome for patient education. Patients and family members have anxieties and other concerns that greatly interfere with the effectiveness of education. Timing of the educational intervention is critical to the patient's readiness to learn. If patient education is to help the patients use information, then perhaps it is reasonable to assume that the process must involve more than giving information to a passive patient. Disseminating information, facts, or consequences alone does not constitute quality education.

USING INSTRUCTIONAL AIDS

It is a well-established fact that people can only remember approximately seven pieces of information at a time (2); this means that any time the patient educator asks the patient to learn new facts, this limitation must be taken into account. Additional studies have found that patients in an outpatient setting remember only half of what the physician tells them (3). The amount of information retained by patients of catastrophic injury is probably even less.

The method used to increase patient recall, as well as saving staff time, is the use of instructional aids. These include everything from the handwritten note to elaborate closed-circuit television systems. However, educational research has confirmed that even though some patients may state a preference for watching technologically sophisticated instructional methods, less sophisticated methods such as pamphlets, charts, and the like are equally effective (4). The teaching aids and instructional materials should be selected on the basis of cost, convenience, and dependability, rather than on the expectation of effectiveness in a learning environment. It cannot be overstated that teaching aids must supplement, not substitute for, the personalized education efforts of the health care staff.

SOLUTIONS

How are these obstacles overcome in patient education for the high quadriplegic patient? Today's health care organizations are so complex that the patient's path through the organization is mapped by handbooks and catalogues.

The solution, in my mind, is one of personal resolve within the individual who has the enormous responsibility of teaching the necessary regimen to the high quadriplegic patient and family. The very character of the health care setting throws obstacles in the way of quality individual teaching. Too frequently the patient must contend with listening to many lectures or viewing videotapes. Individual teaching—personal instruction—must be preserved even in large health care settings. The course content, the information, and the curriculum are there, so what needs remain? One primary need is for patient education to be dynamic and enjoyable.

SOLICITING PATIENT FEEDBACK

Is there really any hope that a health team member can improve and continue to improve his or her teaching? Let's take an example: Nurse Mary, B.S.N., M.S. Mary was a graduate student and was an expert clinician. In all her academic work she was outstanding. There was no question that she knew all the components of nursing. After she had completed her work with the first five high quadriplegic patients she was responsible for teaching, the students were asked to evaluate Mary's teaching. Here are some of their comments: "Mary has convinced me that she knows her stuff, but she is way over my head." "I had no idea what I was supposed to be getting."

Naturally, Mary was concerned about these responses. There was no doubt that Mary was prepared for her teaching; however, it was obvious to her that she had to change the level of her information. We decided that she needed more feedback from her patients if she were to keep the presentation at their level. Perhaps if the students participated more, their discussion would provide clues to their understanding of the materials. "If I let my patients participate, how can I cover the material? I'm rushed for time now. Still, I guess it doesn't do me much good to cover the materials if the patient and family don't understand it. Maybe I shouldn't worry so much about covering everything."

Mary devised questions to focus on major points in the information. She handed these questions out in advance. These questions came up again during the teaching demonstration and stirred up discussion. The point of Mary's experience is not to suggest that everyone should use study questions; rather, it is intended to indicate how improvement can result by getting feedback from the patients themselves.

If the purpose of patient education is to bring about change in patients, the information from patients is required to provide a basis for improving teaching.

SELF-EVALUATION

Since care of the high quadriplegic patient is so demanding, there is a natural tendency to routinize and automate the teaching process in the interest of increased efficiency. As members of the health care team, we incur a heavy responsibility to analyze more carefully the manner in which we spend our patient education time. Here are some questions to ask yourself: Do you teach differently to different patients? Are you making optimal use of time and using teaching aids creatively? Can you honestly say that a change in your teaching approach would be less effective or enjoyable without trying it? Strive to keep enjoyment in teaching and not lose that enjoyment to a rut of daily tasks.

Enjoyment of teaching patients is important, not only for the enthusiasm that the team member communicates to his or her patient, but also in fostering continued improvement in patient education as a whole. Both of these values are likely to be lost if patient teaching becomes routinized and depersonalized to the point that it is no longer fun.

HELPING THE PATIENT INCORPORATE

Patients are pretty good judges of when they have been taught effectively, and my guess is that most teachers are fairly accurate in their estimates of which patients they are most effective with. This, however, should not be taken to mean that teaching is always pleasant and satisfying. When the health care member touches a patient deeply, the patient may face a painful recognition of his/her definition of themselves, their lives, and their relationships with others. Their method of thinking, their conception of life, even their belief in the value of life may be challenged. For patients, the choice is between incorporating the learning into their reorganization or ignoring the content so that it has minimal effect. The patient educator, and other patients, can be important allies of growth if they are able to respond to a patient about the problem of incorporating and learning.

Real success in teaching depends on continual reevaluation and modification of one's teaching. There is danger that we in the health care environment will abandon all pretense of two-way interaction and subvert patient education into a one-way communication of information. Thus, it may well be up to the individual health care team member to fight to preserve personal patient teaching and the time needed to get satisfaction from teaching, rather than letting technology substitute for teaching.

As patient educators, our goal is for the patient and family member to absorb the information and decide to make behavioral change. To meet this goal, our message must get through short-term memory to long-term memory and into long-term storage.

Three factors interface to support comprehension—logic, language, and experience. Patients must see that what you suggest makes sense, fits within their current lifestyle, can be achieved, and is worthwhile to pursue. They must find the language you use to explain your point to be close to their own vernacular, so that they encounter few stumbling blocks in learning. Patients must have personal experiences similar to those you mention so that they can "put it all together" in their minds.

Teaching patients who are high quadriplegic about their injury is indeed "teaching as if their lives depended on it." And that may just be the case. The focus is on the information needed to solve problems the patient may have in carrying out the required regimen. Emphasis should be on patient participation, encouraging the patient to think through solutions or to find ways of coping with problems that the regimen may present.

Rewards through words of support and encouragement are of critical importance in any learning environment and are monumental for the quadriplegic. It is especially important for this patient, who may feel out of control in many areas of life, to have successes acknowledged and encouraged.

It is easy to believe that patients can learn if they really want to. The assumption is that all you have to do is present the information to the patients. The conclusion is that comprehension will occur when information is given. In fact, receiving the message has little to do with understanding the message.

As mentioned earlier, readiness on the part of the patient is crucial for him/her to learn what you have to teach. You will have greater success in your educational efforts when you make the effort to interest the patient, because usually patients tend to respond positively to someone who wants to help them understand.

SPECIAL EDUCATIONAL CONSIDERATIONS FOR THE HIGH QUADRIPLEGIC PATIENT

The emphasis in this chapter has been on the importance of creating a successful learning environment. For the high quadriplegic patient, it is also important to identify specific areas of learning. Obviously, the high quadriplegic person should receive information and training that is applicable to the general spinal cord injury population, but in addition to the general core curriculum on spinal cord injury, special attention should be given to the following educational needs of the high quadriplegic patient.

1. *Respiratory management.* The patient and family members need to understand the basic fundamentals of respiratory functions so they can adequately address and manage respiratory treatments should problems arise. This should include instruction in nebulized treatments, postural drainage, chest stretching, suctioning, etc. The patient and family members need to know how to identify respiratory complications and learn which treatment modalities can assist in relieving symptoms or respiratory complications.

2. *Autonomic dysreflexia/hypotension.* Autonomic dysreflexia and hypotension are two potential medical emergencies that the patient and family members need to fully understand. The patient and family need to be able to identify symptoms and direct others in taking necessary actions to alleviate potentially life-threatening situations from occurring.

3. *Tracheostomy*. The proper care, cleaning, and management of the individual's tracheostomy, including cleaning of the stoma and inner cannula, should also be a part of the specialized curriculum for the high quadriplegic patient.

4. *Equipment*. Equipment management should be a major educational component because of the high quadriplegic patient's dependence on specialized equipment. The patient and family members need to understand the basis of how the equipment operates, how to identify malfunctions, who to contact as problems arise, and what types of preventive maintenance they can take care of themselves.

5. *Feeding*. Meals involve several safety issues for the high quadriplegic patient. The patient may need to be in a supine or half sitting position to avoid hypotension. Most prefer not to eat while being ventilated on the pneumobelt because of the pressure on the abdomen. This situation requires either switching to trach positive ventilation or eating several small meals during the day. The family must also learn to make sure the patient's head is not positioned in hyperextension because this may increase the chance of aspiration. Families must also be instructed to observe for signs of food aspiration when suctioning the high quadriplegic person.

6. *Positioning and range-of-motion exercises*. It is necessary for patient and family to fully understand how to do the various positioning and range-of-motion exercises. The emphasis should be on using these techniques as part of skin and respiratory care and to prevent contractures.

7. *Transfers and patient handling*. Teaching transfers for patients with high quadriplegia is similar to what is taught with any other spinal cord injury patient. However, there may be more need to consider using mechanical lifts, depending on the size of the patient and primary caregiver.

8. *Maximizing function*. It is of primary importance to encourage this patient to develop and use his/her remaining skills to the fullest. Work in this area needs to continue on the patient's return home. The patient should be encouraged to continue the endurance training started in the hospital. Patient and family should both be made aware of the community resources available to promote vocational and leisure activities. Computerized environmental control units and entertainment systems are available to provide this patient with maximum independence and enjoyment.

CONCLUSIONS

The process of patient education involves more than imparting information concerning what the patient must do. Instead, the successful educational process is an interactive effort that enables the patient, or his or her significant other, to assume responsibilities for the patient's care and independence. Ideally, educational experiences should be planned *with* the patient, based on an assessment of his/her present and potential health status, strengths, liabilities, learning capabilities, and emotional needs. The plan for patient education that derives from such an assessment reflects the content to be taught, sequence and duration of instruction, instructional strategies, and evaluation methods.

Successful patient education depends on the patient's interest in and acceptance of the material presented. As patient educators, we cannot rely on bigger, better, or flashier tools to do our jobs for us. The personal, one to one, communicative approach is the key to motivating the patient to learn. Fostering our own energy and enjoyment of teaching, and interacting with the patient in an individual personal mode, are the best ways to ensure a successful patient education program.

REFERENCES

1. Buscaglia L (1982): *Living, Loving and Learning* (Short S, ed). New York: Fawcett Colunbine.
2. Miller GA (1956): The magical number seven, plus or minus two. *Psychol Rev* 63:81–97.
3. Levy P, Spelman MS (1987): *Communicating with the Patient*. St. Louis: Warren H. Green.
4. Young M (1968): Research and studies related to health education (1961–66) patient education. *Health Educ Monogr* 1:26.

19

Psychological Aspects of Discharge

Lester Butt

Craig Hospital, Englewood, Colorado, U.S.A.

As noted in all chapters, there are a myriad of issues with which the high quadriplegic person must contend to maximize a successful outcome. These issues are diverse in nature and pervade physical, psychological, and social areas. For example, in the physical domain, the high quadriplegic person must contend with a multitude of sensory and motor alterations, bowel and bladder dysfunctions, sexual changes, pain, muscle spasms, autonomic dysreflexia, poor temperature regulation, and respiratory problems. Within the psychological domain, the high quadriplegic individual faces an altered self/body image, role changes, the emergence of heightened emotionality, the presence and necessity of substantial medical equipment, apprehension regarding mere survival, the lack of physical contact with significant others, a heightened degree of chronic stress, and significant dependence on others for the most basic of needs. In the social sphere, the person is confronted with the necessity of acquiring predictable and reliable attendant help, fear of isolation and/or vulnerability, vocational ambiguity, and needs for multiple support systems.

It is truly remarkable that more high quadriplegic persons do not simply capitulate to their injury and become psychologically inert. The process of adapting to this massive catastrophic injury is a continual challenge. This process illustrates a dynamic, not a static, quality. Certainly the high-level quadriplegic person does not achieve a level of adaptation that reflects an end of the adaptive process. Much to the contrary, the individual is confronted with a changing array of pressures. Using this conceptualization can be helpful in understanding adaptation's dynamic nature. Each phase of rehabilitation and adaptation presents unique stressors. As shown in the earlier chapters, the initial reactions and tasks reflect the profound and unpredictable nature of the spinal cord injury. Throughout the initial stages of the injury and the rehabilitation process these stresses wax and wane in terms of their impact on the individual and family. As rehabilitation proceeds and discharge approaches, some of the person's initial concerns can be rekindled and amplified. Consequently, the discharge phase can illustrate both a reemergence or continuation of earlier issues in a different form and emergence of new challenges. The specific issues related to the discharge phase will be addressed; however, understanding crisis theory will enable the health care professional to more fully appreciate the person's psychological responses to stress, specifically inherent in the discharge phase.

CRISIS THEORY

All individuals attempt to achieve a state of homeostatic balance; that is, physical, social, and psychological equilibrium. Toward this end people employ characteristic behavioral patterns to reduce stress and resolve problems. Typically, people can contend with daily life without incapacitating lability and deterioration of problem-solving skills. These behaviors allow for tolerance of frustration, resolution of problems, and discharge of accumulated tension, thereby leading to maintenance of one's equilibrium. However, an individual can face an obstacle to important life goals that is for a period insurmountable through the use of customary methods of problem solving. A period of disorganization ensues, a period of upset in which many abortive attempts at solutions are made. This constitutes a crisis wherein no effectively learned coping strategy is available. Consequently, crisis can be defined as an emergency plus a sense of incapacity. If crisis is successfully managed it can add to one's coping repertoire, or conversely, can reinforce maladaptive trends. As a result, crisis possesses growth-promoting potential. An individual in crisis is searching for a solution in an attempt to regain balance/equilibrium/homeostasis. Again, this balance can represent a healthy adaptation that promotes growth or a maladaptive response that signifies psychological deterioration and decline. There are various types of crises but the onset of high quadriplegia represents an extratemporal crisis in that it occurs independent of a specific time frame in the course of one's life. Spinal cord injury is most certainly an "upset in one's steady state." Additionally, given the fact that stress can be defined as the demand on the organism to change, adapt, or modify itself, stress is most assuredly a component of high quadriplegia. Therefore, the clinician can observe that the spinal-cord-injured individual presents with a level of stress that can potentially reach crisis proportions. Because the discharge phase of rehabilitation demands that the individual confront new challenges and modify him or herself, this period of transition requires a more detailed understanding to maximize the possibility of a positive outcome.

OUTCOME FACTORS

Toward this understanding, there are several main issues that should be broached. Common to all individuals who are ready for discharge is the completion of a formal rehabilitation program. This is mentioned in that outcome is a complex interactional equation of (a) background/personality factors (including age, intellectual capacity, philosophic and religious beliefs, emotional level, family structure, previous losses and coping abilities, academic background, quality of interpersonal relationships, and the symbolic and connotative meanings of the spinal cord injury); (b) illness-related factors (including type and location of the symptoms, the developmental timing of the trauma, the rate of onset, the course of the trauma and potential complications, and coping abilities as influenced by medications/hormonal changes, etc.); and (c) physical/social environment (including both the degree of afforded privacy and stimulation as well as the general ambience of the treating institution). As a result, it is impossible to speak of a predictable, uniform, solitary psychological course when discussing adjustment and accommodation to high-level quadriplegia. What the clinician can do is speak to potential issues confronting the patient on discharge with full awareness that the psychological reactions, given the above equation, are highly variable in nature.

With the above in mind, certain pivotal issues should be further explored. Most assuredly, the rehabilitation hospital is viewed with ambivalence by the patient. However, in spite of these mixed feelings, it can and most often does reflect a psychologically safe environment. Within the hospital walls are staff who are familiar with disability, as well as with the necessary medical equipment and concomitant procedures. Additionally, within the rehabilitation center, the high-level quadriplegic person often does not feel alone or markedly different given the other disabled individuals who surround him or her. Typically, caregivers respond with understanding and acceptance of the disabled individual. Consequently, in the process of obtaining requisite education by the staff, the quadriplegic individual, in spite of the existing physical and psychological crises, can progressively feel less vulnerable and more secure during the inpatient stage of rehabilitation.

As the formal inpatient phase of rehabilitation draws to a close, many psychological issues can emerge. Often, newly injured quadriplegic persons, to varying degrees, maintain the belief that they will achieve full neurologic return. As the discharge date approaches, however, there can be a deterioration of denial as a psychological defense. This dissolution of denial can cause the individual a heightened degree of affective expression. The staff can observe this in a variety of ways, e.g., increased lability and/or irritability, withdrawal from the therapy program or interpersonal contact, acting out behaviors, increased despondency, methods to postpone the discharge date, etc. Obviously, with the inevitability of the approaching discharge date coupled with erosion of denial as a psychological defense, the individual is more fully aware of the potential permanence of the disability. Although disconcerting to patient, family, and staff, if adaptation to disability is seen as a process, the prospect of discharge and contending with its implications is certainly another facet in the eventual accommodation to high-level quadriplegia.

SELF/BODY IMAGE

Another central issue that may emerge as the high-level quadriplegic person faces discharge revolves around self/body image. It goes without saying that high-level quadriplegia represents a dramatic, massive metamorphosis in the appearance and functioning of one's body. During the initial stage of rehabilitation clinicians expect the newly injured individual to exhibit marked concern and apprehension regarding their bodies. As in other aspects of rehabilitation with quadriplegic individuals, issues do not necessarily vanish as they are faced; in contrast, issues that are a concomitant facet of this disability can change form contingent on the timing of the problem. For example, the issue of body image can reflect different connotative, subjective meanings at different stages of rehabilitation. Immediately postinjury the issue of survival of the body itself is a frequent and understandable preoccupation. However, as medical stability becomes more the norm, other bodily worries can present. As the discharge date approaches, apprehensions can most assuredly become manifest regarding how the general public will view the disabled individual. Questions of how people will react to physical atrophy and necessary medical equipment as, for example, an electric wheelchair, a ventilator, and a leg bag can become prominent. Often individuals can question whether they will be accepted by others or whether their disability and unique demands will be far too unusual and threatening. Consequently, concerns of interpersonal isolation may be expressed as discharge approaches. In contrast, disabled individuals may feel so different and infer that others will treat them accordingly that they may cloister themselves under the inferred belief that they are somehow unacceptable. It is psychologically remarkable that high-level quadriplegic individuals successfully incorporate the ventilator into their self-image. Given that body image is one aspect of self-image, it is understandable how an altered body can have an impact on how the individual generically reacts to him/herself. Possible behavioral sequelae could be avoidance of public exposure or interpersonal contacts that could affirm the preconceptions that they are discardable, defective, or unworthy. Adding weight to this potential self-concept is the ventilator-dependent quadriplegic person's compromised communication ability. Due to the ventilator, the individual may be forced to communicate his/her physical and/or psychological needs via lip reading, eye blinks, an alphabet board; or with a voice that may be quite different in quality, volume, or tempo. With certain individuals, this may render them reluctant to communicate and thereby expose their deficits. These concerns may become exacerbated as discharge from inpatient hospitalization approaches and contact with people unfamiliar with disability increases. Accompanying the aforementioned possible dissolution of denial may emerge rumination regarding quality of life. High quadriplegic persons confronting discharge from the familiar and supportive environment of the rehabilitation hospital may question the efficacy of life with a disability. Not all high-level quadriplegic individuals manifest the above, but the clinical staff should be sensitized to such possibilities.

STAFF AND ATTENDANT CARE FACTORS

The clinical staff may also detect possible concerns regarding physical status and stability. During the course of rehabilitation, the disabled individual, family, and/or other support personnel are trained and educated regarding the specifics of quadriplegia. Hopefully, this allows quality care and support outside the confines of the hospital. However, in spite of the rehabilitation hospital's best efforts, it is entirely understandable that medical apprehensions can become manifest before discharge. Concerns about any aspect of physical status may be implicitly or explicitly verbalized. However, most often the concerns involve the respiratory system. Additionally, supplemental worries may focus on equipment failures, especially regarding the proper functioning of the ventilator.

Central to a positive outcome is the availability of attendant personnel who maximize the quadriplegic person's quality of life. These attendants need to be sensitive to the quadriplegic person's idiosyncratic physical and psychological needs. Additionally, the attendant staff and/or family should exhibit consistency and predictability to allow the high-level quadriplegic person comfort and security. As discharge approaches, the disabled individual can direct attention toward the quality of support personnel. This can take the form of how knowledgeable and/or responsive the staff will be. The issue of how to successfully contend with interpersonal disputes with attendants on whom the disabled individual is dependent can become manifest. Lastly, within the postdischarge setting or community, will there be accessible opportunities for growth or will life reflect a sedentary and overly circumscribed style?

FAMILY SYSTEM

Most assuredly, it would be remiss to exclude the family as an important variable in the rehabilitation of the high-level quadriplegic individual. An effective family can be conceptualized as a system of complex, mutually interdependent relationships. Inherent within the family are duties and responsibilities that are essential for its functioning and survival. These duties and responsibilities constitute role behaviors and allow the family system to endure. High-level quadriplegia forces massive changes in the roles typically displayed by all family members. Given the fact that the family system is an interdependent system, an alteration in the disabled individual's role behaviors necessitates concomitant behavioral changes within other family members. Any change in the family system has a cascading, rippling impact on the remainder of the family. Consequently, the emergence of high-level quadriplegia creates the need for adjustments of roles both for the disabled and nondisabled family members. Certainly the combination of these role changes coupled with the discharge from an inpatient rehabilitation hospital can prove highly stressful. The disability can prove problematic in that not only are premorbid roles often rendered impossible, but also there is ambiguity or uncertainty regarding new roles the disabled individual may play within the family. Both the dissolution of premorbid roles and the ambiguity of future roles can prove to be emotionally disquieting for all family members in their own idiosyncratic ways. For example, if the male breadwinner within the family incurred the quadriplegia, he may feel as if his roles as provider, husband, and father are severely threatened. Correspondingly, his wife may feel under stress in her roles as a businesswoman, wife, and mother in that the disability necessitates the additional time-consuming role of attendant. Additionally, the children may feel the shift in the family equilibrium given the dramatic changes in the parental roles. Certainly all families' reactions to these role changes can be unique and variable, contingent on their inherent structure. However, this example was used to illustrate the reverberating impact of the disability. Families who are responsible for a degree of attendant care can often feel stress because life–death decisions came become manifest postdischarge. As a result, as actual discharge approaches and these role changes become a reality, the entire family may express ambivalence. The clinical staff should understand these family issues and address them as they emerge. It is important that staff understand that to only rehabilitate the disabled individual is to treat in a vacuum. Given the aforementioned mutual interdependencies and role interactions within the family, factors of the disabled individual and the extended family should be considered as they relate to the rehabilitation process.

INTERVENTION STRATEGIES

Given the aforementioned complexity of an individual's response to high-level quadriplegia, it would be inappropriate to recommend generic intervention strategies. Therapeutic recommendations should be tailored to the disabled individual and his or her family. However, some guidelines can be offered to maximize the chance of a successful outcome. Comprehensive education regarding the various aspects of the spinal cord injury form an essential foundation for rehabilitation. This allows the family system to feel more comfortable in contending with potential complications that may arise. It is imperative that successes occur within the rehabilitation process to reinforce the desire to persevere. Outings within the community are important to appreciate that successes can be achieved beyond the rehabilitation facility's walls. Both patient and family support groups can be useful therapeutic modalities to enhance peer interaction and explore common difficulties. Additionally, leisure activity possibilities illustrate that vocational interests can still exist postinjury. Lastly, on the individual level, it is imperative that staff considers and contends with the unique impasses that prohibit the disabled person from further accommodations to his/her injury.

CONCLUSIONS

As noted, there are a myriad of potential problems that can emerge as the disabled individual nears discharge. The issues mentioned above reflect only central predischarge concerns and are not presumed to be exhaustive. To minimize these problems, the rehabilitation hospital should be one component of a total system of care. Consequently, education and training of the patient's extended-care family should be addressed. Anticipation of potential breakdowns, including the family matrix, is a task for every member of the patient's hospital team. The rehabilitation hospital should allow the patient to understand the hospital's availability should difficulties become evident on return to the patient's community. Typically, complete rehabilitation does not occur during the initial phase of hospitalization and, as such, follow-up care should be made available. Most importantly, it is understood that accommodation to high-level quadriplegia is a protracted process that involves a multitude of factors. Consequently, each new phase of rehabilitation can reflect diverse issues that are highly individualized in nature. As previously stated, the prominent concern for patient and staff is to address to specific connotative meanings that the injury manifests at different stages of adaptation to the spinal cord injury. To do otherwise would be tantamount to regimenting treatment and obviate the appreciation of individual differences. Only by attention to our patients' connotative, individualized interpretation of their disabilities will we, as caregivers, maximize the possibility of a positive outcome in this most problematic of physical deficits.

BIBLIOGRAPHY

1. Aguilera D, Mesgick J (1978): *Crisis Intervention: Theory and Methodology.* St. Louis: CV Mosby.
2. Blank H (1975): Crisis consultation. *Int J Soc Psychiatry* 21.
3. Brandon S (1970): Crisis theory and possibilities of therapeutic intervention. *Br J Psychiatry* 117.
4. Brandon S (1975): Crisis therapy. *Curr Psychiatr Ther* 15.
5. Carroll PF (1986): When your patient must depend on a machine. *RN* 49.
6. Charles R (1985): Coping with life on a portable ventilator. *Home Healthcare Nurse* 3.
7. Davanloo H (1978): *Basic Principles and Techniques in Short-term Dynamic Psychotherapy.* SP Medical and Scientific Books.
8. Epperson M (1977): Families in sudden crisis. *Soc Work Health Care* 2.
9. Gale J, O'Shanick G (1985): Psychiatric aspects of respirator treatment and pulmonary intensive care. *Adv Psychosom Med* 14.
10. Gipson TW (1985): Mechanical ventilation in the home. *Cleve Clin Q* 52.
11. Griffith J (1985): Structural family therapy in chronic illness. *Psychosomatics* 28.
12. Kardener SA (1975): Methodologic approach to crisis therapy. *Am J Psychother* 29.
13. Lamid S, et al. (1985): Respirator-dependent quadriplegics: problems during the weaning period. *J Am Paraplegia Soc* 8.
14. Langley D (1978): Crisis intervention: managing stress-induced personal and family emergencies. *Behav Med* 5.
15. Lindemann E (1965): Symptomatology and management of acute grief. In: *Crisis Intervention* (Parad HJ, ed), New York: Family Service Association of America.
16. Locker D, et al. (1987): The impact of life support technology upon psychosocial adaptation to the late effects of poliomyelitis. *Birth Defects* 23.
17. Luthman S (1974): *The Dynamic Family.* Science and Behavior Book.
18. Marinelli R, Dell Orto A (1977): *The Psychological and Social Impact of Physical Disability.* New York: Springer.
19. Parad HJ (1965): *Crisis Intervention: Selected Readings.* New York: Family Service Association of America.
20. Rappaport L (1965): The state of crisis: some theoretical considerations. In: *Crisis Intervention* (Parad, HJ, ed), New York: Family Service Association of America.
21. Robinet J, et al. (1987): Facing down the fear of ventilator patients. *RN* 50.

22. Schwartz D (1969): Therapeutic intervention in crisis. *Int Psychiatr Clin* 6.
23. Spector G, Claiborn W (1973): *Crisis Intervention.* New York: Behavioral Publications.
24. Stewart T (1988): Psychiatric diagnosis and treatment following spinal cord injury. *Psychosomatics* 29.
25. Textor M (1983): *Helping Families with Special Problems.* New York: Jason Aronson.
26. Trieschmann R (1980): *Spinal Cord Injuries: Psychological, Social, and Vocational Adjustment.* New York: Pergamon Press.

20

Leisure Options for the High Quadriplegic Patient

Sam Andrews and Cindy Kelly

Craig Hospital, Englewood, Colorado, U.S.A.

During the rehabilitation process, the high quadriplegic patient goes through a difficult period of psychological and physiological readjustment. Through recreation and leisure planning, independence and quality of lifestyle can be restored to the high quadriplegic individual. Therapeutic recreation can help to ease the traumatic adjustment process. The overall goal of therapeutic recreation is to encourage each person to reach his/her fullest potential no matter how limited their abilities may be.

With high quadriplegic patients this goal is accomplished by introducing new activities in which they can successfully participate or by reintroducing some of those activities they enjoyed prior to their injury. It should be demonstrated to patients and their families that they are still very capable of participating, using a few appropriate modifications. One focus of therapeutic recreation intervention is to promote self-acceptance and confidence by helping individuals develop skills and talents to compensate realistically for the disability. Success is an essential part of the implemented program. A high quadriplegic patient's involvement in recreation must provide a measure of success with a minimum of frustration. Enjoyment, fun, and accomplishment are obvious rewards for participating in recreation.

EVALUATION

Early evaluation of the patient is essential, not only to obtain important information about his or her leisure background but that of friends and family as well. Typically, the therapeutic recreation specialist makes early acquaintance with the patient and family, stating the purpose of that type of intervention, and, when the appropriate time comes, what therapeutic recreation entails. It is generally believed that a patient with a relatively new injury and his or her family are understandably preoccupied with the severity of the medical situation and not very receptive to much more than words of optimism and encouragement.

Additional information can be obtained from family at appropriate times. They are often very willing to at least discuss the leisure and sports activities the patient enjoyed before injury.

ACTIVE INTERVENTION

After the patient has become medically stable and settled into the routine of daily therapies (usually 1–2 weeks) the time is typically appropriate for the therapeutic recreation specialist to begin working in earnest to implement leisure assessment modalities. Long-term (discharge and postdischarge) and short-term (main amount of time of patient's initial stay) goals can be established. Almost invariably the physician, nurses, and other therapists and counselors will be able to provide information to assist the therapeutic recreation specialist in determining the proper timing and intensity of therapeutic recreation intervention. Standard assessment instruments for people with lower-level spinal injuries work just as effectively for the high quadriplegic patient.

During the time of the assessment it is important to review with the patient and family members the exact role of therapeutic recreation so that realistic expectations of recreation staff are formulated. Recreation has such broad and general meaning to people of varied backgrounds that it cannot be assumed patients and family will automatically understand the role therapeutic recreation staff intend to play.

Early intervention with the high quadriplegic patient is frequently and effectively enhanced by strong, active physician support. Furthermore, initiating activity in conjunction with other therapy activities and/ or appropriate nursing functions also greatly enhances the relationship between the therapeutic recreation specialist and patient and family. Therapeutic recreation specialists should be adequately and properly trained in suctioning techniques, basic ventilator troubleshooting techniques, and any processes essential to the general safety and comfort of the patient. Whereas other staff generally work with the patient when all the specialty support disciplines are more readily available, the therapeutic recreation specialist often works with the patient during times or in locations when/where those services are somewhat reduced or limited. *This is not to say that the therapeutic recreation specialist should go beyond what is deemed reasonable by the attending physician,* but more to say that functions that will be ordinarily expected to be performed by the family should also be performed in competent fashion by the therapeutic recreation specialist. This clearly enhances patient availability for therapeutic recreation activities and sessions. It also serves as a positive example, often encouraging family to become proficient in those functions sooner.

The skill training phase of therapeutic recreation intervention is seen to include four general components. Values clarification is a very important component because oftentimes it provides the high quadriplegic patient enhanced insight into the types of events and activities most important to him/her. Patients can often learn not only what aspects of their lives are important but, more importantly, *why.* A clearer understanding of why certain events, thoughts, and activities are important greatly enhances a perception of needs. When needs are more clearly understood, it obviously becomes easier to identify those needs that must be met. The therapist and the patient can then more easily set out to meet those needs rather than expend unwarranted time and energy trying to duplicate activities in which the high quadriplegic patient engaged before injury. The patient's time with the therapeutic recreation specialist is very limited and it is essential to make the most of it through a process similar to the one just described.

It is important to review communication skills of the patient and family. There is not time to completely review and make major changes in the high quadriplegic patient's communication techniques with family and friends, nor is it practical to attempt to make major changes in the family's communication style with the high quadriplegic individual. It is important, however, to review with each the value of communicating needs beyond basic survival needs in such a way that positive outcomes from such discussion are enhanced. All rehabilitation disciplines should strive to encourage all parties to clearly communicate values and needs while at the same time the same parties remain open about hearing and understanding the values and needs of others. The recreational setting is an excellent medium in which to review and possibly refine such skills. It is a more realistic or practical setting with real issues in value judgment, community interaction, and interpersonal communication among family members and friends, which constantly but naturally occur.

Clearly sharing needs and desires with others, assertive behaviors, and realistic expectations of others (meaning family or friends accompanying the high quadriplegic person) are extremely important tools for successful social and leisure encounters. Therapeutic recreation specialists should dedicate substantial time and effort in communication skill enhancement training.

EQUIPMENT/RESOURCES

The high quadriplegic person typically uses a great deal of adaptive equipment. It is extremely important that the therapeutic recreation specialist work closely early on with other treating disciplines so that basic equipment will also meet as many recreational needs as possible. Some examples of these considerations would be: electrical outlets and receptacles for the wheelchair; brackets and wheelchair superstructure allowing for bipod mounts; appropriate main tires and casters. This can reduce long-range costs to the high quadriplegic patient as well as third-party payers. Furthermore, early coordination of customizing equipment can reduce the need for additional specialized equipment that would represent additional bulk and increase the user's vulnerability to equipment malfunction.

Specialized equipment for recreational activity is often needed. It is very important that any equipment should not be recommended until thorough investigation into its practicality has been made. Too often in their enthusiasm for the patient's success, staff assist in the acquisition of specialized equipment without enough consideration to such issues as storage, maintenance, and installation away from the rehabilitation setting. The danger of the equipment becoming a useless reminder of the disability for the high quadriplegic patient must be carefully avoided.

Resource exploration is an essential component to any recommendation the therapeutic recreation specialist might make to the patient. As patient values and needs are explored, immediate consideration for resources to meet those needs and values should be made. Consideration for such things as transportation resources, human assistance resources, financial resources, and accessibility for the highly specialized wheelchair should be given for both the short haul (i.e., during the rehabilitation process) and the long haul (subsequent to discharge). Even under the very best of conditions in resource planning for leisure activity after discharge, resources often break down. The therapeutic recreation specialist must be prepared to follow up in some fashion to attempt to assure that planned resources have, in fact, been placed in effect and remain so.

PRECAUTIONS

Precautionary considerations for leisure activity should be taught by therapeutic recreation specialists as well as members of other disciplines. Beyond general safety and precautionary considerations for the high quadriplegic patient there are three categories of additional consideration that play an important role in the success of leisure pursuits.

From a *social* standpoint, certain considerations by high quadriplegic patients can truly enhance their recreational experience in a number of ways. One example is when high quadriplegic patients clearly communicate to other participants of a social situation, beforehand, what physical needs they will have during the event and how they intend to handle them rather than asking for assistance continually from those who would not know what is to be asked next. Often that type of situation can be easily remedied by having an attendant accommodate needs. Another example of a difficult social situation is one in which full consideration for those attending an event is not given, such as the noise a ventilator or suctioning equipment might make during a movie in a theater. Practical remedies might include prearranged seating by theater management, or placement in an area of the theater next to an exit with easy entry and exit so that the quadriplegic patient could quietly and quickly be moved outside to a part of the lobby where suctioning would be much less of a spectacle. Advising those seated nearby of unusual sounds or excessive noise should be done as a courtesy so that those who might be disturbed would have the opportunity to move away if they so choose. Remedies to these situations can create a more acceptable and, therefore, more satisfying recreational situation.

The second category concerns *mechanical* considerations. The therapeutic recreation specialist can give a great deal of information on the use of backup mechanical equipment by demonstrating its use in recreational activities. One example of a simple mechanical adaptation for safety backup would be a connection to the electrical system of a vehicle that would allow for auxiliary electricity to operate the ventilator or the mechanical components of the wheelchair, especially suctioning equipment, in case of power failure. Systems such as this might eliminate the need to carry along extra batteries. Ideas such as this tend to remove some of the factors that may serve as deterrents to leaving the comforts of home to participate in recreational activity.

The third category is *environmental* conditions. The therapeutic recreation specialist should spend educational time with the patient discussing the effect of various environmental conditions. Through close collaboration with the physician and nursing staff, information should be shared on the effects of such conditions as dust, heat, sun, cold, altitude, and humidity, to name a few. Again, the aim of such education is to give the high quadriplegic patient the opportunity to enjoy the success of the activity rather than suffer negative consequences of preventable environmental problems.

It is extremely important to identify individual needs when designing individual programs. The individual's interests, values, recreational needs, leisure resources, and capabilities must be taken into consideration so that realistic goals can be set with a high probability of achievement in preparing the high quadriplegic person for effective leisure time use.

ACTIVITIES

Socially, high quadriplegic persons need to nurture a sense of belonging, of being accepted by society. When they are able to accomplish a project or fill a role successfully, they will then have an opportunity to build self image. This may be accomplished through such activities as decoupaging with a paint brush in the mouth or becoming a licensed ham radio operator using a puff-and-sip Morse coder. A device such as the puff-and-sip Morse coder can be designed on the same principle as the puff-and-sip control of the electric wheelchair. All activities that can be accomplished with head, mouth, or chin control should be explored.

Simple table games with magnetic pieces moved by a mouthstick can be used. These games can be played with a friend, family, or a staff member. Card games can be played by cutting holes in the upper middle portion of the cards so a mouthstick can be inserted to move them. Cards from any type of table game can be arranged in a simply constructed card holder along with the use of a bird beak device with which to pick them up and/or move them.

Electronic video games and personal computers can be adapted with a chin control and/or pressure-sensitive switch that allows high quadriplegic individuals to operate them independently by themselves or with a partner (Fig. 20-1). Various brands and quality levels of stereo cassette players, compact disk players, and AM/FM receivers have total pushbutton or remote switching and controls allowing for adaptive operation. These units are also configured in such a way that the use of bird beak devices and adaptive storage libraries gives high quadriplegic persons the capability to insert or remove disks or cassettes themselves.

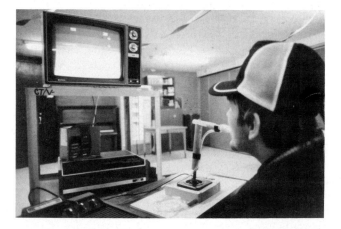

FIG. 20-1.   Homemade mouth-operated video game joystick adaption.

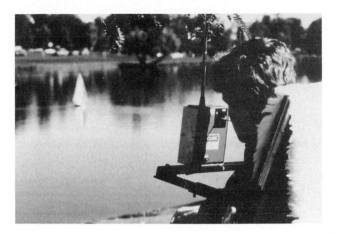

FIG. 20-2. Mouth-operated, radio-controlled transmitter placed on adapted frame operating sailboat in the distance.

For fishing, there is an adapted fishing reel that is operated by disengaging the drive belt of the electric or puff-and-sip wheelchair. By installing the rod in a bracket and engaging the reel to this belt, the fisherman can reel in fish by simply operating a switch, thus creating opportunities to fish with casting assistance or fishing off the side or back of an appropriately configured moving boat. More sophisticated casting and reeling devices are being tested at the time this chapter is being written. Expectations are high that a device that is totally chin or puff-and-sip controlled and will work off the electrical system of the electric wheelchair will open many new horizons for high quadriplegic fishing enthusiasts and their family and friends. They will use the same amount of effort to operate the fishing device that they would to operate the puff-and-sip electric wheelchair.

Aquatic activities can also provide an environment for socialization and some independence. Radio-controlled sailing is one type of aquatic activity. The same skills are needed to operate a model sailboat or a full-size boat. A control is positioned so that the two radio-controlled joystick levers are within the range of the high quadriplegic person's mouth, chin, or mouthstick. When the boat is in the water the high quadriplegic individual is the sole controller (Fig. 20-2). Family and friends can also participate in this type of activity and no previous sailing experience is required because the basic skills can be learned quickly. This type of activity also provides an avenue for competition through model yachting clubs across the United States that organize races featuring these radio-controlled boats. In a case such as this, the disability presents no disadvantages or handicaps to competition. Even with mouth controls, a high quadriplegic person can compete on an equal basis with any able-bodied person. The same operational principles for the sailboats apply to radio-controlled cars, airplanes, gliders, and power boats. Activities such as these lend themselves to valuable family activity (especially with youngsters), affording a wide spectrum for activity involvement.

Other aquatic activities to consider are rafting and sailing. These are extremely high-risk activities and not generally recommended because much preliminary work must be done to ensure appropriate safety conditions. However, under exceptional circumstances even the ventilator-dependent quadriplegic person might be a candidate for rafting if proper attention is given the many safety considerations that can be controlled. Each situation presents its own safety considerations. Some common ones are the recruitment of highly qualified rafting specialists, highly stable rafts, well-studied appropriate waters, ideal weather conditions, spare manual ventilating equipment, and appropriate protection for ventilator equipment (to name just a few). The high quadriplegic person can exercise mental strategies for tactical maneuvers and be very actively involved in operations such as judging weather conditions and other essential variables critical to operation. Again, these are activities in which family and friends can be involved.

Camping is another activity for high quadriplegic individuals. They can provide themselves the opportunity to be with family or friends away from the typical home or institutional environment. Although they will be dependent on others for their care, they can be responsible for making such decisions as campsite selection, weather-related contingencies, and campsite arrangement. They might even participate in hauling firewood by towing it with the electric wheelchair.

In all activities the physical aspect is only one part. There are also mental, social, and emotional aspects of intervention to be considered. Recreational outings offer a means of testing out self-image in public, and they can be a time for socialization. A successful experience on an outing can encourage high quadriplegic individuals to try that experience or others similar to it again. Challenging outings can expose them and their family and friends to situations that might be encountered at home. They can begin to problem-solve on their own or with others so that these challenges are less threatening to them later. As families get more opportunity to problem-solve, especially with the assistance of staff, the outings subsequent to discharge will be less of a burden, thus enhancing the probability of the high quadriplegic person getting out into the community on a more frequent and probably healthier basis.

Activities once thought impractical, if not impossible, are, in fact, "doable" with appropriate planning and coordination with the members of

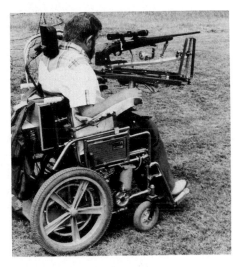

FIG. 20-3. W/C SR-77 rifle mount with rifle and scope fully operated by chin and mouth control.

the other disciplines of the rehabilitation program. Activities of an "adventuresome" nature include such events as kite flying, ocean cruises, hot air ballooning, and big game hunting (Fig. 20-3). They are highly popular and are becoming less difficult to conduct as experience is gained. Again, it must be emphasized that a great deal of planning, ingenuity, safety consideration, and resource analysis, all of which the high quadriplegic person should be highly involved in, are essential components to short- and long-term success.

Music and drama also serve as important therapeutic modalities as well as pleasurable activities. The coaching and cheering at athletic events should also be considered as opportunities to allow the high quadriplegic person a means for creativity, self-fulfillment, and expression. Creating or participating in skits, talent shows or dramatic productions, and athletic or other spectator events are an opportunity to escape the physical confines of the wheelchair. They may even be able to build lung capacity and strength as they strive to sing or project the voice.

Yet another activity for major consideration is photography. There is such great latitude for creativity and self-expression. Today's cameras can be purchased with the specific automatic features to meet the needs of each individual, easily accommodating specific preferences. The use of bipod or suspension equipment attached to the electric wheelchair places the camera in a desirable position for operation by the high quadriplegic individual. Further adaptations of camera controls such as manual focus and light aperture can be made to suit individual desires. The activity can easily be carried on to the darkroom for additional creativity in photocomposition.

CONCLUSIONS

This chapter has discussed experiences that have been demonstrated to be effective in therapeutic recreation intervention. Following a basic format of introduction and assessment, skill training, and resource exploration as previously described provide increased opportunity for high quadriplegic persons and their families to use recreational skills and resources to add strong incentive to live in as healthy and independent a condition as possible after all the effort, energy, and resources have been expended to return the individual to a healthy state.

Once the high quadriplegic person is discharged, follow-up and re-evaluation are essential in assuring that appropriate leisure skills are commensurate with the desires and abilities of the individual as conditions in their lives change.

21

The Lifetime Care Process

R. Edward Carter

The Institute for Rehabilitation and Research, Houston, Texas, U.S.A.

Plans for the follow-up care of a patient with high quadriplegia and ventilator dependency begin early in the course of rehabilitation at a spinal cord injury center. Initial thoughts toward home programs and home management generally begin during the initial evaluation. After the initial evaluation at the spinal center, each discipline attempts to set their goals for discharge and begins to plan for the patient's existence in the community. As the initial rehabilitation process begins to draw to a close, more formal plans are necessary.

During the rehabilitation process the family and patient are involved in a formal spinal cord injury education program, the patient is elevated to his/her highest level of functional independence possible within medical constraints, and the home programs for maintenance of physical and occupational therapy are planned. The predischarge stage is one of individualization. It involves a shift to the patient of as much responsibility for their own physical well-being as they can assume. They may be able to do this physically or only vocally, as in directing their care. Medications that initially were necessary for the management of the patient should again be reviewed and streamlined or minimized to decrease home cost and, hopefully, to increase adherence to the prescribed program. The patient is usually given a 3- or 4-week supply of medications so that (s)he may be discharged and get settled into home before having to worry about refills.

If the patient has gone home on a weekend pass or leave of absence, the necessary environmental modifications can be planned from this experience. If not, sketches and measurements can be brought in by the family from which home modification plans can be fabricated. The feedback from many families has demonstrated that it is most cost effective to initially make only the minimal and/or simple home modifications necessary to manage the ventilator-dependent patient immediately after discharge. If families wait approximately 4–6 months after being home with a ventilator-dependent relative, they have a much better idea of the types of refinements they personally would like in terms of the home modifications. Many times, families, in their desire to assist the patient, launch into major home modifications which, after a 6–10-month period, are found to be unnecessary.

EARLY DISCHARGE PLANNING ACTIVITIES

The predischarge plan should begin with a complete assessment of the patient's medical and functional status. First and foremost, of course, is the accurate documentation of the neurological level, strength of musculature, and sensory level. This is used as a baseline in the event of decreasing strength or changing neurological levels at a later date, which may be indicative of such things as a spinal cord cyst, etc. General nutrition is checked not only by following the patient's weight, but also with both hemoglobin and hematocrit, and total protein and albumin. Major efforts at improving nutrition during the acute care phase may have been overachieved and now nutrition may require adjustment to keep the patient's weight stable, or if necessary, reduce the patient's weight. If there is any hint of aspiration, swallowing studies should be rechecked as well. The respiratory system is checked by means of a chest x-ray film, arterial blood gases, repetitive tidal volumes, and an evaluation of culture and sensitivity from tracheal aspiration. In the event of subsequent home problems, antibiotics can then be started more rapidly. A recheck of all respiratory equipment and back-up equipment is also essential.

Both renal and hepatic functions are again checked, particularly with patients receiving dantrolene sodium (Dantrium) or other types of hepatic toxic drugs. Final urinary recommendations are made on the basis of urodynamic studies and the type of urinary drainage to be used at home is agreed on between the patient, family, urologist, and spinal cord injury physician. Many patients with high-pressure bladder systems need to be followed much more closely because of the possibility of renal damage secondary to bladder hyperactivity in the absence of infection. A urine culture, sensitivity, and colony count is also obtained and the family is rechecked in their training of the urinary drainage system management. A urethral or suprapubic catheter may be more desirable than the use of intermittent catheterization for bladder drainage. Because the family has other medical issues to address, particularly the respiratory management of the patient, a less time-consuming method for bladder drainage is helpful.

From the skeletal viewpoint, an x-ray film of the fracture site should be obtained and checked for evidence of late instability and as a baseline for future use. In addition, a 36-in gravity loaded, anteroposterior (AP) and lateral spine x-ray film series is useful, particularly in the prepubertal group, as a baseline for the evaluation of long-term development of scoliosis.

Family and/or attendant training should be completely reviewed and the family instructed in the total home program. Resources should be checked for sponsorship of medications and supplies on discharge and for equipment repair and maintenance, especially repair of the wheelchair, ventilator, environmental controls, etc. Contacts for immediate repair or exchange of equipment in or near the patient's home should be arranged predischarge if the patient lives out of the rehabilitation center's service area. An aggressive approach is necessary to call, recruit, and encourage a family physician to participate in the follow-up care of the patient. At the same time the center should offer support and consultation in person or by phone to both the family and the family physician. Local medical care should also be arranged through a private physician, who is sent copies of the medical records in advance of the patient's discharge. Advance arrangements need to be made for change of tracheotomy tubes and/or gastrostomy tubes, change of urinary devices, etc. Visits by local public health or visiting nurses associations can be arranged particularly for review of the program and to help the family settle into the home after discharge, provide moral support, etc.

A discharge equipment checklist is prepared and discharge transportation is arranged in advance. The patient should be counseled concerning the necessity to return for reevaluation and the timing of the reevaluation. Goals for the estimated time before return to school or a vocation, even on a part-time basis, can be planned before the next admission. For those patients who are completely ventilator dependent, a prearranged phone call is scheduled by respiratory therapy to monitor respiratory status monthly for the first 6 months followed by a call every 3–4 months.

With the complete return to strength and full endurance of muscles present, the state of physiologic balance and return of host resistance is 14–18 months from injury for the majority of high-level quadriplegic individuals. Because of this, hospital admissions should be shortened and completed on an intermittent schedule. The initial rehabilitation hospitalization, in our experience, usually averages 4–6 months for the ventilator-dependent group. The second admission should be ~6–8 months after the first discharge.

Because of the increased incidence of early complications, the endurance of the patient during the first rehabilitation admission is often inadequate to accomplish as many functional activities as (s)he will

ultimately be capable of performing. These activities are addressed in
the second hospitalization. In addition, there are a number of diagnostic
studies that need to be repeated ~1 year postinjury to evaluate the patient for negative medical changes that can be successfully treated. Particular among these studies is the recheck of the spine x-ray film for
late instability, the intravenous pyelogram (IVP) for evidence of hydronephrosis and the respiratory system with respect to blood gases, ventilator settings, etc. Historically, ventilator-dependent patients like to
hyperventilate and tend to maintain this type of setting on their ventilator. In the days of poliomyelitis a certain percentage of ventilator-
dependent patients were found to periodically become hostile, anxious,
or fearful and increase their ventilator settings. However, when the need
for increased ventilation passed, the patient did not return the mechanical settings to a normal breathing rate and depth. Then when the next
episode occurred, there was a further increase in the ventilator setting,
and the patients ultimately put themselves in a constant marked hyper-
ventilatory state.

MAJOR MEDICAL SYSTEMS DISCHARGE REVIEW

A medical check list is automatically considered at discharge for baseline determinations as mentioned and also during follow-up sessions.
For patients who are geographically accessible, office visits initially every
4–6 weeks and, later, every 6–8 weeks for the first year, then quarterly,
and then semiannually in the absence of problems will probably suffice.
Detailed follow-up of the major functional systems and potential problems will be addressed in the following paragraphs.

Motor and sensory levels of the neurological system are evaluated at
6 months and annually, with the patient instructed to contact the center
if any variation in either the sensory levels or motor strength occurs.
Potential problems include late instability or the development of a spinal
cord cyst. Follow-up evaluation of the skeletal system includes flexion
and extension views of any previously fractured spinal areas. This is
done at 6 months, 1 year, and annually for several years and then as
needed for evidence of any late spinal instability. As mentioned earlier,
until prepubertal patients pass through puberty, an annual 36-in grav-
ity-loaded AP and lateral spine x-ray film is obtained for evaluating
changes towards scoliosis.

The skin and nutritional system is checked primarily by observation
of the skin with close attention paid to the patient's weight. The initial
attempt at a high-calorie, high-protein diet is necessary to replenish the
depleted protein stores. Later a secondary set of problems may occur if
caloric intake exceeds the caloric output. A different type of counseling

is necessary from a dietary standpoint to maintain weight at an appropriate level. Hemoglobin and hematocrit should be followed at each follow-up visit until the patient's values reach normal. Normal hemoglobin and hematocrit values are fairly good indexes to signal that a patient has reached the final stage of the recovery program. With any hint of a skin problem, total serum protein and albumin should also be followed until they approach normal. Serum calcium level checks are repeated if indicated to monitor or rule out hypercalcemia, which most frequently occurs in youngsters.

From a vascular standpoint, the patient's thighs and calves should be monitored for symmetry and/or change in size as an early clue to potential deep vein thrombosis or heterotopic ossification. Reinforcing instruction on autonomic dysreflexia should also be given to patients and families.

From a gastrointestinal standpoint, in addition to recognition of possible aspiration, an adequate bowel program should be maintained. Preferably this will occur no less frequently than three times per week. If the patient is receiving tube feedings, the gastrostomy tube should be checked and changed periodically and the contents of the tube feedings checked according to the patient's state of nutrition.

From a genitourinary standpoint, renal functions are checked with blood urea nitrogen and creatinine at 6 months, 1 year, and then annually. Urine culture and colony count, depending on the type of urinary drainage, needs to be monitored. Evaluation for evidence of back pressure resulting in hydronephrosis, urinary tract infection, and/or stones should be done. IVPs are generally performed during the first admission, at return after 6 months, and then annually for the first 2–3 years, during which time the patient is most vulnerable to complications that can increase morbidity and decrease life span. After the first 3 years, IVPs should be performed every 2–3 years unless the patient has problems that necessitate returning for annual evaluations. After enough IVPs are obtained to document the patient's architectural uniqueness, a change to a renal scan may be made. Renal scans reveal the same information in addition to identifying the individual's renal blood flow and measurement of glomerular filtration rates. This data is quite helpful in the later years when some patients become hypertensive as a symptom of renal vascular involvement that may be treatable, resulting in reversibility of the hypertensive state.

The neuromuscular system should be followed from the standpoint of the level of spasticity and hypertonicity. Hypertonicity frequently leads to skeletal and joint contractures. Sudden increases in the level of spasticity can be associated with a spinal cord cyst, bladder stones, and other types of sensory irritation. Hepatic function studies need to be checked periodically on those patients taking skeletal antispasmodic drugs, particularly dantrolene sodium.

The major problem system is the cardiorespiratory system. This follow-up can be carried out by respiratory therapy at least monthly by telephone during the first 3–6 months. Home respiratory programs, if they included intermittent positive pressure breathing, chest physical therapy, or suctioning, should be rechecked and modified as necessary. Arterial blood gases and recalibration of the ventilator settings should be performed at least every 3–6 months. The patient should be scheduled for routine tracheotomy changes every 3–4 months. Flu shots should be considered for the fall and early winter seasons. Pneumococcal vaccines should also be considered, particularly with those patients who may have had a splenectomy after their initial injury.

DISCHARGE FOLLOW-UP AND CONTINGENCY SUPPORT PLANS

It is important that patients and their families feel as secure as possible when they are at home and that their questions and needs be met on a timely basis. The ventilator-dependent quadriplegic patient should be encouraged to reintegrate into the community and participate in activities that, if they feel secure in their care, will tend to occur more often. A desirable feature of the spinal cord injury center is to have a follow-up nurse or designated individual who becomes the single contact person for patients and families whether their problem involves equipment, medications, supplies, medical problems, emergency situations, or otherwise. A designated responder and phone number at the spinal cord injury center can be similar to the "911" emergency number. The designated follow-up individual then acts as a triage point, referring questions and problems to the appropriate source within the facility and assisting the patient in solving problems that arise. It is this type of follow-up program, together with patient and family education, that minimizes recurrent unplanned hospitalizations and complications, assists the patients and families in becoming more secure in their environment, and allows the return of the patient to full participation in their community.

IV

The Real World

Introduction

Robert Menter

Craig Hospital, Englewood, Colorado, U.S.A.

The real world is where each person was before their injury and where they will return after their injury. Hospitalization is equivalent to a timeout in the life story, during which there is a change in costumes, props, and scenery. The timeout or transition is temporary, giving way to resumption of the unique life each person was leading when they were injured.

In the first three sections of this book, we discussed survival, medical stability, equipment, education, and discharge planning. In this section, we return the individual to the community and all of its varying resources. Although the information covered in the first three sections is specific and has changed very little over the past 10 years, much of the information in this section is still evolving and is the subject of ongoing investigation.

Transition into the real world brings many changes, but foremost is the change in decision-making from a staff of experienced professionals to a layperson who has just completed a brief course in spinal cord rehabilitation. When the individual is back in the real world, the medical treatment team becomes just another resource on the sideline. The individual becomes the expert and we, the treatment team, learn from him or her what the real world is like. Only by learning from the experiences of our former patients can we better prepare others for the resumption of their life activities.

The second striking transition in going from the hospital back to the real world is the transition from uniformity of daily routine and resources to great variation in solutions and resources. Great disparity exists in attendant care and family and financial resources. As a result of these disparities, people in the community have greater variability in lifestyles and quality of life than in the hospital.

This section introduces and shows us the perspectives of three very active individuals with high-level quadriplegia. Some of the basic ethical issues from the perspectives of the patient, various family members, and the medical treatment staff are discussed. Some perspectives of the insurance industry will be covered along with the results of a multicenter follow-up study relating to many quality-of-life issues.

22

Ethics

Robert Menter and Sam Maddox

Craig Hospital, Englewood, Colorado, U.S.A.

Ethics is the study of conduct and moral judgment. It is a subject both old and new, particularly in the delivery of health care—old in that it dates back to pre-Greek civilization, and new in that it is a central issue in modern medicine.

Two terms, paternalism and autonomy, dominate discussions in biomedical ethics. Paternalism, a system of decision making similar to that of the family, relegates authority to a central figure. In the medical context, the control figure is the physician, who decides what is right for the patient in the style of "Father Knows Best." In recent years, the concept of paternalism has come under close scrutiny and is changing, both in the family and in the health care environment.

Autonomy is the principle of self-governing or self-determination. It has many biomedical implications, such as the right to informed consent, the right to refuse treatment, the right to competent care, etc. In recent years the concept of autonomy has gained much strength, and with the assistance of court decisions, has assumed a preeminent role in the delivery of health care.

In medicine, the concepts of autonomy and paternalism must take into account a series of conditions, some of which are: (a) competence—the mental capacity of a person to make a decision—entails the person possessing a set of values, the ability to communicate and comprehend information, and the ability to reason and deliberate; (b) informed consent—the consent given by a competent individual after receiving adequate information; (c) beneficence—the duty to protect the well-being of the individual; and (d) quality of life—the daily pattern of life activities and how they fit in with the individual's values and expectations.

Most problems in ethics arise out of disagreement as to which principle—autonomy or paternalism—should govern a situation. At what point is a patient able to make a valid judgment? Illness or disability may foster psychological contraints—fear, anxiety, depression, denial—which may in turn affect deliberation and reflection. Because there are many perspectives and interpretations of ethical problems and because consensus is so elusive,the courts have increasingly been thrust into the mediator role.

An August 1987 article by Chaplan et al., published by the Hastings Center, an organization founded in 1969 to study ethical problems in biology, medicine, and the social and behavioral sciences, adds some clarity to the ethical problems particular to rehabilitation medicine (1). The discussion notes that in the traditional acute medical setting, patients are depicted as passive agents of medical interventions. In the rehabilitative setting, patients must change from passive agents to active participants in their own care. A model of interaction (the education model of ethics) between provider and consumer is suggested. A brief summary follows.

The educational model is one way of dealing with the ever-changing issue of patient competence after a serious injury requiring rehabilitation. In the acute care and treatment setting, many factors such as pain, medication, depression, or lack of knowledge often combine to interfere with the patient's competence. Therefore, it is appropriate that during acute care, paternalism, with minimal autonomy, is the acceptable way of intervention. The physician's goal should be to maintain life until conditions of autonomy can be restored. As medical stability returns, an educational program is initiated to develop knowledge and understanding so the patient can make a meaningful assessment of his or her disabling condition. Patient values regarding quality of life are fully considered; the participatory model also typically includes family members. As the education process unfolds, and competency becomes clearer, beneficence should yield to autonomy. In this evolving model, it is the physician's initial responsibility to provide a caretaker role; thereafter, it is a moral imperative to return control to the patient as competency returns.

An earlier Hastings Center report (August 1982) features an article by Terrence F. Ackerman entitled "Why Doctors Should Intervene" (2). Ackerman focuses on why patient autonomy is compromised by severe illness: "Ethnicists typically condemn paternalistic practices in the therapeutic relationship, but fail to investigate the features that incline physicians to be paternalistic," says Ackerman. For example, psychological issues—denial, depression, guilt, fear, and anger—obscure a patient's ability to make a competent decision. Other patients, falling back on the culturally reinforced "sick role," yield to the discretion of medical providers, and do not wish to participate in decision making.

During the rehabilitation process, strategies may have to evolve beyond the mere provision of information. Ackerman argues that information the individual minimizes (as in denial) or falsely emphasizes (as with acute anxiety) must be discussed in greater detail, and set in proper perspective. The physician may have to alter the tone of discussion with the patient—emphasizing a positive attitude with the overly depressed or anxious patient, or a more realistic and cautious attitude with the denying patient—to neutralize psychological constraints. It may also be necessary for the physician to influence the beliefs of people close to the patient. It is imperative that physicians carefully assess the psychological and social profiles and needs of each patient; adequate intervention, then, becomes a matter of assisting patients to restore maximum control over their lives.

Perhaps the most difficult of all ethics controversies is the termination of life. An April 1988 article in the *New England Journal of Medicine* examines the ethical uncertainties specific to discontinuation of mechanical ventilation (3). The authors, Schneiderman and Spragg, suggest a hierarchy of decision making. The first consideration for withdrawal of ventilator support is the medical indication: whether or not the device will indeed contribute to preserving life. "If its appropriateness is unclear, mechanical ventilation should be started with the knowledge that if it proves to be futile or not beneficial or disproportionately burdensome, it can later be stopped."

Next in the hierarchy is patient autonomy. Informed and competent patients, argue the authors, "have the right to refuse ventilator care. . . . If the patient's wish is to withdraw the ventilator, that wish must be honored." And if that wish is granted, it is the physician's obligation to ensure that the patient has no discomfort.

The next level of the decision process is to consider the patient's best interests. But what determines a person's best interests? Schneiderman and Spragg suggest this is a much more complicated problem than simply prolonging life. What are the burdens of continued treatment? Can the patient be expected to return toward a functioning, integrated existence, free of pain and suffering? How does anyone weigh the burdens of continued life against the benefits of that life?

The last of the authors' hierarchical judgments of this ethical framework involves external factors. How will decisions regarding treatment affect family and intimate friends? What about financial considerations? The authors suggest that decisions based on external factors, such as institutional or budgetary limits, be made as a part of public policy, not on a case by case basis.

Few areas of medicine combine, as does high quadriplegic spinal cord injury, the overwhelming effects of a disabling illness, the lack of understanding and knowledge by the patient, and the institutional nature of the illness to thoroughly interfere with the patient's competence. With time, and with the assistance of the treating team, competence returns. And in almost all cases, the patients want to survive and carry on with their lives.

There are, to be sure, cases in which individuals determined to be competent choose not to continue life. What are the responsibilities of the physician, the treating staff, or the institution in responding to the patient's wishes? In these situations the rehabilitation team members each have philosophical perspectives and ethical references that may impede their ability to meet the patient's request. If the physician, other treating staff (nurses, therapists, etc.), or the hospital administration do not feel they can comply with the patient's wishes, it is appropriate to transfer the care of that individual to others who can.

Beyond the acute and intermediate ethical problems, there are longer-term issues in high quadriplegia. Some higher-level patients who do not require mechanical ventilation occasionally have respiratory infections that require ventilator assistance for the acute pulmonary toilet. Unfortunately, some will not be able to wean again and will become ventilator dependent. This dependency, therefore, may loom ahead for some people who avoided it in the early rehabilitation stage. It is not possible to predict when and to whom this additional disability will happen. Therefore, it is important for health care providers to discuss these possibilities with patients so they can make clear, informed decisions when such conditions arise.

Another future ethical dilemma may evolve out of lifelong active medical management and intervention. In our best intentions, we program patients to seek medical treatment each time a medical problem develops. Indeed, those who do not pursue intervention are frequently labeled as bad patients. It never occurs to most patients that they have a choice; they seem unthinkingly to follow the program of intervention. Many health providers, therefore, are not prepared for those patients who make the ultimate choice—to stop living. How and when do these people decide? Although it may go against the expectations of survival and the fundamental basis of the healing arts, it is necessary for physicians and providers to respect the autonomy of the individual. If the hospital is considered an inappropriate location to grant a patient's wish to die, it will be necessary to create alternative locations of care where the processes of life can be gracefully resolved; these would perhaps be similar to the hospice facilities for terminally ill persons.

Termination of life creates a series of ethical dilemmas for all of the parties involved. Many states consider assisting an individual with terminating his life a punishable crime. To protect all of the parties, it is imperative to follow a process of deliberation and documentation. Whenever any doubt exists as to the competence of the individual, the consequences of the request, or the means of carrying out the request, it is imperative to call in others experienced in ethics of termination of life issues.

Two important tools have evolved to help deal with ethical issues in the health care setting: the living will and the biomedical ethics committee. The living will is a legally binding directive activated by an individual in a stable, competent psychological state outlining the perimeters of health support measures to be taken in the event of a change in competence or a changing medical state. The living will can limit use of cardiopulmonary resuscitation, ventilator support, artificial nutrition, and other life-sustaining measures in the event that illness and factors associated with illness create a state of incompetency. The bioethics committee serves as a resource for both individuals receiving care in the program and for health care providers participating in that care. The committee acts to reflect philosophical guidelines, legal and religious expertise on bioethical issues represented by the broad perspectives of the committee, thus eliminating personal bias.

The following is a summary of several ethical problems discussed by three persons with experience in biomedical issues. The discussants comment on a situation involving a recently injured young man who decides he wants to die rather than continue life as a ventilator-dependent quadriplegic. Also, the group discusses the situation as if the individual were a teenager, were 65, or were counting on his life insurance policy to provide for his family.

The group includes Chief Judge Charles Buss, of the 21st Judicial District in Mesa County, Colorado. Judge Buss presided over a widely reported case in 1986 and 1987 involving a severely disabled man who wished to be allowed to die. Hector Rodas, almost totally paralyzed, unable to speak or swallow, used a letterboard to tell the court, "I don't want to live like this anymore." The American Civil Liberties Union argued on Rodas's behalf that the Hilltop Rehabilitation Hospital in Grand Junction should allow him the final choice. The hospital, fearful of further litigation, contended that its staff would be participating in a suicide. Judge Buss accepted the principle that "suicide does not occur where the natural consequence of a person's illness is death."

Judge Buss says his was a difficult decision, with little case law to rely on. When he made his ruling, however, the judge says he was confident he was doing the right thing. First, there was some precedent affirming patient autonomy in other jurisdictions; second, Buss says, "I relied on my sense of what this country is all about—we all have a free choice as long as that choice does not harm others." Finally, says Buss,

"I was satisfied this guy knew exactly what he was doing. Moreover, he had 10 to 14 days after my ruling to change his mind." Rodas did not change his mind.

Also included in the discussion are Giles Scofield and Kathleen De-Silva. Mr. Scofield is affiliated with Concern for Dying, an educational council on ethical issues of death and the originators of the Living Will. Ms. DeSilva, who is high-level quadriplegic (see Chapter 23), is the in-house counsel for The Institute for Rehabilitation and Research (TIRR) in Houston.

What follows is the hypothetical situation the group responded to.

A 25-year-old man is 8 weeks postinjury. He is ventilator dependent, having fractured C2/3 in a diving accident; he is neurologically a C2 complete, Frankel class A. Vital capacity is 300 ml. He is medically stable but has atelectasis and requires suctioning; he has just come out of a halo vest, which makes clear to him the reality of his injury. He believes there will be no further recovery. He is involved in a rehabilitation program, is up in his reclining wheelchair ~4 h a day. He can vocalize using a Jackson tracheostomy tube, but requires frequent suctioning. Medications include Valium 5 mg p.o. q.i.d. for spasms, a bronchodilator for atelectasis, an anticholinergic for his bladder, and a stool softener for his bowel program. Today the patient refuses treatment, and asks that someone make arrangements to "pull the plug." A psychological evaluation has been ordered.

The patient was a carpenter who was unemployed at the time of his diving accident. He has a high school education, is married, and has two children ages 3 and 1 years. The family lives in a rental home. His wife has never worked and is very dependent on him; she fears being left alone if he were to die. Before his injury, the patient, when drinking socially with friends, commented he would not want to live as a severely disabled person.

The ethical questions, and the responses of the discussants, follow.

In performing a psychological evaluation, how does one determine competence?

Judge Buss: I think the value of the psychological evaluation for a person in the above situation is to determine whether he has the cognitive faculties intact. We need to know whether or not he has a value system, whether he is able to understand his physical and mental condition and the prognosis for recovery, and whether or not he understands the decisions he has to make to receive or terminate treatment. The psychological evaluation might also help in determining whether or not he understands and values other competing interests, particularly as those interests might encourage his receiving treatment.

Mr. Scofield: The traditional notion of competence, with its specific legal connotations, is increasingly being replaced by the notion of capacity, which is more flexible and consonant with reality than the customary view of competency has been. I take competency for the purposes of this case to mean decision-making capacity, however that concept may be defined.

In assessing a patient's capacity, especially when it involves the capacity to refuse life-sustaining treatment, a necessary but often overlooked preliminary step is some sort of self-assessment by the evaluator, to determine what he or she brings to this process. The failure to take account of one's own biases, attitudes, fears, and other feelings on such issues, especially in the area of terminal care, can be detrimental to a fair evaluation. If we are to judge or assess the decision-making capacity of others, a step which necessarily implies the possible limitation or curtailment of a patient's self-determination, we must acknowledge our role in that process, and how we may bias the outcome.

With those caveats in mind, it is appropriate to select a test of capacity or incapacity. Decision-making capacity involves something more than the mere ability to communicate a preference about treatment; we seek to ascertain the patient's understanding about the information he has been given about his condition, prognosis, and options. Is he able to reason and deliberate about this information in a way that is consistent with his or her own values and beliefs—is he able to process information about his condition into something that makes sense for him as a person? The mere fact that someone reaches a conclusion we might not have reached or makes a decision in a way we would not have does not alone justify our invalidating that choice by declaring it to have been made without proper decision-making capacity.

To know whether the patient has reached a decision that seems consonant with his or her own beliefs, it is essential for us to become familiar with that patient's belief system. Some of that information, but surely not enough, is contained in the patient history; more would be in the medical chart, with the family, and obviously, with the patient. We would certainly want to explore this patient's previously expressed sentiments about not wanting to be kept alive if he were severely disabled, to know why he thought that and whether he still does. It may be useful to ask the family how the patient seems to them.

While taking this and other information into account, we have to ascertain the ways in which the setting and/or medication may affect the patient's deliberative processes. If it is possible to alter the medication without increasing the patient's discomfort, this probably should be attempted, though we need to avoid manipulating the medication in order to manipulate the outcome.

Finally, we need to make certain that the patient has the capacity to understand the information that he is being given.

Ms. DeSilva: Competence is based on many factors and would appropriately be determined by a psychologist or psychiatrist. In this case, a psychological evaluation has been ordered, apparently because the patient has refused treatment and wants to end his life. I do not think that competence is necessarily an issue here because if the man was competent before his injury, there is no reason to believe that he is now incompetent after his injury.

What are the salient issues in this case?

Judge Buss: I think the first issue is to determine whether or not he is competent to make decisions regarding treatment. Competency is not easily defined or determined and the legal definitions of competency vary depending on the purpose to be served by determining competency. Competency of one to determine for themselves whether to accept life-sustaining treatment is and should be a higher degree of competency than a competency level to determine whether to accept mild forms of treatment such as pain relievers, for example. Colorado law and medical ethics probably do not coincide as to standards for competency.

A second issue raised by the problem is determining that the patient is completely informed as to his decision and also to the alternatives available to him and others involved, such as his family.

A third issue is whether or not the medical staff, including the doctors, hospital, and nursing staff, have certain rights and privileges that might interfere with his decision to terminate treatment. Doctors and nurses, particularly, have a set of professional ethics and personal ethics that might give them a personal right to refuse to honor this patient's request to terminate treatment.

Another issue is whether or not he has a right to terminate treatment. Also at issue is whether he has a terminal illness and whether or not it is suicide for him to terminate treatment and murder for those who assist him in doing so.

Mr. Scofield: The issues commence with the choice faced by the patient, in terms of prognosis, length of life, and the quality of life that he would have with his disability. Because it is unlikely that the patient's acceptance of treatment will prompt any further assessment, we should consider the implications of his decision not to receive further care, assuming that refusal is deemed to have been competently made. For the patient who, understanding his condition, has elected to forego further care, the courts have generally considered whether the presence of any of four other factors bars honoring that choice. These include: (a) the prohibition against suicide, (b) the preservation of life, (c) the interests of third parties, and (d) the maintenance of professional integrity.

The first two factors generally consider whether the patient somehow intended to be in this situation. Although consideration of the first of these two questions might get into an interesting inquiry about how accidental this accident was, it isn't likely to provide any useful guidance on this case. The courts, in addressing the requests of relatively young patients who can be maintained on life-support systems for several years, have considered the prohibition against suicide and the interest in preserving life. Although those cases have generally involved patients in persistent vegetative states, the courts have uniformly honored such requests, concluding that a request for treatment to stop is not a willful taking of one's own life and that the withdrawal or withholding of treatment, even where it would preserve a patient's life for an indefinite number of years, is merely permitting the natural processes to run their course. Whether the fact of this patient's present vitality would cause a court to view this case differently is unclear, but that was not the case in the Rodas case, which was decided in Colorado.

According to the American Medical Association, it is not unethical for physicians to honor a competent patient's request to be taken off life-sustaining treatment, including artificially provided nutrition or hydration. The Association's position addresses only patients who are terminally ill, a category this patient doesn't easily fall into, and those who are in an irreversible coma. Since it is believed, however, that patients have the right to refuse consent to treatment (or that they may not be treated against their consent) any likely concern over this patient's wishes is going to arise out of the implications rather than the mere fact of this refusal. In either event, there is no obligation that physicians participate in the actual withdrawal of such treatment and doctors have, on grounds of personal conscience, refused to go along with such wishes. Some institutions have adopted policies prohibiting the withdrawal of certain types of treatment, such as nutrition and hydration; these have not always been upheld by the courts. On the other hand, in a recent trial court decision, a family did not contest or seek to have a court overturn a rehabilitation hospital's decision that it could not have a patient carry out his treatment refusal plan at its facility because it would have a demoralizing and adverse impact on a staff dedicated to overcoming physical adversity. Even assuming, however, that the staff or hospital might wish to take such a position and that neither the court nor family would contest it, the staff optimally ought to consider how the patient would be impacted by a decision that he be discharged to a new, strange facility in order to die.

The interest of third parties also concerns the wife and the children. In the Farrell case—in which a 37-year-old mother of two, who because of her ALS, wished to stop treatment—a psychologist spoke to the children, who were somewhat older than the children here, to ascertain their feelings about their mother's wish. That psychologist found no reason to deny the mother's request. We may well ask if the interest of any third party ever compels the conclusion that the life of another be maintained even when the patient has no further interest in that life. Do we postpone death until the family is ready or willing to accept it? Until the children can "understand" it?

Ms. DeSilva: Important issues include the following.

1. Quality of life. Quality of life can only be assessed by the individual involved. It is a personal decision based on many factors, including intellectual, emotional, moral, spiritual, and others. A person's quality of life is often measured in terms of one's ability to deal with the problems of everyday living in spite of one's limitations. I think "quality of life" essentially defies measurement; it involves one's innermost reason for existence and sometimes cannot be explained to others. Quality of life is certainly not based solely on one's physical condition. Just because a person is endowed with a fully able body does not mean that he or she will possess "quality of life" in terms of that person's perception of life and its fulfillment.

2. State of mind. In this situation, the patient's state of mind at this time is extremely important. He has not yet lived with his injury long enough to know what his situation will ultimately be. He is obviously depressed and it is not clear whether his physical condition will improve. He has not had time to adjust to a daily lifestyle outside the hospital and to interact with his family and friends in his home environment. His state of mind also indicates that he has not had sufficient time to think about all the ramifications of a decision to pull the plug.

3. Individual rights versus societal standards. This may ultimately be the most difficult problem if the man continues in his wish to die because of the evolving nature of the "right to die" issue. I believe very strongly in the individual's right to make such a choice, but in this situation, the man has not been given an adequate opportunity to understand and accept the consequences of an irreversible decision, nor has he had enough time to find out whether his life is worth living.

4. Options for the future. This man may have several future options he has not thought about which might affect his current thinking. He probably will increase his sitting time and may also have other respiratory options later. Once he returns to home, he could arrange a living situation with his wife and in-home attendant care. Although he only has a high school education, he may still have a great deal of vocational potential which he has not yet explored. He also continues to have viable roles as a father and husband.

5. Motivation. In my opinion, individual motivation is a key factor in any person's ability to live with a disability. It goes along with quality

of life and is another term that is not easy to define or describe; it comes from within the person. This case does not give enough facts to know what this man's inner strengths and motivations are and whether he will utilize these personal resources.

What if this man said he had $300,000 in term life insurance and wanted to die now while the insurance is valid to provide his family some financial security rather than devastation?

Judge Buss: This additional fact might come into play and have an effect on termination of treatment when determining his value system in the process of determining his competency. Ultimately, a decision as to competency would take into account whether or not the individual has a socially acceptable value system. If he does, his motives for terminating treatment might be less significant. If he does not have a socially acceptable value system that guides him in his decision-making process, then ulterior motives such as insurance might be looked at as indicating he is not competent to make a decision.

Mr. Scofield: This raises an interesting question in terms of the interests of third parties, since they will be provided for, in the financial sense, if the patient's request is granted, and will be devastated if the request is denied. Does this mean that if the patient had no insurance his request would be denied because he had not made suitable provision for his family, even though he is no longer able to? If, on the other hand, the patient had a pension worth $125,000 now, but would quadruple in value in six months, could we deny his request until he became a better provider? If we are able to consider financial considerations here, why do we not consider the cost of continued care in deciding whether it should continue or not?

Ms. DeSilva: This fact would at least show that the man had given more thought to the situation as it affects his family, but a decision to end one's life should not be based primarily on financial considerations. Furthermore, it is not even clear whether the insurance would be paid under such circumstances. Again, while this may seem like a prudent decision, the man may still change his mind and may decide that he is more important to his family than the money. Although finances would be an issue to be addressed at some point, I do not believe that it is relevant at this time.

Assume the case involves a 13-year-old boy (similar medical information and time sequence) and that the parents are requesting the plug be pulled. How would the issues differ?

Judge Buss: Colorado case law, I believe, gives a 13-year-old child significant rights to make his own decision. No case has specifically been decided by a Colorado court on this issue, but other cases of the Colorado appellate courts could be interpreted to provide that a 13-year-old child has the right to make the decision. If the child has this right, then the parents would not have that right to decide. If the parents have the right to decide, then this adds the issue of substituted judgment.

Mr. Scofield: This raises perhaps the most vexing of questions. Traditionally, parents have been given decision-making authority over their children's medical care, because it is presumed that children lack the capacity to make such decisions and that their parents will decide matters in the child's best interests. This tradition has been substantially eroded over the years, with recognition of the "mature minor's" ability to reach decisions including, as was recently decided in the case of a 17-year-old Jehovah's Witness, the refusal of medical treatment viewed as life-sustaining. Studies of children with diseases such as leukemia show that they have some understanding of what is happening to them, though this may not be at the level we would equate with actual capacity. There is, therefore, no reason to leave the child totally out of this process.

We should explore the reasons why the parents do not wish to have treatment continue, and see in what way those reasons can be accommodated without stopping treatment. Depending on what those reasons may be, we may wish to provide them with information about the types of support available for them to deal with this tragedy. It may be necessary, if the parents insist that treatment stop, which in essence reflects their desire to abandon this child, to see what steps can be taken to continue treatment, if that seems to be what the child wants as well. Is it, however, proper for us to insist that this life be maintained, in the event that both family and child wish treatment to stop, to the point where we feel comfortable with the decision reached, as we might if the patient were 25? Is our reaction to this case one that stopping treatment is unreasonable, as in the "objective" sense that some patients with this disability have survived or that we are simply uncomfortable with letting a 13-year-old who can live, with enormous disability, die?

Ms. DeSilva: This case differs because the parents are making a decision about their son's life based on their feelings and beliefs rather than those of their child. A 13-year-old boy has his whole life ahead of him, and he, not his parents, is entitled to find out what kind of life he may have and whether he is able to live with his disability. In many ways, I believe it is easier for a younger person to adjust to a disability because children are extremely adaptable to difficult situations—they are not burdened by preconceived ideas of what life should be. If this boy's parents cannot cope with his physical situation, I believe that either they need counseling to determine whether they are willing to raise a handicapped child or they should give their son the opportunity to live his life with someone else.

What if this man were 65 years old, retired, and had grown children? How would the issues differ?

Judge Buss: Again, this changes the facts slightly and changes certain considerations. If the test of whether or not life-sustaining treatment should be terminated or continued is a balancing test of competing interests, then the fact that a patient's children are grown and no longer dependent on him becomes an important consideration.

Mr. Scofield: The issues are somewhat different since the interest of third parties in this man as a "provider" are irrelevant, assuming that they have any relevancy at all. The other issues, about capacity, etc., remain. Are our feelings about this decision influenced by any sense that, at 65, the patient has lived a "full" life, and that his choice is more "acceptable" to us than it is in the case of the 25- or 13-year-old, even though, medically speaking, there may be little difference among the cases? (I acknowledge that the complications of continued care may be different for patients in different age groups, but it is not likely that our view of the reasonableness of a patient's choice is going to depend on whether he is willing to accept or forego some sort of infection associated with receiving continued care.)

As with other patients, we would want to know what has prompted this patient to make this decision, whether it is because he fears a continued existence of disability, does not wish to be a burden to his family (or use up assets which would go to the children if not spent on expensive care), or because he thinks he has simply lived long enough. Is depression present? Can the patient be taught to live with this disability? Need he live with it simply because we have made it possible for him to do so?

Ms. DeSilva: The only major change in this case is the age of the person with the disability. Although the employment and family status are different, this man would also face the same issues described in question 2. It is still entirely possible for a 65-year-old man to live his remaining years as a severely disabled individual, although it might be very difficult and he may decide it is not worth it at his age. While this situation seems to lend itself more readily to the right of an individual to end his or her own life, it is still a personal choice that should be made when the individual has had a sufficient chance to examine and reflect upon all of the factors involved.

CONCLUSIONS

As health care providers strive to meet the needs of chronically ill or disabled people, they must recognize the limits of their mission—chronic care is more a negotiation than a triumph. This understanding requires a redefinition of the doctor–patient roles, respectful of autonomy and mutuality. But even as medicine affirms the need to treat the individual with dignity and justice, ethical questions foster continuing and confounding issues. When is a patient competent to join his or her physician as a partner? When can patient-centered autonomy be challenged? What determines quality of life? How do a patient and physician decide to terminate treatment? What if a patient chooses to die, against the moral reluctance of the medical staff? What about the interests of families and friends? Who pays if the patient cannot? These and many other ethical issues are not often decided as part of public policy. Sometimes the courts must intervene to sort out conflicting values. Meanwhile, the issues will intensify in coming years. Medicine in general, and rehabilitation medicine in particular, must continue to address these complex problems in an open, participatory way.

REFERENCES

1. Caplan AL, Callahan D, Haas J (1987): Ethical and policy issues in rehabilitation medicine. *The Hastings Center Report,* August 1987.
2. Ackerman TF (1982): Why doctors should intervene. *The Hastings Center Report.*
3. Schneiderman LJ, Spragg RG (1988): Ethical decisions in discontinuing mechanical ventilation. *N Engl J Med* 318(15).

23

Consumer Perspectives

Sam Maddox and Robert Menter

Craig Hospital, Englewood, Colorado, U.S.A.

Surviving a high cervical injury is a new phenomenon in modern medicine. Less than a generation ago, the odds were very slim that these people would live much past the intensive care unit, but quicker and better accident-site management, effective trauma care, and quality rehabilitation not only preserve lives but allow the high quadriplegic person to reintegrate into the community and in most cases regain a fulfilling and productive lifestyle.

This chapter is told in the voices of three such survivors, Brian Hogan, Kathleen DeSilva, and Les Peer. Each is a tribute to the rehabilitation resources of a spinal cord injury specialty center (Hogan, from Santa Clara Valley Medical Center, San Jose, California; DeSilva, from The Institute for Rehabilitation and Research, Houston; Peer from Craig Hospital, Englewood, Colorado).

These three are known in the medical community as "consumers." That they are—they consume the resources of the best spinal injury treatment available. They consume equipment and medical products unique to their life circumstances. In many ways these people represent the most desired outcome of the rehabilitation "product." But Brian, Les, and Kathleen will be the first to tell you they do not see themselves as models for what is expected after a life-changing disability. They were chosen for this discussion not as prototypical high quadriplegic individuals, but because they are all articulate and resourceful, and on their own terms, quite successful. They discuss a wide spectrum of issues and problems, but they speak only for themselves.

Brian, Les, and Kathleen responded to a set of questions intended to explore issues of their "quality of life." The questions explored many areas. What makes life worth living since your spinal cord injury? Do you feel you have control over your life, and in what ways? What is your greatest satisfaction? What do you want or need to accomplish in this life? What are your greatest fears? How does the medical community help or hinder your life? What advice would you give to health care professionals who interact with you? How soon can people make informed decisions about wanting to live after an injury such as yours? Did you have feelings of wanting to die that the staff should or should not have responded to?

The purpose of this chapter is to personalize the topic of high quadriplegia in a way that helps people better understand that a life with a severe disability is not without special problems, but that it is not a life without options, choices, and possibilities. The panelists vary in age and in length of disability. Each sustained a cervical fracture at the C1/2 level, although each has a different respiratory situation. Each panelist is an active member of his or her community; each has a lifestyle that is by no means oriented around medical issues. None of the panelists is religious in the organized church-going way. None is banking on regeneration research to make much of a difference in their lives, although each expressed interest in the topic of "cure" work. Each attests to being happy and has a view of the world unclouded by self-doubt or retrospection.

THE CONSUMER PANEL

Les Peer

Les Peer, 42, was injured in a skiing accident on Thanksgiving Day, 1982, in Aspen, Colorado. Les, who broke his neck at the C1/2 level, still lives in Aspen. He is able to wean from the respirator 6 h a day, and has been off the machine as long as 14 h, using his neck muscles for respiration. This allows greater freedom during transfers. He is attended by registered nurses 24 h a day. He uses a chin control for his wheelchair; he hopes to obtain a computer when voice activation is more advanced. Les is not working, but reads voraciously, writes poetry and short fiction, and hopes one day to pursue some business ideas, to use what he describes as his "good judgment." In describing life with high-level quadriplegia, Les is quick to note there are no broad-based answers or solutions for people in his situation.

"What makes life worth living since my spinal cord injury? This is simple. I can smell. I can taste. I can query. I can read. I can listen. I can argue. Life is not a fearful thing. Not thinking. Not smelling. Not tasting. Not laughing. Not living—those are my fears.

"I'm reluctant to give any advice, but what people in an identical situation might do is look out through the haze after getting through the first few months. Recognize what you can do and what you can enjoy. Then to the greatest extent possible, explore and understand and pursue those things.

"As for the things you can't do, you can't close them out of your mind, but you have to set them aside, put them back into a slight fog. You must dance with a new devil now, but I see no pleasure in dwelling on what I cannot do. That's a scab over a sore I shall not pick. My outlook is this—if I can't run down the road, I can wheel down it. That's better than not being able to go down the road at all.

"The term 'quality of life' can carry with it all of the abstractions that a Madison Avenue executive could ever hope to conjure up. From the joy of a cornflake that won't wilt in milk to alfresco candlelight dinners in the Himalayas. As a respirator-dependent quadriplegic I can practice in some of our ad men's fantasies and not in others. I must find my interpretation of quality of life somewhere within. I believe that the secret to finding a fresh existence within the posttrauma framework is somewhat akin to studying microbiology. Learning to distill down your existence or focus to the smaller framework set before you. Finding wonder and pleasure in the minute so that it takes on the aspects of a fresh world.

"I have learned to take joy in that which I can enjoy and regard that which I cannot participate in with somewhat scholarly distraction. I've also learned that I must be wary of extreme passion, for I am better suited, at this stage, with a level plane rather than the risks of peaks and valleys. As for relationships, I still share my life with lady friends, and I'm even closer to some than I was before, but I've made it clear that I don't expect someone else to constrict her life because of my limitations. Sex is no longer an issue; it's easier at this level, when one is not even able to touch, to have fond memories that stir up passions.

"I believe each and every high quadriplegic must learn to create a fresh framework for his/her life and once in place, he or she must fill that framework to its maximum. The fuller the framework the higher the quality of life. Never mind those things outside the framework. Never mind that this may seem at times parochial and tunnel visioned, for we all, handicapped and whole, have our limitations.

"Once within the framework we have to deal with the bits and pieces. It is very appropriate that we are termed the 'consumers,' since our day-to-day existence involves massive consumption. We consume our time, our attendant's time, our nurse's time, our doctor's time, in disproportionate amounts compared to the world at large. We consume Chux, Chix, swabs, gauze, night bags, day bags, pads, pills, ad infinitum. And as casually as we use these items and services, we must give thanks for a society that can afford this extravagance. But at the same time, grateful as I am to be alive and somewhat independent, I have to learn to be overbearing and pedantic for there is no detail of my care that, if neglected, cannot cause traumatic results. The high quadriplegic person is defenseless from mistakes, so day to day I must ask my competent and caring nurses to pay attention to what must seem to be the most trivial and tiny of details. I've become a bit like the time traveler who must not disturb a blade of grass in the past lest it negate his existence in the future. Being a successful high quad requires almost a sixth sense, in that you must try to anticipate not only what is going on and where it can lead but what can go wrong and its prospects. And at the same time not offend your caregivers.

"Part of my sense of self-worth, the satisfaction I glean from life, is rooted in being able to help others. I hope that along with this condition comes a certain amount of objectivity as related to friends and loved ones. Perhaps it's the distance that comes with being somewhat isolated physically from the day-to-day world. I believe that I have been able to lend an unprejudiced ear to the problems of my friends. There is value in that, and perhaps a touch of voyeurism, but it generates value and comfort.

"I have not lost control over my life. I am able to supervise those that care for me; also, I am able to adapt the limited timetable of my day to those things I can enjoy. As for my needs, perhaps tap dancing with Gregory Hines to the strains of the Blue Danube wouldn't be too much to ask, but wishful thinking aside, I plan to maintain my mind and my body in hopes of a cure or advancement, experiencing the joy of day-to-day living, albeit somewhat confined. I pay attention to the news on regeneration research, though not as closely as I should. There is a lot of chaff among the wheat, but do I have hope? Absolutely. I believe firmly there is something down the road, in my heart as well as my mind. I'd have to be crazy not to believe. There are indications there is a window of opportunity for the research to pay off. I'd just as soon look out the window, even though it be a small one.

"I am alive because of the medical community. From the ski patrolman who kept me alive going down the mountain, to the flight nurse who bagged me, to the hospitals, to the doctors, to the respiratory therapist, to the ICU nurses. The machinery, the wizardry, and the magic of modern science, I am grateful for them all.

"I am not grateful for those in the 'medical community' who market some of the toys and geegaws that when they work are wonderful but all too often only serve to frustrate. My experience with wheelchairs, van conversions, control units, etc., is that quality control is a significant problem. Equipment is unreliable—which can be a life-threatening thing for me—and it's expensive. The device is worth fifty cents if it's in a toy, but it's $100 if it is in a piece of rehab equipment.

"I'm alive, I'm whole, and I'm 6 years posttrauma. That is an accomplishment I must share with the health care professionals around me. Still, from my perspective, it seems there is a lingering sense of guilt or self-agonizing attached to the process of saving a spinal cord injured individual's life. Almost as if the doctors, nurses, medical technicians who save the life anguish over their responsibility for it. I've arrived at this conclusion, unscientific as it is, simply by looking at questions posed for me. There seems to be a constant theme of euthanasia running through your thoughts.

"Well, let me let you all off the hook—I am happy to be alive. Whether this apparently deluded euphoria will continue is perhaps the source of the answers you seek. But for now and for the past 6 years I think and delight and despair like a functioning soul.

"Medical professionals must realize they are in a different form of medicine in spinal cord injury. They shouldn't be afraid that the door can close in their face, that the patient will not heal, that they can't do as much; their practice may not be satisfying as when the cripple walks, or when the cancer patient goes into remission for 20 years. This is medicine by bits and pieces; the doctors have to listen to the patients, and work with them piece by piece. They should remember there are lots of us out there, happy as hell, despite the fact we can't walk on water.

"On the flip side, I don't know how soon people can make decisions about wanting to live after severe injury. It was not a question I asked myself. In fact, it was brought up extraneously by those concerned for my welfare. I think that it is a one-by-one situation. No touchstones. No guideposts. Another cross for the attending physician to bear. I would only counsel the professional to watch, listen, and listen, before anyone leaps.

"In the long term, hope, be it wildly optimistic or controlled optimism, is a major factor. I believe I would not be sane if I did not hope for the future. It is what makes the short term a foundation of the long term. Each brick of short term is two parts maintenance and one part tomorrow—meaning that I must keep the machine intact while expanding that part of me that will grow—thought, knowledge, friends, and family.

"In the end I am alive. I see, I smell, I taste, I am happy in moderation and anguished in staccato bursts of mood that pass. These are attributes that I owned before the trauma and still own today. How I exploited them before contributed to my quality of life then, how I exploit them now is the quality of life for me now."

Brian Hogan

Brian Hogan, 28, was injured in his hometown of Stockton, California, 5 days before his 16th birthday; his bicycle hit a hidden rock and threw him into a tree. He broke his neck at the C1/2 level, and had a passerby not been trained in emergency care, he would have asphyxiated, Brian says. At the time, he had planned to enter dental school. Now, Brian is a law student at the University of California at Berkeley, hoping for a career in environmental law. To study, Brian uses a special chin-level shelf system, set up by an attendant with his required reading. He uses a mouthstick for page turning and typing, etc. Brian uses some strategically placed switching devices, but other than an IBM computer for taking notes and writing, he employs no exotic high-tech solutions for his day-to-day activities. He uses a pneumobelt for respiration during the day, and phrenic nerve pacers at night.

"When I was first injured, the hospital rehabilitation staff was the exclusive source of my physical and psychological needs; without them, I assumed, I would deteriorate. My disabilities, I believed, were much too severe to allow me to once again become self-sufficient. During this acute stage, I lived in fear for my very life, often thinking death was a better alternative than permanent disability. This shouldn't happen to me, I felt. I was not made to be completely paralyzed from the neck down, unable to breathe, dependent upon the willingness of others to help me with my bladder and bowel care. I ought to be dating girls, playing tennis and waterpolo—living as other suburban California teenagers. But here I was, at 17, dealing with issues I thought I would be free from until I was 71. I was angry at myself for allowing this situation to occur.

"Clearly, I remember being told by a rehab nurse that I would 'see' home, but never 'live' there again. This reinforced all of my stereotypes of the limitations and 'strangeness' of disability. Disability was synonymous with inability; a disabled lifestyle offered no lifestyle at all. The word 'disabled' implied sickness, weakness, infirmity, dependence.

"The proposition 'I am severely disabled' frightened me, underscoring a sense of 'badness'; I searched for some reason something so 'bad' would happen to me. This was the 'tragedy' aspect of my injury, filling me with a sense of loss over my 'other' body, my 'good' and 'healthy' body. The body society 'wants' me to have.

"In retrospect, however, I see that many of my feelings sprang from images of disability perpetuated by an idealized version of the American teen. I know now these feelings were wrong. All types of severely disabled persons, including high quadriplegic individuals, have great potential. This potential must be realized through independent living and complete community integration—but there are many problems.

"After I left the rehab unit, my family was the source of my success. They knew that I was, in most respects, still the same human being I was prior to my injury. With their encouragement, physical as well as psychological support, and financial assistance, I returned to high school, then attended a college in my home town for a short time. I felt a need to move away from my family, to explore a sense of freedom and self-reliance. So I moved to Berkeley to attend the University of California.

"I was extremely fortunate to find U.C. Berkeley and its Disabled Students' Program (DSP). DSP had many resources, one of which is a dormitory program which provides special assistants, or SAs, on duty 24 hours a day. These SAs help the severely disabled students, train and manage attendants, tap community resources, and assist with adaptive aids in the dorm rooms. This program stresses the importance of independent living, which means managing your own life as much as possible, on your own terms. I graduated in 1986 and I am currently living in my own apartment and attending law school at the Berkeley campus.

"Many unique issues confront the high quadriplegic individual. Respiratory concerns outweigh any other physiological problems I may encounter. Therefore, close management regarding potential respiratory problems must be stressed early in the rehabilitation process. Technology—phrenic nerve stimulation and the pneumobelt—enables me to live independently. Still, many high quadriplegic individuals live in more dependent situations than they ought to; the burdens of respiratory care, in some instances 24-hour care, may be financially distressing.

"Financial resources ought to be made available for this group to stimulate increased independence; in the least, we ought to be able to pay skilled personal care attendants a 'fair' wage. There are sound political reasons to provide these financial resources—independent living is a 'good' economic and social outcome. The dependent lifestyle of 'burdening' family and friends with a quadriplegic's daily living needs is both inefficient and psychologically undesirable.

"The high quadriplegic person must 'learn' the system to use it, but at the same time resist being paternalized by it. Major decision-making power over my life is made by others who have neither seen me nor made any effort to get my consent. For example, in California's system to fund personal attendant care, a case worker visits my home to determine the income necessary to sustain a minimum lifestyle. Monthly payments are then made to me, based on the minimum wage; I manage this allotment among my attendant staff. The minimum wage, however, is inadequate for skilled attendants, since most are paid between $5 to $7 per hour. Therefore, I must reimburse them from my personal monthly income.

"What's more, the state's determination process for an individual's needs reinforces dependence and weakness. Because the wage is so low, the disabled person must 'act' more helpless than is actually the case. When a caseworker visits me I must act 'totally' dependent upon my attendants to maximize my monthly stipend. However, in reality, I use atten-

dants for personal care and cleaning and I have built adaptive aids to
feed myself, manage appliances, take care of paperwork, etc. The social
worker never sees my true level of independence because the system
forces me to maximize my resources by simultaneously becoming completely dependent.

"The political and economic aspects of disability become moot points
if the patient, during rehab, does not want to live. This is a major ethical issue for medical professionals, who may supercede the will of the
patient and paternalistically preserve the patient's life. There are many
variables to consider in determining the patient's right to die. We may
talk in terms of professional responsibility to see that all of the patient's
fundamental health needs are met. Of course, a physician's responsibility is loaded with moral, legal, and unspoken personal criteria encir-
cling this issue.

"But, the brute reality is that some high quadriplegic individuals do
not want to live, and after many hours of psychological counseling ought
to be granted their death wish. The Hippocratic Oath has not kept pace
with the life-sustaining machines we have developed. I argue that death
is also part of the health care profession; we beg the question by saying
a physician ought not to be able to provide a comfortable death for any
patient who wishes this. Of course, for the high quadriplegic individual,
the removal of the respirator is a passive invasion of the patient's body
and this leads to suffocation. I do not understand the distinction between this act and the infusion of quick life-ending medication. I have
experienced the sense of suffocation and it is very unpleasant. If I ever
decide to end my life, I would not like to die in this manner. It would be
excruciatingly long. We treat our pets with more comfortable forms of
death.

"The introduction of lethal medication puts the burden of care onto
the patient's shoulders by recognizing that this is the patient's final act.
The patient makes the decision that life ought to be ended and is assisted by the professional, in an atmosphere of care and trust. A prohibition against active euthanasia is paternalistic and simply does not
recognize the diversity of lives among us. Passive euthanasia mystifies
the death process by placing the dying process in the hands of God or
natural forces. Death must be treated with a modicum of awe and respect, but in a fashion that does not alter the will of the patient. Some
people choose to live in a society that views permanent disability with
repugnance. Others, however, do not and must be given the opportunity,
with informed consent, to a comfortable end to their own torment.

"I knew that if I chose suicide during rehab, death would be painful.
This was a deterrent. This option, however, would be available in the
future, if I really wanted to end my life. But, as time went by, I became
more independent and comfortable with myself. At one level, my mind

changed with the passage of time, and no professional could have predicted this. Yet, at another level, some patients express an emotional and physiological 'need' to die, and medicine may best serve them by acceding to their wishes.

"True social change, with full acceptance of all types of disability, is the crucial next step. We must demystify disability and recognize all human potential; afterward, the high quadriplegic individual may not feel such a psychological urge to end life. The severity of my disability ought not hamper interaction with my community—my disability is a rather meager piece of my being. I should be judged on the merits of my full personality.

"As I compare my thoughts about high quadriplegia now with thoughts I had 10 years ago, I feel both inspired and saddened by how much more work we have left. I have become comfortable with my present lifestyle, insofar as my daily relationships with others are concerned. But at another level, I have missed many experiences of 'common' Americans, and in this way, I will always be different.

"My disabilities follow me wherever I go. Oftentimes, I am disabled in my dreams, or quite ironically, I am an attendant for someone else. Psychologically, this may indicate that I have completely accepted my disability, or it may signal further denial and refusal on my part to actually come to terms with myself. At times, I feel remorse for my 'old' body image and how much easier things were before injury. I feel as if I would be completely accepted—a white male coming from a middle-class background. On the other hand, my disability has given me fresh insights that I could not otherwise have had. My injury has sensitized me to human issues and has provided me insights into real prejudice. I now realize that the world must change and all forms of racism, sexism, and 'able-ism' must end.

"I argue that many subcultures, especially including high quadriplegic individuals and other severely disabled members of society, must invoke their personal and legal voices to attain their rightful status among all other social classes. It is incumbent upon the disabled community to speak for itself and initiate a dialogue within a diverse, fully integrated society. People with disabilities must become more visible, since greater visibility erodes stereotypes and encourages interaction."

Kathleen A. DeSilva

Kathleen DeSilva, 36, was injured in 1968. A high school sophomore in Shreveport, Louisiana, she was practicing gymnastics and slipped on the uneven parallel bars, fracturing her neck at C1/2. Shortly after, her parents moved to Houston so Kathleen, the oldest of seven children, could go to The Institute for Rehabilitation and Research (TIRR). She gradu-

ated with her class in Shreveport in 1970, then moved on to Rice Univer-
sity where she graduated in 1977. Kathleen, who once wanted to be a
doctor, began law school at the University of Houston even before getting
her B.A. and obtained her J.D. in 1980. Kathleen is now the in-house
attorney for TIRR. She is married to Peter Simmons, a C7 quadriplegic
who had been her tenant for 4 years. Kathleen had phrenic nerve pacers
implanted in 1970; she rents a ventilator only when she has a respiratory
medical problem.

"Since my injury at age 16, there have been many things that have
made my life worth living. I was fortunate to have wonderful, loving
parents who cared about me and my future and who always gave me
their utmost support and encouragement. We've always been a close-
knit family. Since my parents' deaths, I married a kind and loving person who makes every day worthwhile. I have a good job and enjoy my
work and the people I work for at the hospital (TIRR). I believe I am a
very fortunate woman and know that the people around me have made
my life worth living. I'm a very happy person.

"I also think that there is a motivating force within one's self that
cannot be explained but that makes a person decide to get on with life
because of those tangible and intangible factors that make it worth living. We are shaped by factors that have nothing to do with disability;
this force, this will, is something you just have to possess within you. In
my case, I always had the desire to achieve, to be someone.

"Ultimately, the choice about whether life is worth living is a very
personal and private decision. In my case, I never seriously questioned
whether life was not worth living because there was always a new ad-
venture to look forward to—going home from the hospital, graduating
from high school, moving into my first apartment, graduating from college, designing and building my own condominium, graduating from law
school, opening a women's gift store business, starting my first job, getting married, taking trips, etc.

"When can a person make an informed decision about wanting to live
following an injury such as mine? This would vary from individual to
individual, depending on that person's age and circumstances, moral and
spiritual values, and ability to adapt and adjust to a new lifestyle. Essentially, it remains a very personal and private decision based on a
variety of factors that are different with each individual.

"Although my injury was over 20 years ago, I'm sure I experienced
thoughts of death and expressed wishes to die during moments of
depression; I didn't want to discuss these feelings with the staff. This
wasn't an issue to be responded to by the staff. It was a personal matter
involving me and my family. I still believe that the staff should respond

to such thoughts and wishes only if the patient requests or seeks their help; otherwise, the patient should be allowed to deal with these feelings in his or her own way.

"In many ways my disability was more difficult for my parents. It had to be awful—there was nothing they could do. I was still in my own world, still thinking about boys, the prom, who's dating whom, passing the finals, etc. When I see parents of newly injured people today, I try to encourage them, and tell them this isn't the end of the world. People with severe disabilities do accomplish many things, and find things that are satisfying and fulfilling. After a time, my parents never questioned that I would go on and reach my goals, that I would fall in love and get married. It's real important for family members to recognize the injured person's goals and dreams are not all washed down the drain.

"Of course, like most other people, I sometimes question my self-worth or value to others because I feel like there are so few things I can do for others. I basically know, though, that I am a good wife, sister, friend, and person. I may have occasional doubts about my abilities in the workplace, but I also believe I am a self-motivated, intelligent individual with sufficient knowledge and training to apply my skills in my profession. Doubts about my self-worth or value usually occur when I am worried or frustrated about other matters.

"I can become frustrated when I have to ask someone else to do something for me, or for example, if I have my house cleaned, and it's never done as well as I would do it. But for the most part I have control over my life because I do control most aspects of it through management of my household, finances, personal care, work environment, leisure activities, etc. Although I depend on others to do the physical work involved, I direct them to carry out my needs. I make my own decisions and choices based upon the options that are available to me. Controlling one's life is essential to maintaining personal dignity, independence, and quality of life. It is sometimes difficult to feel you are in control when you are so physically dependent on others for very basic personal needs, but I still maintain control over my life by making the decisions myself.

"My attendant care is provided in a shared situation with several other people in a 20-unit condominium complex we designed and built in 1976. We have a nonprofit group, Independent LifeStyles, that manages the attendant services. This allows us to keep the costs down because we share the services. My husband Peter is president of Independent LifeStyles.

"My job at TIRR involves corporate counsel, risk management, contracts, insurance, liability, etc. It's challenging and presents different problems every day. I never get into a rut. I've worked there 6 years. I use a computer at work, with a mouthstick.

"Over the years people have told me I am inspiring to them; that makes me uncomfortable, because I don't really know what that means. People may imply I'm somehow better than the rest, which is certainly not true. My life experience is different, my coping mechanisms are different, but oftentimes, people see my situation as one they themselves could not cope with. They don't see how a person who cannot move anything can function as an ordinary human being.

"Of course I am an ordinary person. My greatest satisfaction is that I have my husband to share my life with and that we love each other for who and what we are. I lead an independent life in my own home and enjoy looking forward to each day. I was raised as a Catholic, and though I question organized religion now, I still have a strong sense of spirituality, that there is a force bigger than we are. I have in the past considered the 'why me' of my situation, but I don't dwell on that sort of metaphysical question.

"As for the topic of regeneration research, this is something I don't think about much. If there is some breakthrough, I can get the information from people at the hospital. Even if there were to be something, after 20 years of being so physically limited, what would it mean for me? It's a matter for me of directing my thoughts. There are some thoughts I just don't seek.

"I've always been an ambitious person. I set high goals for myself and strive to achieve them. Even before my injury, I wanted to have both a career and a family; my desire to accomplish these goals has never changed. I need to work at a job that I consider to be worthwhile. I like to be successful at what I do and the personal satisfaction I get from doing a good job is far more important than monetary rewards. The most important thing I want in this life is happiness, and I have succeeded in being happy despite the sadness I still experience from the loss of my parents. I also need a sense of security about my life in terms of home, job, attendant care, etc.

"My greatest fear is losing my husband. I also fear losing my independence and the ability to exercise control over my life. I worry about not being able, for whatever reason, to receive the attendant care necessary to function daily. Becoming more disabled as I grow older is a concern, as is becoming senile and mentally impaired, or losing the ability to communicate with others. Being alone for the rest of my life is another thing I fear. Most of my greatest fears are essentially no different from those of other people.

"Generally speaking, my interaction with the medical community is limited to absolutely necessary occasions—it is important to me that my lifestyle remains nonmedically oriented. The biggest help I get from the medical community is having a primary physician who has treated me and followed my care for many years, thus enabling him to know and understand me better as a whole person. He trusts my judgment and listens to my opinions because he believes that his patients know their limitations better than anyone else. The professionals in the medical community also help by providing me with the latest information on medical treatment, new equipment, technological advances, research projects, interesting publications, etc.

"The medical community also hinders my life in several ways. There are typically very lengthy waiting periods for appointments, accompanied by the requirement for extra hospitalization for illness or surgery because of my physical condition. Also the cost of medical care and equipment for a high-level quadriplegic person is very expensive.

"It is very important that health care professionals involved in spinal cord injury act as a team and know what the other members are doing. I would advise such professionals to listen to their patients and learn each person's individual wants and needs. I would also suggest that they keep up with the latest developments in patient care, research, and technology so they can serve as competent sources of information to their patients. I also hope that as their patients leave the hospital environment, the professionals view them more as clients or patrons rather than as patients."

24

The Insurance Industry Perspective

Rene L. Monforton

Automobile Club of Michigan, Dearborn, Michigan, U.S.A.

The increase in high-level spinal-cord-injury survivors has created for insurers a number of concerns about the availability of care, dissemination of information within the medical profession, and financing of products, services, and accommodations. These are important issues that have an impact on the goal of successful rehabilitation. Open communication between insurers and care providers will help everyone in reaching that objective.

WHO SHOULD PROVIDE THE FOLLOW-UP

One of the primary concerns for insurers is the tremendous variation in outcome, which influences long-term funding. Derivative questions arise, such as why is it that if a patient receives acute care and rehabilitation at a specific facility, the follow-up care will frequently be provided by the same facility? Although this is acceptable for individuals being treated within a reasonable distance of their residence, patients frequently are transported long distances for acute care and primary rehabilitation services. Recognizing the uniqueness of this type of injury, the medical needs throughout the rehabilitation process may be best served by a limited number of facilities. However, the long-term follow-up care should be provided in a facility close to the patient's home, if adequate resources are available and the case is properly managed.

We have the technology to transport this patient population long distances, but it is not cost-effective to transport patients back to the primary care facility for follow-up care. There is a need for facilities specializing in the care of high quadriplegia to develop transfer agreements and to train remote care providers. Because of our ability to transport seriously injured individuals, it becomes necessary that the knowledge and skills be shared on a more global basis. If not, the few facilities providing services will become overburdened with follow-up patients. This "disbursement" of knowledge to a broader base will help assure that local facilities will have the ability to provide the necessary care and the expertise to identify potential medical problems before they occur. Continued communication and coordination with a well-trained case manager is equally important in assuring a positive result.

THE NEED FOR CONSISTENCY

As previously indicated, there are substantial variations in outcome depending on the facility that provides the acute care and rehabilitation. It defies logic that individuals with similar levels of injury will ultimately require significant variations in attendant care based solely on where the treatment was rendered. Some facilities encourage significant others to participate as caregivers, with support from attendants and periodic visits by a registered nurse. Other facilities do not encourage family participation and recommend the use of licensed practical nurses and/or registered nurses as caregivers on a 24-h basis. There have even been instances in which more than two caregivers were prescribed for a 24-h period.

These tremendous inconsistencies in recommendations for attendant care cause insurers to have legitimate questions about what is unreasonable or excessive care. Frequently, this situation results in insurers encouraging families of injured persons to transfer their loved ones to facilities where outcome is generally predictable. Short of this occurrence, these conflicts will most likely result in frustration for the medical profession and family and ultimately will result in unnecessary litigation.

Medical staffs from facilities specialized in the care of high-level quadriplegic patients must standardize a range of acceptable long-term care. Variations in individual lifestyles and questions concerning living arrangements have an impact on the decision-making process and may prevent the possibility of developing specific outcomes. However, standardization could be developed in the form of acceptable ranges of home care, such as 24-h attendant care, with an additional 4–6 h of professional services by a trained L.P.N. or R.N. Considerations concerning an individual being maintained in a private residence, with family, or independently, is a variable that can be quantified.

Home care is the most expensive long-term consideration and must be reasonably addressed to the understanding and agreement of all persons. Additionally, lists of required equipment and/or optional equipment should be developed. Home modifications should be based on barrier-free and/or quantifiable square footage for additions to a primary residence.

THE NEED FOR COMMUNICATION

These concerns, if addressed appropriately by the medical professions, would alleviate unnecessary litigation and lead to a better understanding between insurers, medical professionals, and the injured person. After all, we are all working to the benefit of the injured person and any barrier we can remove to allow us to work in an effective manner is beneficial to the care, recovery, and rehabilitation of the patient.

Injured persons can achieve their maximum potential in a cost-effective manner when all parties concerned work together toward that end. For this reason, it becomes of paramount importance for medical professionals and families to include insurers in the rehabilitation process. Funding for the care, recovery, and rehabilitation of an injured party has a significant impact on the decision-making process for the medical profession. Without the knowledge of the funding mechanism available, it becomes extremely difficult for medical professionals and family to examine available alternatives to make an appropriate decision.

INSURERS AND PROVIDERS WORKING TOGETHER

Insurance comes in many forms and sizes and is administered on the basis of contractual responsibilities. Within the health insurance industry alone, we have private corporations and governmental agencies providing funds for medical services. Each health insurance contract has unique limitations, based on the needs or desires of the subscriber or insured. Contracts vary from limited lengths of stay and/or limited services through catastrophic forms of insurance. In addition, there are long-term disability insurance, Worker's Compensation, no-fault insurance, and reinsurance. Without the involvement of an insurance representative, it is virtually impossible for service providers to be aware of contractual limitations affecting the decision-making process. In addition to the various insurance programs, there are social programs, such as Medicaid, providing benefits. These programs, administered through individual states, develop their own limitations and/or schedules for the funding of medical care. Funds allocated for services are generally approved through a legislative process and frequently result in annual changes in the level of compensation. The claim payment process of each of the various forms of funding differs widely. Health insurance plans and Worker's Compensation rely, for the most part, on schedules of payments for various services, frequently based on prevailing rates in an area. These plans are somewhat rigid and codified and to move beyond these barriers, a great deal of justification is required of the claim representative.

The no-fault auto insurers and some of the health or long-term disability insurers provide more latitude in the administration of the benefits. The terms "reasonable" and "necessary" become key words and their interpretation depends on overall company claim philosophy and the experience and judgment of the claim adjuster. Understanding the nature of the treatment or rehabilitation plan is important for the adjuster and frequently involves requests for substantial documentation or explanation. In addition to the individual contract ramifications, large cases frequently lead to the involvement of a reinsurer who pays for benefits beyond a certain monetary limit on behalf of the insurer. In some instances, the reinsurer becomes directly involved in the management of the claim and can increase or decrease the complexity in resolving problems.

There is also concern about the role of liability insurance in the overall management of these cases. Unfortunately, the small limits of most liability policies make the insurer's role relatively insignificant. When liability is clear, their interest is simply paying the claim and having it resolved. In the instance of a high-limits policy, insurers are hesitant to become involved because such activity can be interpreted to be an admission of liability. It should be kept in mind that the primary responsibility of an insurer handling a liability case is to protect the rights of the insured. In some cases, it is in the best interest of the insured that the insurance company become involved in the funding of care for the injured person.

A further complication involving a liability insurer is the time delay when the judicial system enters into the equation. If a liability case is not quickly resolved, it is not unlikely that 2–3 years may pass before the liability is resolved in the courts.

Insurers are acting within contractual responsibilities and guidelines established by their company, and when the treatment or service is outside of the norm, delays occur.

The delays are frequently problems for all parties involved. The medical professional's biggest complaint is that the insurers are slow to respond and complicate establishment of appropriate courses of action through the slow approval process. In fact, this can be quite true and the insurance industry has to develop a higher level of sensitivity to these problems.

Concurrently, the medical professionals can facilitate benefit requests through a combination of educational programs and through more precise documentation that considers the contractual concerns of the insurers. A major step in unraveling this communication road block was the creation of the Insurance Rehabilitation Study Group in 1965, which enhanced communication and provided a forum for sharing information. Unfortunately, only approximately 50 companies are involved, a small representation of the insurers involved in these cases.

The many forms of funding mechanisms negate the opportunity to understand each and every form of insurance contract available in today's market. Similarly, the many treatment options are difficult to understand even by the more sophisticated administrators of the various funding plans. Consequently, it has become more important for medical professionals to encourage insurer representation during the rehabilitation process. With the availability of an insurance representative, questions concerning funding can be resolved long before decisions are made by the medical professional. This is not to say the medical decision will differ, but rather, to suggest that the need will exist to identify a separate funding mechanism for a particular service and/or product.

The entire area of available funding lends itself to misunderstandings and suspicion, but if all parties communicate honestly, and with respect, appropriate alternatives generally can be identified. Openness, honesty, and respect lead to a lasting trust, removing unnecessary barriers.

Once the barriers have been removed, each subsequent involvement between the insurer and facility builds on this trust and proves beneficial for all persons. We can all win.

THE PROBLEM OF DEFINING "MEDICAL NECESSITY"

If we were to collectively attempt to identify areas of concern, I believe funding for *medical needs* would be lowest on the list. Conversely, highest on the list would be quality-of-life issues. This is due to the fact that in most cases, insurance mechanisms provide funding for reasonably necessary medical care, services, products, and accommodations. Most frequently, our concerns are about medical necessity versus quality of life. We would all agree there is medical necessity for alarm systems to alert personnel when an individual requires assistance. However, serious questions arise when we speak of the need of an environmental control system to remotely operate various functions (open drapes, operate TV or radio, etc.) not specifically related to the care of the individual. Attendant care is a medical need. Is an environmental control system a medical need, or a quality-of-life issue? Although there may be philosophical differences as to quality of life and its impact on future medical needs of an individual, the fundamental question is whether such devices qualify for reimbursement as a medical necessity.

Technology has and will continue to create areas of disagreement. It is not an insurer's responsibility to provide funding for equipment characterized as experimental. The efficacy of new devices must be subjected to specific research procedures and independent certification. Such procedures would document indicated use and justify the need.

THE MARKETING OF QUALITY CARE

The last concern is the marketing of acute care and rehabilitation services for the spinal-cord-injured population. There have been tremendous advances in medical treatment and technology resulting in meaningful independence for catastrophically injured persons, but it continues to be one of the best-kept secrets.

Specialized care facilities and professionals need to market the services they offer to hospitals throughout the United States. We continue to hear of those horrendous cases involving complications that could have been avoided had the person been transferred to an appropriate facility. Timely transfers will occur when specialty program providers communicate the availability of their services nationwide. Even though many insurers and case managers representing insurers have knowledge of specialty programs, few know their specific locations. Utopia would be the development of a national network with multiple centers participating with literally thousands of hospitals; this may be the ultimate answer to quality care for this population.

Opportunities to encourage insurer use of specialty programs and participation in the rehabilitation process have been overlooked. Written communication to corporate executives that detail the positive humanitarian impact, cost savings, and gratitude for their involvement has positive results. This type of compliment will create good will and generally stimulate increased use of specialty programs. You will also instill confidence in corporate management that their employee or case manager has acted in the best interest of all persons. Ultimately, future patients will benefit from the air of trust and confidence created by your communication.

When we communicate with honesty and respect, we can best discharge our respective responsibilities. Barriers of any shape or size can be overcome and the insured/patient is the recipient of the benefit. After all, we are trying to help the injured person succeed, and working together assures the best opportunity for success. We can all win.

25

Working Effectively with Insurance Case Managers

Dolores Hynes

North American Reinsurance Corporation, New York,
New York, U.S.A.

To work effectively with insurance case managers it is necessary to understand the total concept of case management and the diversity of roles the case manager plays. It is also important to recognize that changes in our health care delivery system, and the roles of other participants, have had an impact on the traditional view of medical case management.

MANAGED HEALTH CARE

The concept of "managed health care" has emerged as costs have continued to escalate, employers have become rationers of health care, and government moves further away from responsibility in financing health care needs. This new managed case approach, however, focuses more on mechanisms of cost containment such as preadmission screening, utilization review, second surgical opinion, hospital bill audit, etc., rather than a comprehensive approach to the needs of the whole person. It is not intended to suggest that cost containment mechanisms have no merit, but in and of themselves they do not eliminate duplication and fragmentation in our health care system, nor do they address long-term issues and quality of life.

For those persons who have been involved in rehabilitation, especially specializing in catastrophic injury, the real concept of medical case management has been a comprehensive approach that entails the earliest possible evaluation of the individual's condition and current treatment program, referral to and use of appropriate resources, participation in the treatment process whereby the lines of communication are kept open and there will be ongoing reviews of the effectiveness of the treatment program, the follow-up to assure maintenance of the goals that have been achieved, and detection early on of any changes or complications that may compromise health maintenance. To achieve this process it is necessary for the case manager to interact effectively with all participants including patient and family, physicians and other members of the treatment team, social services, employer, attorney, and community resources.

GOALS OF MEDICAL CASE MANAGEMENT

Effective interaction with case managers requires a realistic look at, and understanding of, the goals set by all participants (both short- and long-term) during all phases of care: acute, subacute, rehabilitation, and long term.

The insurance carrier's goals are dictated by coverage obligations that may vary from those mandated by Worker's Compensation statutes to those stated in health and disability contracts purchased on a group or individual basis. There is a considerable variable here in that the obligation at one end may be for the lifetime of the individual and at the other end coverage based on a very limited dollar amount. Early clarification of coverage issues is essential and the carrier will then determine its goals, whether for a one-time evaluation or for continuing intervention and the determination of both short- and long-term needs.

Ideally, the insurance carrier's goal, especially in addressing a catastrophic loss such as spinal cord injury, is to see that maximum medical improvement can be achieved in a timely manner while at the same time preserving benefit dollars. This can be achieved by early intervention to assess the patient's needs, coordination of an appropriate treatment plan, use of the best resources available to maximize an early return to home and community, and follow-up to assure stability and health maintenance.

The goals of a private provider of case management services should reflect those of the carrier who has contracted for these services. Sometimes, however, the focus may be somewhat different in that a more parochial approach is used rather than a national perspective of the availability of more appropriate resources. The case manager, although well informed on local facilities and resources, may not have a larger geographic focus, even though employed by a national organization, or perhaps in recognizing the desire of the carrier for cost containment, sometimes may be reluctant to push for a move outside the immediate area to a more specialized facility. Also, the issues of short-term versus long-term involvement may have an impact on how the case is handled.

It is imperative that all case managers have the opportunity to become knowledgeable about treatment trends and resources over a wide range through educational programs, whether they be in-service through their own organizations or attendance at outside seminars. This is especially important in dealing with the many complex issues that arise in the management of the high quadriplegia patient.

The goals of the treatment team are both individual and collective. Each team member, encompassing the various disciplines of care—including physical therapy, respiratory therapy, occupational therapy, speech therapy, recreational therapy, social service, nursing, and medical—will set his or her own goals but must interact with all of the members to effect the common goals required for the patient to achieve maximum potential. In so doing there must be ongoing dialogue with the case manager as well. We must recognize that in a treatment setting there are a variety of patients with various insurance coverages. Communication with the insurance case manager can help eliminate confusion and discord in the decision-making process regarding equipment, supplies, home modifications, and all of the many facets of discharge planning, all of which are all the more complex in the high quadriplegic population.

The goals of patient and family must also be considered and options discussed. The case manager as facilitator can help guide patient and family through the maze of an often unknown system. Is the patient realistic in his/her expectation regarding outcome? Does the patient's fear of dependence jeopardize his/her ability to become more independent? Are the patient's questions being answered? Does he/she even know what to ask? Is it more important for the patient and family to remain in a geographic area near home or how do they make the decision on choosing an alternate, sometimes distant facility that may be more suitable to address the medical and rehabilitation needs?

Interaction with the family in the home setting can help determine what the support system has been and will continue to be. Is it the goal of parent/spouse to be caregiver? Is that person capable of assuming that role and what other outside resources will be required? Will the issue of role reversal have an impact on family stability? Support services for patient and family must be investigated and initiated on a timely basis to prevent breakdown. Continuing dialogue between the case manager, health care professionals, insurance carrier, and patient and family can help eliminate crisis intervention and demonstrate that crisis prevention is ultimately more beneficial.

It is important for the case manager to know and understand the medical issues as well as the psychosocial issues that will affect goal setting and decisions regarding long-term management.

Advances in medical technology, from accident scene to evacuation to

trauma centers, specialized intensive care units, and appropriate rehabilitation facilities have increased the number of survivors of traumatic
injuries who are ventilator-dependent. An increasing expansion and
support of outpatient services have opened new options for care of these
persons and many would opt for home care, or group home care, rather
than the alternative of institutional care. Availability of appropriate durable medical equipment and ancillary services that can be provided in
the home setting indicate that we are capable of providing this care for
an extended period.

However, there are ethical issues that arise and these must be presented and discussed openly by and with patient and family, medical
and rehabilitation professionals, and case managers.

Practical issues such as the physical layout of the home environment
necessary to support the amount of equipment needed for care and the
willingness of family to participate in that care may be limiting factors
in and of themselves. Experience has shown that in the best of circumstances what may initially appear to be a positive, stable situation can
turn into disillusionment, guilt, and anger. The case manager must stress
and support the need for open dialogue and family counseling before
discharge and continuing heavy psychological support postdischarge.

Case examples will illustrate that various factors such as the patient's
age, medical stability, and family and community support have an impact on how "success" may or may not be measured.

Steven, an 8-year-old boy struck by a car while riding his bicycle,
suffered a C1 avulsion, is now 18 years old, and has remained home
since his discharge from the rehabilitation facility. The consistent determination of his mother and the guidance of a knowledgeable case manager, as well as funding for what was considered reasonable and necessary, have been the prime factors in this continuing success. In fact,
Steven was eventually mainstreamed from home tutoring to public school
education and in 10 years has not had an acute hospital readmission.

John, at age 54, sustained a C2/3 complete lesion as a result of a
work-related injury and remained ventilator-dependent. With appropriate equipment, supplies, and nursing support he was eventually discharged home with his wife. However, this man had many postdischarge
complications necessitating an average of six emergency room visits per
year, at least two inpatient hospital stays per year, and many prescriptions and supplies. John died at home, 6 years postinjury, apparently of
a myocardial infarction while being suctioned.

Although in each case there was success in achieving a return to the
home setting with all appropriate services in place, stability was not the
same, but perhaps there was still a better quality of life in both cases.

Does the employer have a role in setting goals of medical case management? If the individual has sustained a work-related injury there is immediate communication with the employer as part of the insurance process. The case manager, however, will meet with the employer to keep them informed of the injured worker's status and progress. The feasibility of a return to employment may be viewed as an impossible goal, but any possibility of success will require education, innovation, and imagination, and certainly the need to keep the employer an active part of the rehabilitation process.

If the injury is non-work-related and the individual is insured under group health benefits the employer still plays a part, but may have very different goals. As employers have turned from the role of "passive payers" of health care to "active purchasers" they have also been viewed as "rationers" of health care with the major focus on cost rather than on what constitutes quality. Third-party administrators and benefits managers on behalf of the employer can work along with case managers to address the needs of the employee or his/her dependent, and within policy limits, help to better use and preserve benefit dollars. Researching alternative services and identifying areas as options for ultimate cost effectiveness, even though not covered in the contract language, should be presented to the employer for their consideration.

WHO IS THE CASE MANAGER?

Case managers may be directly employed by the insurance carrier, may be self-employed, or employed by a company that contracts with a carrier for its services, or, most recently, an "internal" case manager employed by the rehabilitation facility. With each of these comes different philosophies; however, in all instances this person must act as a liaison between all of the parties involved, including the insurance claims handler. It should not be intended, or misconstrued, that medical case managers be "investigators" but, rather, facilitators to communicate, coordinate, and educate.

More traditionally, medical case management services had been provided by registered nurses employed directly by an insurance carrier. However, because of increasing need and use of these services there are now many private providers who contract with carriers on an individual basis. Along with registered nurses there are now occupational therapists, physical therapists, social workers, and vocational counselors among those in this field. Knowledge of medical issues plus good communication skills and the ability to interact well with people are essential qualities that the case manager must possess. There is no specific training for persons in case management. Typically, it is a matter of on-the-job training and, often, good common sense. It is extremely important that case managers develop "field" experience under the supervision of someone with a knowledge base and expertise to impart the important elements of this multifaceted approach in health care management.

With the increasing number of persons entering the field of case management has come "credentialing." The primary sources are: CIRS, Certified Insurance Rehabilitation Specialist; CRRN, Certified Rehabilitation Registered Nurse; and CRC, Certified Rehabilitation Counselor. All of these have certain basic requirements, including education and vocational experience, to sit for the certifying examinations, and all require continuing education credits to maintain status.

Again, the need for case managers to have exposure to educational programs dealing with the complex medical and psychosocial issues of the severely disabled must be emphasized. Many case managers have no first-hand experience with catastrophic injury management and may find themselves groping for guidance. The need to refer to a more experienced person, or work with another person, should be addressed honestly to enhance the best possible outcome.

THE PROCESS OF EFFECTIVE CASE MANAGEMENT

Effective case management starts with early identification of serious injury or illness cases. Most insurance carriers have developed some type of "red flag" system whereby the claims handler—who must be properly trained—can identify even a *potentially* high-cost claim. The imperfect mechanisms used may be by diagnosis, length of hospital stay, multiple complications, dollar amount already spent, etc. But perhaps the important issue is that the claims handler *act* on this information as quickly as possible.

There are various components of the case management process and these have been described in different ways, using different terms. Encompassing these are the following: (a) assessment of the individual's condition to determine what services are necessary and how to most appropriately provide them; (b) coordination of the many facets of the treatment plan, ranging from referral to a different physician or facility to arranging transportation, durable medical equipment, home care needs, therapies, etc., so that there can be a combined effect to ensure success; and (c) intervention by the case manager to ensure interaction between patient and family, physician and treatment team, and the insurance carrier so that all can have a better understanding of each phase of the treatment and rehabilitation plans.

The case manager continues to participate to evaluate progress, assess changing needs and appropriateness of services, and coordinate discharge plans. To ensure continuing success, follow-up becomes extremely important. Once the disabled person has been removed from the protective and structured environment of the rehabilitation facility, it may be all too easy for breakdown to occur in areas of service, family support, compliance, etc. It now becomes even more important for the case manager to continue the relationship not only to anticipate and prevent complications, but if any should occur, have them addressed efficiently and effectively.

THE MEDICAL CASE MANAGER AS AN EDUCATOR

There are many issues to be addressed, some small, some significant, as patient and family move through the maze of the health care system. It is not unusual that there be distraction, confusion, fear. The initial contact of the case manager with family should be one of support. This is extremely important so that a rapport can be developed in which there is trust that this person will be available to assist, answer questions, and offer guidance.

Coverage Issues

The major lines of coverage include Worker's Compensation, auto/no-fault, accident and health, liability, and long-term disability. Depending on the coverage, unique concerns arise over dollar limits involved, specific contract language, time frames, terms such as "reasonable," "necessary," and "customary," discontinuation of benefits and extracontractual issues. Because there can be many variables involved, questions should be asked and answered on an individual basis, and not by drawing comparisons between one patient and another or one coverage versus another.

Although the case manager must be knowledgeable about insurance coverage issues, it is the responsibility of the claims handler to make decisions on interpretation of the insurance contract. The flow of information from the claims handler to the case manager to patient and family and all those who provide services is an integral part of the case manager's role as educator.

Medical Issues

Education regarding terminology, skin care, dietary habits, exercise, and recognition of signs and symptoms of complications can be reinforced and carried on from facility to home. Physicians and other medical personnel should not view the case manager as an intrusive person just seeking out information, but rather as a link between all parties to effect better communication. Ongoing dialogue should encourage questions from patient and family and be directed toward the appropriate resource so that these may be answered plainly and fully.

Legal Representation

Some patients are represented by attorneys who may not understand the role of case management and thus consider it not in the interest of his/her client to cooperate. It often becomes a difficult, and sometimes frustrating, task to convince the attorney that the goal is to facilitate cooperation to maximize outcome. The bottom line is to work together to provide the quality care needed to effect the best possible result for the individual. If this requires a face-to-face meeting in the attorney's office, so be it. Any avenue that may present an opportunity to demonstrate to counsel the goals and objectives of a rehabilitation plan should be used as an opportunity to educate him/her about the resources available to the client, and the responsibility to mutually cooperate.

Coordination of Funding Sources

The family is too often unprepared and unsophisticated about knowing what funding sources may be available to them. Problems regarding loss of income become burdensome, especially when faced with a catastrophic injury that may inhibit return to the work force for an extended period, if ever.

Coordination of resources by the case manager may fall into three categories: contractual—all possible insurance coverages as well as benefits that may fall under the Consolidated Omnibus Budget Act of 1986; legislated—benefits coming under the Social Security System, including Social Security Disability Insurance, aid to dependent children, vocational rehabilitation services, etc.; voluntary—funding that may be available through various organizations such as United Way, the National Multiple Sclerosis Society, the Muscular Dystrophy Association, etc.

Community Resources

Determining what resources can be plugged into, and how to access these resources, can be researched by the case manager. Transportation and recreation opportunities may be available through volunteer groups, high school students, church organizations, and organizations working with the disabled. When resources are not available in the community, the case manager can often be an advocate to develop awareness and possibly help to initiate programs through education.

Employment

Because of the significant physical impairment of the high quadriplegic patient, return to the work force is often not considered a realistic goal. In essence, there would need to exist ideal circumstances for this to be achieved. However, any potential should not be ignored and the case manager's awareness of availability of state and private vocational rehabilitation services should be brought into play so that all possible resources will be used. We should also keep in mind that technological advances in environmental control units may present some options for employment in the home or office heretofore not even considered.

EFFECTING COMMON GOALS

Throughout the entire process of case management run the threads of communication, coordination, cooperation, and continuity. It becomes the responsibility of all persons involved to understand that all of these elements are necessary to effect the common goals that have been established so that the disabled individual is viewed as a "whole person." This is true whether or not the individual returns to home and community or whether alternate living plans are required.

In the "real world" of our health care delivery system, things do not always run smoothly. Insurance carriers and their claim handlers may be viewed as cold and insensitive. However, there is a responsibility to obtain documentation so that claims can be processed efficiently. It is also the responsibility of physicians and providers to interact with insurance personnel, providing them with necessary information on a timely basis. Accountability becomes a requirement of all.

As we recognize that severely disabled persons are surviving longer and longer, and that only a very small percentage of postinjury time is spent in the rehabilitation facility, the importance of the case manager's role in follow-up becomes even more apparent. What must remain paramount is that a "partnership" should exist, thereby integrating individual goals into common goals that ultimately will be mutually beneficial.

BIBLIOGRAPHY

1. Davis DH (1986): Case management—new applications. In: *The Risk Report.* Dallas, TX: International Risk Management Institute, Inc., 4(3):1–7.
2. Deutsch PM, Sawyer HW (1986): *A Guide to Rehabilitation.* New York: Matthew Bender.
3. Haddad AM (1986): Ethical considerations in long term home care for ventilator-dependent clients. *Pride Instit J Long Term Home Health Care* 5:3–7.

4. Hembree WE (1985): Getting involved: employers as case managers. *Business and Health* 2(8):11–14.
5. Henderson MG, Wallach SS (1987): Evaluating case management for catastrophic illness. *Business and Health* 4(3):7–11.
6. Logan JE (1986): Taking advantage of medical case management. *Settlement Forum* 4(3):6–7.
7. Merrill JC (1985): Defining case management. *Business and Health* 2(8):5–9.

26

Government Assistance (Medicaid) for Ventilator-Dependent Quadriplegic Patients

Maureen A. Cox and Conal Wilmot

Santa Clara Valley Medical Center, San Jose, California, U.S.A.

It is the experience of the staff of the Santa Clara Valley Medical Center Spinal Cord Injury Rehabilitation Unit in Northern California that there are major differences in benefits and assistance available to ventilator-dependent quadriplegic patients depending on whether the patient has Worker's Compensation coverage, private insurance, or MediCal, California's equivalent of Medicaid. When planning for acute care, rehabilitation, equipment needs, and future care of the patient after rehabilitation, the differences in benefits become readily apparent. There are also major differences from state to state in the coverage Medicaid/MediCal provides for acute hospital care and rehabilitation, as well as services available after discharge.

Any discussion related to the care of ventilator-dependent quadriplegic patients must endeavor to clarify differences in available benefits between states. Rehabilitation facilities were contacted in Alabama, Texas, Colorado, Pennsylvania, Massachusetts, and Illinois. Many challenges, problems, frustrations, and hopes were expressed by social workers, discharge planners, physicians, nurses, and other rehabilitation staff. Professionals contacted stated that the constraints of providing adequate care to ventilator-dependent quadriplegic patients are not confined to those dependent on Medicaid but often also to those with limited insurance coverage from private insurance companies and health maintenance organizations as well. However, it does appear that private insurance companies typically assign personnel very promptly to become involved with the rehabilitation staff, whereas Medicaid/MediCal personnel are frequently unavailable to work with the staff, particularly the social worker and/or discharge planner, regarding present and future needs and discharge plans.

Among the states contacted, California has the most complete coverage for acute hospital care, rehabilitation, durable medical equipment, medical and nursing supplies, and respiratory equipment. In some states minimal equipment needs are covered; some will provide only a manual wheelchair, not an electric wheelchair. One state does not pay for oxygen nor some nursing supplies and another state will not provide a hospital bed of any type after discharge. Some states have a limit to the number of days of rehabilitation allowed; one state program provides only 12 days' hospital coverage annually irrespective of diagnosis.

Regardless of individual differences in benefits, all those contacted thought the services available *after* discharge are woefully inadequate and this is where the least optimism is felt. Generally there are very few options available in the community for Medicaid/MediCal ventilator quadriplegic persons. Some states elect to participate in a Medicaid-covered home and community-based services waiver program, which is funded by federal and state money. This is also titled an In-Home Medical Care (IHMC) waiver. Those states that have the waiver program may provide up to a maximum of 16 h per day of licensed daily nursing care in the home, except in California, which has a maximum of 24 h a day. However, the latter is rarely provided, and when it is granted, it has become extremely difficult to hire Licensed Vocational Nurses because of the low reimbursement rates paid by MediCal to the home health agencies. This has become even more difficult in the past 2 years due to the severe nursing shortage throughout the nation. It is also apparent that the handling of IHMC waiver applications varies from county to county within California; some county MediCal staff deny the service without explanation. Reportedly, California's MediCal may allow approximately 200 IHMC contracts to be assigned throughout the state at any one time. There are various diagnostic criteria required to be eligible and varying numbers of hours per day of nursing care are granted. It also has to be demonstrated that care in the home with licensed nurses is cheaper than the cost of acute hospital care and that there is no less expensive facility able to provide appropriate patient care. There are stringent requirements regarding the home setting and proof that the family will provide support and often be responsible for a number of hours of patient care on a daily basis. No precise figures are available from the state as to how many IHMC contracts have been issued, how many IHMC cases are currently served, nor the diagnoses or hours of daily care actually granted. It is generally believed that the majority of IHMC contracts are granted for children. The following case example will illustrate the difficulties encountered in trying to implement IHMC for a patient at the Santa Clara Valley Spinal Cord Injury Rehabilitation Center.

An IHMC waiver (Title 22, California Administrative Code, Section 51344) was requested for J., a 26-year-old man, in October 1985. He had a fully accessible apartment prepared for him adjoining his parents' home. The waiver was denied and appealed three times. Eighteen months later, in May 1987, 24-h care was approved for this patient. However, during the 18-month waiting period the nursing shortage had become acute. MediCal's reimbursement to nurses was much lower than that paid by insurance companies and it proved impossible to hire the nurses required to care for J. His plight was appealed by both state and federal legislators and received attention from several television stations, public radio, and three newspapers. MediCal refused to increase their reimbursement rate. The Santa Clara County Legal Aid attorney working on this case, together with several other Legal Aid attorneys, filed a suit in the State Superior Court on behalf of his client and three other ventilator-dependent patients charging that the state had failed to implement the IHMC program in a number of ways. The court ordered the Department of Health Services to find an agency and nurses to be trained and to staff J.'s care so that he could go home within 30 days of the date of the order. MediCal failed to abide by the order and the attorney prepared to file that the Department of Health Services be held in contempt of court. Before the attorney's return to court, MediCal decided to increase the nursing rate for the five San Francisco Bay Area counties, which included Santa Clara County. The home health agency J. had chosen was able to hire the nurses and 3 weeks later he was able to go home. There was no other facility in the state able to provide his care during the period from October 1985 to April 1988. The acute care hospital costs were double those for home health care. Therefore, the 2½ years of delays in this case cost hundreds of thousands of dollars.

Placement options are very limited across all states contacted. Many patients have no suitable home in which to live after discharge. Some states have a very limited number of skilled nursing facilities that will take a Medicaid ventilator-dependent person. It is suspected that many ventilator patients remain in or return to acute care hospitals and that many receive no rehabilitation whatsoever. California has six subacute facilities designated to accept ventilator patients. However, experience has shown that these facilities have long waiting lists, that many of their patients are long-term residents, elderly, semicomatose, or in a vegetative state. There are very few beds available for quadriplegic persons who are young and fully alert. There is no skilled nursing facility in California that will accept MediCal ventilator patients.

No facility contacted was aware of any group-home setting for Medicaid patients, other than the much-lauded New Start Homes in Southern California. The MediCal-funded pilot program has been evaluated and at the time of writing New Start Homes is seeking state licensing. This living arrangement appears to be very successful from the staff's, resident's, and families' perspectives and it is hoped that expansion both in Southern California and other areas of California will be permitted. The houses for New Start Homes are located in several residential neighborhoods and the residents, both adults and children, are able to attend school and pursue a variety of activities. The atmosphere is that of a private family home as opposed to an institutional environment. Staff in the rehabilitation facilities expressed the hope that either their state would be able to develop such a program eventually or that they might be able to transfer ventilator quadriplegic patients from their state to New Start Homes in California.

For those ventilator patients having a home to return to and a family willing and able to provide care, there is a varying amount of attendant care obtainable in most states. In-Home Support Services (IHSS) funds are usually distributed by the county from county, state, and sometimes federal money. These programs generally pay approximately the minimum wage rate for nonlicensed persons to provide attendant care; in some cases this is a family member. It is often very difficult to find and retain reliable attendant care for minimum wage. The hours granted for IHSS services range from a low of 6 h per week in one state to a maximum in California of approximately 60 h per week. The maximum is never granted if there is any other nursing or home care agency providing services in the home.

Some rehabilitation facilities interviewed struggle to supplement the services Medicaid provides by contacting churches, philanthropic groups, women's volunteer services, and encourage family and friends to organize fund raisers. No Medicaid funding is available to assist with home modifications or to purchase an attendant-driven van. There are very few other resources that can provide help with these needs.

The impression gained from contacting other rehabilitation centers is that social workers and/or discharge planners have feelings of isolation, frustration, and hopelessness regarding the discharge and aftercare of ventilator-dependent quadriplegic persons, particularly those with Medicaid coverage. Staff feel the need to connect with other rehabilitation centers in other parts of the country experiencing similar struggles to learn from them how they cope and what they might do to improve the chances of arranging appropriate and adequate care for the ventilator quadriplegic individual. Other comments expressed were that nurses and other staff find it very difficult to encourage patients and families to think positively about return to the community and/or home when the staff know how improbable, perhaps impossible, it will be to find sufficient care for the patient. There seems to be almost a dread of accepting ventilator-dependent patients who have Medicaid or limited insurance coverage. This is due to the knowledge that there may be nowhere to go after rehabilitation is completed and the grim prospect of "warehousing" the patient, perhaps for life. This appears to create much inner conflict for staff committed to the philosophy of rehabilitation; they observe the great disparities between the goals of spinal cord rehabilitation and the Medicaid patient's eventual demise.

It is not known how many people are in this predicament in the United States. There are no precise figures available as to how many ventilator-dependent quadriplegic patients are accepted into rehabilitation centers, how many remain or return after rehabilitation to acute care hospitals, how many go to nursing homes or subacute facilities, and how many return home. How long do these persons survive, what is the quality of their medical and nursing care, and what are the emotional effects of long-term confinement on the patients and families? It has been estimated that approximately 150 people a year (0.64 per million U.S. population—Mike deVivo, University of Alabama, Birmingham, personal communication, 1988) survive the initial trauma and enter a hospital as a ventilator-dependent complete quadriplegic patient (C3 and higher). It appears that approximately 45 of these 150 enter spinal cord rehabilitation programs annually. It is not known what happens to the approximately 105 people not entering rehabilitation programs.

The professionals contacted expressed a need for provision of more family support, especially for those caring for a family member at home. It has been a common experience that families, relationships, and marriages break up under the stress of a major trauma to a loved one, even when there are adequate financial resources and nursing care. This stress on the family is compounded when the family is expected to provide the care with little or no financial and nursing assistance.

Questions raised by the social workers contacted related to how much longer there will be a discriminatory system of health, rehabilitation, and home care. Will there ever be a system of health care for *all* people in the United States or at least mandatory catastrophic insurance coverage? Staff are concerned about when and how families should be told how much care and responsibility they might have to take in the future for their family member and when the patient should be made aware of his/her limited options.

Some staff contacted in states with very limited services for ventilator patients expressed the wish that they had the services other more generous states had to offer. However, the question arises as to whether it is a disservice to provide all state-of-the-art medical technology to sustain a person's life at the time of the initial trauma, to provide acute hospital care and even full rehabilitation to a ventilator-dependent quadriplegic patient, if society is not willing to provide or cannot provide a reasonable quality of life for the survivor's remaining years. It needs to be determined what are reasonable standards for aftercare and how these can be proposed and implemented. It also needs to be determined whose responsibility it is to address these issues and to elicit the cooperation of many different professional disciplines so that plans can be made not only for survival and longevity but also quality of life for the ventilator-dependent quadriplegic individual. Although the number of MediCal/Medicaid ventilator quadriplegic patients is not known, it is recognized that they are generally a young population and have the potential to live long lives.

Is it possible that this population is not only not counted nor organized, but is too small to have a powerful voice to lobby for better lifetime care facilities? Should this population, which appears to be invisible and perhaps devalued by society's present measuring sticks of worth—independence, productivity, glamour, and financial resources—form coalitions with other oppressed minority populations? Are there places in the United States where this is already happening? If efforts are to be made, should they remain at the state level or be nationwide?

It is clear that there are no easy solutions to these problems because of the varying lifestyles, family configurations, and goals of the ventilator-dependent quadriplegic persons affected, as well as the political, philosophical, cultural, and economic constraints that have to be considered. In the survey conducted, it is apparent that there is a strong need to (a) provide more hours of licensed nursing care in the home through IHMC waivers, (b) increase the number of attendant hours and wages paid to caregivers, (c) consider direct hiring of licensed nurses to work in the home, (d) provide specialized training to nurses' aides to care for ventilator quadriplegic patients (present laws do not permit home health agencies to staff at that level of training), (e) provide more respite care for families caring for ventilator quadriplegic persons, (f) promote and develop a group home concept similar to that at New Start Homes in Southern California, (g) develop more accessible low-income housing, and (h) form coalitions with other groups who need long-term home care issues addressed and bring these issues to the attention of policy makers at both the state and federal levels.

Very little seems to have been done to involve and inform the state and federal respresentatives of the struggles for ventilator quadriplegic individuals to receive adequate lifetime care. In some areas of the country television, radio, and newspaper articles have focused on the needs of individual ventilator quadriplegic persons. This has certainly helped educate the public about some of the problems for the severely disabled. The media might well be used more frequently to increase public awareness. There also is a need to seek help from foundations and philanthropic organizations to determine what funding they might provide, especially in the area of equipment and development of accessible housing.

It is acknowledged by all that the problems are not expected to disappear. They must be addressed head-on in an organized, informed manner. It is recognized that given the ongoing advances in medical technology, more and more trauma cases will survive. There is the knowledge and skill to keep those persons alive for many years. However, quality-of-life issues must be considered so that all ventilator quadriplegic patients have the opportunity to live fulfilling lives outside of medical institutions and nursing homes. If the present situtation does not change, more hospital beds will become gridlocked. Those facilities could become warehouses, unable to accept any more ventilator patients, regardless of coverage. Even now, a number of facilities are either not taking Medicaid ventilator quadriplegic patients or are considering refusing them in the future.

Patients and families should not have to carry the burden alone. All staff involved in the care of ventilator patients know that this devastating trauma can occur to anyone. There is a need for a balanced outlook both subjectively and objectively. If it is agreed that medicine should use all available technology to save lives and to rehabilitate those who are severely disabled, then there is a need to work for and establish standards of care that afford the person so tragically affected a safe, fulfilling life with every attempt to maintain the dignity and cohesiveness of the person and the family. It is essential that spinal cord injury rehabilitation staff around the nation share their ideas and formulate plans to assist ventilator quadriplegic persons achieve and maintain a quality of life and endorse the worth of the individual, regardless of that person's insurance coverage and financial resources.

27

Long-Term Outlook for Persons with High Quadriplegia

Gale Whiteneck

Craig Hospital, Englewood, Colorado, U.S.A.

The success of a specialized program in high quadriplegia care cannot simply be measured in terms of the number of cases that survive acute care and rehabilitation for discharge. The true test of success lies in the morbidity, mortality, and quality of life obtained after discharge. This final chapter examines these long-term outcomes for individuals with high quadriplegia treated in specialized programs in the last few years and then speculates what may influence these outcomes in the future.

The opportunity to systematically assess the outcomes of high quadriplegia was provided by a grant from the National Institute on Disability and Rehabilitation Research to the three programs specializing in high quadriplegia care that collaborated in preparing this book. This long-term follow-up investigation of former patients from all three centers was conducted by a team of physicians and researchers, including Dr. R. Edward Carter and Margaret Ann Wilkerson with the Institute for Rehabilitation and Research; Drs. Conal Wilmot and Karyl Hall with the Santa Clara Valley Medical Center; and Dr. Robert Menter, Susan Charlifue, and the present author with Craig Hospital. This chapter highlights the results of the follow-up study reported in detail in 1985 (1).

THE FOLLOW-UP STUDY POPULATION

The study population included all high quadriplegic persons with a complete neurologic lesion at C4 or above admitted to one of the three centers between 1973 and 1983 within 1 year of a traumatic spinal cord injury. Information about the outcomes of these 216 individuals was obtained from extensive medical record review, personal follow-up interviews, and cost data collection from numerous health care providers.

Eighty-six percent of the study group were male and 70% were injured between the ages of 11 and 30 years. Vehicular accidents were responsible for 44% of the injuries. Diving accidents accounted for 19%, gunshot wounds 10%, falls 9%, sport-related accidents excluding football 7%, football accidents 4%, and the remaining 6% of the injuries were caused by other assaults or medical/surgical complications.

All participants in the study had high level quadriplegia with complete neurologic lesions at discharge. Fifty-nine percent were C4 quadriplegic, 17% were C3, 13% were C2, and 10% were C1 or higher-level quadriplegic.

During the spinal cord injury system admission 62% used mechanical ventilator assistance, but by discharge only 35% required full- or part-time ventilator assistance. The remaining 65% were ventilator independent at discharge.

Analysis of residence at discharge indicated that 74% were discharged home, 9% were discharged to other hospital settings, 7% were discharged to a nursing home or extended care facility, and 3% were discharged to other group living situations. The remaining 8% (17) had died before discharge from the SCI System.

Of the 17 who died during the initial hospitalization, four were reported to have died of cardiac arrest. Three individuals, all of whom were not using ventilators, died of respiratory failure and two ventilator-dependent individuals died of pneumonia. Three ventilator-dependent people died from cerebrovascular disease. The remaining five individuals died of various causes, including pulmonary embolism, duodenal ulcer with hemorrhage, an arterial puncture secondary to tracheostomy, and other ill-defined conditions.

SURVIVAL IN FOLLOW-UP YEARS

The long-term survival status of the 199 individuals alive at discharge was analyzed (Fig. 27-1). Substantially different survival rates were found between ventilator-dependent and ventilator-independent cases. At 1, 3, 5, 7, and 9 years postinjury the survival percentages of the ventilator-independent group were 93, 83, 79, 77, and 73%, respectively. For the ventilator-dependent group the survival rates were 86, 70, 63, 63, and 59%, respectively. All calculations were based on the number of cases injured 1, 3, 5, 7, and 9 years previously.

Of the 33 deaths that occurred in the follow-up years postdischarge, eight were due to pneumonia. Cardiac failure or arrest was responsible

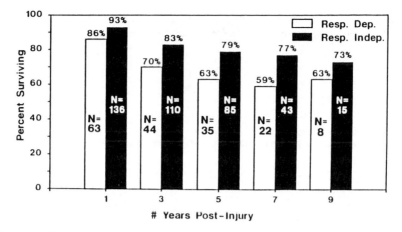

FIG. 27-1. Long-term survival status of 199 high-level quadriplegic persons after discharge. (This figure and Tables 27-1 to 27-4 are reproduced from ref. 1.)

for eight deaths. Respiratory insufficiency was the reported cause of three deaths. Septicemia and pyelonephritis each caused two deaths. Hereditary chorea, malnutrition, gangrene, pulmonary embolism, pulmonary collapse, closed head injury, and a foreign body in the pharynx were cited as the primary cause of death in one case each. Causes of death were undetermined for three individuals.

MORBIDITY AND CARE IN FOLLOW-UP YEARS

During the years after initial discharge a variety of medical problems were experienced by this patient population (Table 27-1). For individuals ventilator dependent at discharge an average of 49% contracted urinary tract infections each year, compared with an incidence of 39% in the ventilator-independent group. Respiratory problems excluding pneumonia were reported in an average of 19% of the ventilator-dependent individuals each year, compared with the ventilator-independent group reporting an average incidence of 7% per year. Reports of pneumonia in the ventilator-dependent group were 15% per year and in the ventilator-independent group were 6% per year. There were relatively small differences between the ventilator and nonventilator groups in the reported incidence of various urinary tract problems other than infections. A variety of operative procedures were reported in the follow-up years, the most prominent of which was external sphincterotomy, performed in 22 cases. Skin surgery was reported in 13 cases. Spine stabilization procedures were performed seven times, tracheotomies were performed four times, and two laminectomies were performed.

Table 27-1. *Comparison of Medical Complications in Follow-up Years Between Respirator-Dependent and Independent Individuals*[a]

	Respirator-dependent (%)	Respirator-independent (%)
Pneumonia	15.0	5.8
Other respiratory diseases	19.4	6.8
Calculus of kidney/ureter	4.4	2.4
Bladder calculus	11.3	10.4
Urinary tract infection	48.8	38.7
Infections of kidney	0.6	1.8
Hematuria	2.5	0.8
Heterotopic ossification	1.9	5.0
Other bone diseases	3.1	2.0
Septicemia	1.3	0.4
Vertebrogenic pain syndrome	2.5	5.2
Decubitus ulcers	25.0	25.9

[a] Values indicate average percent of population reporting the complication per year.

An average of 50% of the study population reported having been hospitalized at some time in each follow-up year. The incidence of rehospitalization was slightly higher for the ventilator-dependent group (57% per year versus the ventilator-independent group at 48% per year). The ventilator-dependent individuals had an average of 22.2 days of hospitalization per year and the ventilator-independent group averaged 10.5 days of hospitalization per year. In the ventilator-dependent group there was a trend of increased length of stay in the later follow-up years; however, there was a trend of shorter hospital stays in the later years for the ventilator-independent group.

Four situations regarding care in the home were examined: (a) paid attendant care; (b) care given by nonpaid person; (c) time spent with someone not involved in care; and (d) time spent alone.

In the ventilator-dependent group, the clear majority of time (59%) was spent with paid attendants. Fifteen percent of the group's time was spent with nonpaid caregivers; 23% of the time was spent with individuals not involved in care; and only 3% of the time was spent alone.

In the ventilator-independent group, nearly equal amounts of time were spent in three categories: paid attendant care (34%), nonpaid caregiver time (28%), and time with persons other than the caregiver (31%). In this group, 7% of total time was spent alone.

The most frequent skill level of paid attendant was an aide, with licensed visiting nurses, family members, friends, and other unskilled individuals also frequently used. Only 19% of the cases used a registered nurse in the care team. In more than two-thirds of the cases, the cost of paid attendant care ranged between $3.00 and $10.00 per hour.

QUALITY OF LIFE IN FOLLOW-UP YEARS

All of the ventilator-independent cases and all but two of the ventilator-dependent cases were out of bed each day. Ninety-two percent of the ventilator-independent cases and 83% of the ventilator-dependent cases were out of bed more than 5 h each day. Frequency of leaving the house was also high among those surveyed. More than two-thirds of the ventilator-independent cases and nearly two-thirds of the ventilator-dependent cases got out of their homes 3 or more days per week.

Table 27-2. *Average Time Use*

Activity	Frequency	Respirator-dependent	Respirator-independent
Go out to eat	Times/month	2.0	4.3
Go to the movies	Times/month	1.2	1.1
Attend lectures, theater	Times/month	0.2	0.3
Attend club, lodge meetings	Times/month	0.4	1.1
Shop	Times/month	2.2	3.5
Participate in sports	Times/month	0.2	1.1
Attend sports activities	Times/month	0.9	1.6
Take rides	Times/month	2.5	4.7
Go to parties	Times/month	1.1	1.1
Go to the library	Times/month	0.5	1.3
Write letters	Times/month	1.6	2.5
Play cards, games	Times/month	6.8	4.2
Community or church work	Hours/week	1.3	1.1
Visit friends	Hours/week	4.1	4.6
Go to school	Hours/week	6.9	5.1
Working	Hours/week	2.9	3.9
Computer activities	Hours/week	3.3	3.9
Work on hobbies	Hours/week	3.4	3.9
Entertain friends	Hours/week	8.5	9.3
Take courses at home	Hours/week	1.0	0.3
Listen to the radio	Hours/week	15.9	16.6
Watch television	Hours/week	39.0	33.1
Talk on the phone	Hours/week	2.6	5.6
Read	Hours/week	8.0	8.7
Just sit and think	Hours/week	13.0	18.7

Ninety-three percent of the ventilator-dependent and 96% of the ventilator-independent cases were living with other individuals. In addition, substantial numbers of contacts were made with family and friends living outside their households. More than two-thirds of both groups saw or spoke with more than five family members or friends each week. Although approximately two-thirds reported having lost friends since their injury, 90% reported making new friends since their injury as well.

The study participants were asked how many times per month or how many hours per week they spent in each of 25 specific activities (Table 27-2). Although the largest blocks of time were spent in passive activities at home including watching TV, listening to the radio, or just sitting and thinking, the data on more active pursuits indicate that many high quadriplegic persons are engaged in varied and vigorous lifestyles. Frequent reports of going to school, working, entertaining and visiting friends, engaging in computer activities or other hobbies, playing cards, writing letters, going to parties, taking rides, shopping, eating out, and going to movies were mentioned. The frequency and hours spent in these activities did not seem to vary dramatically between ventilator-dependent and ventilator-independent individuals.

Relatively high respondent ratings of self-esteem were found using the Rosenberg Self-Esteem Scale. When asked about suicide ideation, half reported considering suicide since injury, but the majority had not considered suicide recently. When asked the question "Are you glad to be alive since your injury?", 92% responded affirmatively. Sixty-four percent of the ventilator-dependent cases and 54% of the ventilator-independent cases rated their quality of life either excellent or good. Only 10% of both groups rated their quality of life poor or very poor.

COST OF HIGH QUADRIPLEGIA CARE

An analysis was made of the cost of high quadriplegia care, both in the initial phases of acute care and rehabilitation and in the long-term phases of follow-up.

The initial cost of care was more than twice as expensive for ventilator-dependent than ventilator-independent cases (Table 27-3). On average, $76,042 was spent on acute care for ventilator-dependent cases in the hospital before their arrival at one of the three participating spinal injury systems of care. For ventilator-independent cases, an average of $38,137 in presystem acute care cost was expended. In addition, the acute care charges at the three SCI system facilities averaged $47,830 for ventilator-dependent cases and $5,337 for ventilator-independent cases. The rehabilitation expenses at the three systems averaged $181,929 for ventilator-dependent cases and $64,553 for ventilator-independent cases. This brought the mean total medical care expenses from injury through dis-

Table 27-3. *Average Acute and Initial Rehabilitation Expenses*[a]

Phase	Respirator-dependent (n = 34)	Respirator-independent (n = 72)
Presystem (mean)	$76,042	$38,137
System acute care (mean)	47,830	5,337
System rehabilitation (mean)	181,929	64,553
Total expenses		
mean	305,801	108,028
median	225,342	93,667

[a]Analysis based on 106 patients for which all cost information (presystem, system acute, and system rehabilitation expenses) was reported.

charge to $305,801 (median, $225,342) for ventilator-dependent cases and $108,028 (median, $93,667) for ventilator-independent cases.

The average annual follow-up care expenses were also substantially greater for ventilator-dependent cases (Table 27-4). The average attendant care cost for ventilator-dependent cases was $34,648 per year, whereas the average for ventilator-independent cases was $12,075. Add-

Table 27-4. *Average Annual Follow-up Care Expenses*

Mean follow-up expenses	Respirator-dependent (n = 24)	Respirator-independent (n = 76)
Attendant care	$34,648	$12,075
SCI system inpatient charges	38,013	2,174
SCI system outpatient charges	33	279
SCI system physician charges	1,849	624
Nonsystem inpatient charges (including nursing homes)	16,980	6,512
Nonsystem outpatient charges	273	382
Nonsystem physician charges	392	776
Equipment charges	1,809	1,801
Modification charges	3,565	450
Medication and supply charges	3,295	1,964
Miscellaneous charges	389	570
Total expenses		
Mean	$101,246	$27,607
Median	$53,481	$21,977

ing the cost of system and nonsystem inpatient, outpatient, and physician charges, equipment charges, modification expenses, medication and supply charges, and other miscellaneous expenses brings the grand total for annual follow-up care to a mean of $101,246 (median, $53,481) for ventilator-dependent cases and $27,607 (median, $21,977) for ventilator-independent cases.

LONG-TERM OUTCOMES NOW AND IN THE FUTURE

The study just reviewed offers several important insights into the present status of high quadriplegia outcomes. Advances in care in recent decades has dramatically increased survival. The medical condition of high quadriplegic persons post initial discharge is relatively stable. Most importantly, the quality of life after rehabilitation can be quite good. The cost of care was extraordinary, and much more expensive both initially and yearly thereafter for the ventilator-dependent quadriplegic individuals.

It is clear that specialized comprehensive high quadriplegia programs can produce positive results. This present capability of success requires considerable resources and an experienced multidisciplinary team, but a satisfying quality of life can be achieved.

As we look to the next decade, several factors are likely to influence future outcomes. As emergency care continues to improve, more high quadriplegic persons may survive the initial trauma. Earlier management in high-quadriplegia-oriented SCI centers may decrease initial complications and leave respiratory function less compromised. The dissemination of existing knowledge, such as this book, may prepare more facilities to offer quality care or encourage early transfer to facilities prepared to manage this catastrophic injury.

Techniques to medically manage high quadriplegia will undoubtedly improve. Advances in high technology rehabilitation may also contribute to better ventilatory options, environmental controls, communication devices, computer interfaces, and other enhancements to independence. It is reasonable to expect slow but continued progress in medical and functional areas.

The real question is whether society can keep pace. Significant changes are needed in funding and support systems if successful outcomes are to be maximized. Creative options for attendant care are required. Adequate funding is necessary for specialized medical care, extensive equipment, and attendant care. Policymakers must recognize the unique problems of individuals with high quadriplegia and commit resources to address these issues. With such support, the pattern of improving outcomes seen in recent years can continue in the next decades.

REFERENCE

1. Whiteneck GG, Carter RE, Charlifue SW, Hall KM, Menter RR, Wilkerson MA, Wilmot CB (1985): *A Collaborative Study of High Quadriplegia* (Rocky Mountain Regional Spinal Injury System, Northern California Regional Spinal Injury System, and Texas Regional Spinal Cord Injury System). Englewood, CO: Craig Hospital.

Index